HEALTH CARE IN TRANSITION

BLOCKCHAIN AND HEALTH

TRANSFORMATION OF CARE AND IMPACT OF DIGITALIZATION

HEALTH CARE IN TRANSITION

Additional books and e-books in this series can be found
on Nova's website under the Series tab.

COMPUTER SCIENCE, TECHNOLOGY AND APPLICATIONS

Additional books and e-books in this series can be found
on Nova's website under the Series tab.

HEALTH CARE IN TRANSITION

BLOCKCHAIN AND HEALTH

TRANSFORMATION OF CARE AND IMPACT OF DIGITALIZATION

JAN VEUGER
EDITOR

nova
science publishers
New York

DOI: https://doi.org/10.52305/PWSO5327

NOTICE TO THE READER

Library of Congress Cataloging-in-Publication Data

ISBN: 978-1-68507-232-2

Published by Nova Science Publishers, Inc. † New York

CONTENTS

PREFACE

The secure storage of medical records is vital to any healthcare system. Relying solely on centralised servers increases the likelihood of sensitive information going public. Transparency and increased security of blockchain technology make it an ideal platform for storing medical records.

Patients can safely store their privacy-sensitive information by securing their data on a blockchain using cryptography. This enables them to share their medical information with any healthcare institution with their approval. The healthcare system is currently very fragmented, but if all users were to use a secure global database, the flow of information between them would be much faster.

A great advantage of a global database is that clients do not have to tell their story every time. A medical specialist, for example, can see exactly what a patient has been through and what treatments and examinations have taken place. The information is also available in real time to the healthcare professional the client has indicated to have access to his file.

A new revolution is taking place that is clearly different from the third industrial revolution (Internet, communication and globalisation). This fourth industrial revolution involves a fusion of technologies such as biotechnology, nanotechnology, artificial intelligence, robotics, the Internet of Things, cloud computing and blockchain. Our healthcare society is also changing fundamentally, also under the influence of COVID-19.

These fundamental changes require an integrated and comprehensive response, involving stakeholders in public and private society. The challenge is how to use innovations from the fourth industrial revolution to take healthcare to a new level and solve at least the most pressing problems in healthcare and society. Blockchain will play a major role in this. It is a core technology that has the potential to combine digital data with physical systems.

The starting point of our healthcare is that patients can choose the care that suits them. But how can a patient do this in a field where the complexity is only increasing? In addition, the ageing population will lead to an increase in the demand for care. Rising healthcare costs and an increase in chronic diseases also require a new approach. And treatment is increasingly taking place in a home environment rather than in a hospital or care institution. So there is a great need for innovation in healthcare.

Healthcare is a high-tech and information-intensive environment. Partly because of this and because of the importance of good communication for the client, you would expect the exchange of information in healthcare to be well organized. However, healthcare is organized in such a complex way that both professionals and clients lack insight. For instance, healthcare professionals describe conditions and treatments in different ways, which makes it difficult to interpret information from different healthcare records unambiguously. In addition, healthcare providers use a variety of information systems, making it difficult to link information. Obviously, security of information is an important issue, which also contributes to the complexity of data exchange.

Digitalization makes it possible to implement fundamental changes in business operations. The trick for administrators is to securely and intelligently connect all the applications and information systems that healthcare parties use. In this book, we elaborate on how blockchain will contribute to these challenges. Blockchain is a decentralized network for storing data. It is designed to achieve integrity, transparency, efficiency and accuracy of data.

With this book in three chapters, we present the impact of blockchain and digitization in healthcare with (1) a systematic literature review om implementing blockchain solutions in health care and organizational consequences, (2) blockchain in health care and (3) transformation of elderly care and impact of digitalization.

Jan Veuger, 2021

In: Blockchain and Health
Editor: Jan Veuger
ISBN: 978-1-68507-232-2

Chapter 1

A SYSTEMATIC LITERATURE REVIEW ON IMPLEMENTING BLOCKCHAIN SOLUTIONS IN HEALTHCARE AND THE ORGANISATIONAL CONSEQUENCES

George Garritsen[1,*], Jan Veuger[2], PhD, and Petra C. de Weerd-Nederhof[3], PhD

[1]Head Lecturer in Business Economics/Business Administration, Graduation Coordinator, Saxion University of Applied Sciences School of Commerce and Entrepreneurship, The Netherlands
[2]Saxion University of Applied Sciences, School of Finance and Accounting, School of Creative Technology, School of Governance, Law and Urban Development, Hospitality Business School, School of Commerce and Entrepeneurship, School of People and Society, The Netherlands
[3]Organisation Studies & Innovation, University of Twente, Faculty of Behavioural, Management & Social Studies, The Netherlands

[*] Corresponding Author: PhD candidate. E-mail: g.a.g.garritsen@saxion.nl.

Abstract

This Systematic Literature Review provides insight into the development, trends, and impact of implementations of blockchain solutions in healthcare. To introduce the subject of blockchain, an image of the essences of blockchain as a technique to realise digital transformation was obtained from scientific literature. The purpose of this review is to focus on the current use of blockchain in healthcare and the direction of development. Background information on the characteristics of blockchain as a technology has been provided to give information about the context. To carry out this Systematic Literature Review, a methodology has been described, in which four research questions have been formulated, which deal with the developments, trends and adoption process of blockchain solutions in healthcare. The Scopus Database was used. Both the number of publications and citations show a strong increase from 2018. Publications are particularly prevalent in the research areas "Computer Sciences" and "Engineering". This indicates that the focus in terms of blockchain is mainly on technology. China is currently the country with the highest citations per scientifically referenced publication with the topic "blockchain in healthcare". Both the research field and the stage of implementation give an indication of the developments in the field of blockchain solutions. This Systematic Literature Review indicates that an important field of research concerns the sharing of data and healthcare information within and between healthcare institutions. Many blockchain solutions are in the planning and development phase. To gain a clear picture of the trends within the implementations of blockchain solutions in healthcare, an analysis was carried out by type of initiative. Blockchain solutions that have as their initiative the improvement of transactions between organisations and initiatives that are disruptive to existing business models, show an increase. An in-depth elaboration of the TOE framework has given insight that the availability of blockchain as a technology, the organisational readiness and the pressure from competitors are important considerations of adoption.

Keywords: blockchain, healthcare, systematic literature review, inplementations, adoption

Introduction

Blockchain is a technology to realise digital transformation in healthcare. (Veuger & Woldendorp, Blockchain in healthcare, 2021) This Systematic Literature Review examines what is known within the research literature about terms "implementations of blockchain solutions in healthcare and the considerations of adoption". The aim is to provide insight into the development, trends, and impact of blockchain implementations in healthcare and the considerations for adoption. A systematic literature review is to be conducted to gain insight into the global adoption phase of blockchain in healthcare. The goal is to gain insight in the extent to which blockchain in healthcare has already led to implementable solutions.

In its article on the health (care) future of the Netherlands, Deloitte outlines that, due to falling costs of technology and new developments, future care will be organised more outside the hospital and therefore closer to the patient. Examples are remote monitoring, diagnostics, and consultations. This will make personal interventions possible, and the patient will not have to visit the hospital immediately. (Luijs, Bergen, & Engelen, 2020). Moving care from the hospital closer to the patient means a transformation in which technological development and digitalisation are the triggers. According to Beijen, digital transformation is characterised by a transition from product focus (the provision of care) to a focus where the customer (the patient) is at the centre. Organisations that place the focus on the patient are characterised by a continuous openness to change, are insight-driven and have access to platforms that enable cooperation between various stakeholders from a technological perspective, without this leading to a loss of quality (Beijen, 2020). Blockchain is a technology that can be used to facilitate such a transformation. What is blockchain? In essence, blockchain is a data structure - a kind of database - to which only digitally signed data can be added collectively by the peer-to-peer network (without a central party). However, it is necessary that this data meets certain conditions (rules), which is also verified collectively. (Goossens & Verslype, 2019). A blockchain does not grant administrator rights to change or delete data. A change can only take place by carrying out a new transaction, whereby the consensus protocol applies. (Nakamoto, 2008). When making a change within a block, the hash value of the block also changes, which results in the chain being interrupted. This means that changes within a block are not possible, which reduces the vulnerability to fraud. Blockchain has the technological advantage of increasing transparency and strengthening trust. Transparency and trust are particularly important aspects to realise value creation in the longer term. (Berns, et al., 2019). In the healthcare sector, it is important that data transactions between different entities can take place in a secure manner, due to the high degree of privacy sensitivity. This is because the data in question is confidential. It is a trend that more stakeholders play a role in healthcare, including large technological companies such as Google and Apple (Luijs, Bergen, & Engelen, 2020). This will free up more capital to invest in new technologies that make transformation possible. Also J. Veuger and H. Woldendorp, in the book 'blockchain in healthcare', outline the role and importance of digital transformation to enable a shift from healthcare to health. (Veuger & Woldendorp, Blockchain in healthcare, 2021) It is strange that adoption of blockchain in healthcare is insufficient, given its potential to strengthen trust and increase transparency, with privacy sensitivity being a key issue. Many studies have been done on the adoption of blockchain in healthcare and the considerations for not yet using blockchain as a technology for digital transformation. Many studies deal with the technological aspects of blockchain. Important technological considerations mentioned in the literature for not immediately applying blockchain are about the lack of standards for information exchange (Boulos, Wilson, & Clauson, 2018). In addition, aspects such as scalability and working from different platforms are mentioned as considerations for not applying blockchain. Scalability is about the speed of processing data. Platforms are about technical suitability

(Griggs, et al., 2018) (Liang, Zhao, Shetty, Liu, & Li, 2017). These literature reviews show that little is known from an organisational perspective, what are now important considerations for adopting blockchain, as a technology to achieve digital transformation. Clohessy & Acton confirm this in their study on the influence of organisational factors on blockchain adoption. (Clohessy & Acton, 2020) Pawczuk, Massey and Holowsky indicate that contextual factors such as people and culture can be critical success factors for an innovative technology (Pawczuk, Massey, & Holdowsky, 2019). These critical success factors are part of Weiner's conceptual model (Weiner, 2009). This model provides insight into which dimensions are important when measuring organisational readiness for change. In a study by Jouade & Saade on the use of blockchain in various domains, a gap is identified in healthcare regarding the barriers to blockchain adoption by users (patients), but also service providers such as doctors and hospital administrators. (Jaoude & Saade, 2019) Tandon et al, confirm this gap in their publication, blockchain in healthcare; A systematic literature review, synthesising framework and future research agenda (Tandon, Amandeep, Najmul Islam, & Mantymaki, 2020). This gap indicates that little is yet known from an organisational perspective about the adoption of blockchain in healthcare. Research and ideas from "The Duality of Technology" by Orlikowski (1992), assume that changes need to be made to organisations as technologies change. The degree of change depends on the complexity of the technology being adopted. (Orlikowski, 1992) Holotiuk and Moorman confirm that blockchain is a complex technology, which presents organisations with several challenges. Cooperation between organisations and early involvement are important aspects in the development of ideas, adoption, and application of technologies. (Holotiuk et al., 2018) In Bailey's AMO framework, collaboration and engagement are important components for determining organisational capability (Bailey, 1993).

The objective is to gain insight from literature research into which indicators from an organisational perspective influence the adoption of blockchain as a technology for digital transformation within the healthcare sector. To realise this objective, more insight is needed into the use of blockchain in healthcare. A Systematic Literature Review can provide valuable information on the current knowledge in a research area. It places the subject of blockchain in a broader context and shows why the study is timely and important (O'Reilly, 2012). Furthermore, a Systematic Literature Review makes it possible to identify existing gaps in knowledge to carry out further future research. (Gopalakrishnan & Ganeshkumar, 2013) In order to gain a better understanding of the use of blockchain in healthcare and the adoption of this technology, the following four research questions were posed:

1. What has been the development of implementations of blockchain solutions in recent years within the healthcare industry?

2. What are the main trends of implementations of blockchain solutions within healthcare?
3. What distribution is visible within the phases of adoption regarding blockchain solutions in healthcare?
4. What factors are considered in the adoption of blockchain solutions?

This publication is structured as follows: Chapter 2 covers motivation and contribution of the literature review. Chapter 3 provides background information on Blockchain technology. Chapter 4 deals specifically with blockchain as a technology within healthcare. Chapter 5 discusses the applied methodology for conducting a literature review. Chapter 6 presents the results of the literature review. Chapter 7 answers the research questions. Chapter 8 formulates the conclusion, and the discussion. Chapter 9 presents the agenda for the continuation of the research.

Motivation and Contribution

In contrast to the mentioned articles, this work presents a Systematic Review and Analysis of the state-of-the-art concerning blockchain research, in the field of healthcare and then specifically focused on the realisation of implementable solutions. The aim of this paper is to indicate the use of blockchain in healthcare and to show the initiatives and possible directions of blockchain research, concerning implemented solutions.

Background Information

This chapter provides insight into the most important characteristics of blockchain as a technology. Blockchain is basically a distributed ledger with the ability to exchange data between individuals, who are part of the network (Swan, 2015). Blockchain technology was introduced at the same time as the introduction of Bitcoin. Blockchain as a technology has ensured that duplication of transactions with cryptocurrency is no longer possible. Bitcoin uses the consensus mechanism where the majority (51%) decides whether a transaction can be validated or not. Mining nodes are those that can create a new block to store the data and perform the transaction. It is not always necessary to introduce a cryptocurrency where blockchain is used as a technology, working on a decentralised application (Raval, 2016). The remainder of this chapter describes the fundamentals, characters, and key elements of blockchain, to provide the reader with an understanding of how the technology works.

Types of Networks

There are various types of networks on which a blockchain operates. For example, there is a public, private, 'permissioned' and 'permissionedless' network (Dai & Vasarhelyi, 2017) The choice of the type of network depends on the purpose for which the technology of blockchain is deployed. A 'public permissioned' blockchain is best suited for ensuring client privacy (Nordrum, 2017) and therefore applicable within healthcare, where privacy is an important issue.

Consensus Protocols

Blockchain makes it possible to carry out transactions between two different entities without the need for a third party to validate the transaction. The consensus mechanism takes care of obtaining validation. There are different protocols for obtaining consensus. What is the added value of a protocol within a Blockchain? The added value of a protocol is that it provides the validation of transactions. In doing so, Blockchain network peers must agree on the exact state of the shared ledger and order in which new blocks are added to the ledger (Aste, Tasca, & Di Matteo, 2017).

7 different consensus protocols can be distinguished namely (Janse & Lin Lim, 2020):

1. Proof of Work (PoW)
2. Proof of Stake (PoS)
3. Delegated Proof of Stake (DPoS)
4. Proof of Importance (PoI)
5. Proof of Activity (PoA)
6. Proof of Burn (PoB)
7. Proof of Deposit (PoD)

The most used protocols are Proof of Work and Proof of Stake (Janse & Lin Lim, 2020). In Proof of Work-consensus protocol, as set up for Bitcoin for example, a data block may only be added to the blockchain if a valid hash of the block is found. With Proof-of-Stake, being allowed to produce a block depends on (a) a random selection process and (b) a stake, for example based on the number of coins held by an entity. There are several possible variants of the Proof of Stake protocol (Zheng, Xie, Dai, Chen, & Wang, 2017). The most well-known form is the Delegates Proof of Stake. This protocol is best compared to a continuous representative democracy where everyone who has a coin can vote for witnesses and delegates. The role of witnesses is to validate transactions and to be allowed to produce new blocks. For providing this service, witnesses receive a reward per block produced. Delegates have no role in verifying transactions and validating and producing blocks. The role of delegates is to oversee and monitor the governance structure of the blockchain protocol (Janse & Lin Lim, 2020). The entity with the highest importance score can validate transactions by producing new blocks (He, Guan, Lv, & Yi, 2018). The Proof of Activity protocol assumes those nodes that are most active within the network. The more active nodes are within the network, the more secure the network is. Initially, the Proof of Work protocol is executed to produce the block, where in terms of validation, a choice is made from those nodes that are most active (He, Guan, Lv, & Yi, 2018). In a Proof of Burn, an entity is given the right to add and validate a block at the time when cryptocurrency has been sent by this entity to a nonspendable address and destroyed. (Gourisetti, Mylrea, & Patangia, 2020) The last consensus protocol is the Proof of Deposit. In this protocol, each node that participates in validation must pay a deposit to earn the right to create new blocks. The deposit can be forfeited and the right to make blocks can be restricted if certain conditions are not met. (Hölbl M., Kompara, Kamišalić, & Zlatolas, 2018).

Smart Contracts

Blockchain makes it possible to automatically execute transactions using Smart Contracts. But what are Smart Contracts? Cieplak and Leefatt describe in their publication "Smart Contracts as; "A smart way to automate performance". In general, Smart Contracts are computer protocols that implement the terms of a negotiated contract in a self-executing way (Cieplak & Leefatt, 2017). Smart Contracts can take place in two ways. First, there can be deterministic contracts; here the program code does not rely on information outside the blockchain to initiate the execution of the contract. All the necessary information is stored in the blockchain itself. Secondly, there may be non-deterministic contracts. In this type of Smart Contract, information from outside is needed to execute the Smart Contract. By outside, another data source is meant, for example, the Internet or another database. (Hewavitharana, Nanayakkara, & Perera, 2019)

Rules for Validating a Blockchain

Validation rules are the set of rules within the network that are used to validate transactions and update the ledger (Janse & Lin Lim, 2020). The sender starts a transaction by creating a message, which contains; the 'public' address of the recipient on the network, the value of the transaction and an encrypted digital signature. The sender then sends the transaction into the network. The blockchain records the time when the transaction was created, the so-called timestamping. The nodes (computers/users) decipher the encrypted signature and thereby validate the message. They compare the time of creation of the transaction with earlier times to avoid double spending. The message then enters a queue of transactions to be processed. The transactions to be processed are collected by one of the nodes and placed in a block. The node sends the block within a specific time interval to the network for validation. The computers in the network can validate a block. They do this through an iterative process that requires consensus from the network. The validation process depends on the type of consensus protocol used. The type of consensus protocol used depends on the network in use. The common denominator is that it must be possible to determine that a transaction is valid and that corrupt transactions are rejected. Once the transactions in a block have been validated, the block is fixed in the blockchain and the new updated status of the ledger is sent to all nodes again (Muzammalab, Qu, & Nasrulin, 2019)

Blockchain in Healthcare and the Need

When looking at the healthcare sector, a study by Pessin, Shanler, Cole, & Stevens shows that there is a growing interest from the healthcare sector in blockchain technology worldwide. (Pessin, Shanler, Cole, & Stevens, 2019). The research by Pessin, Shanler, Cole, and Stevens shows that 55% of the institutions surveyed (n = 204) are interested in using blockchain as a technology. The following areas are mentioned as interesting for using blockchain as a supporting technology.

- Medical records management.
- Medical claims management.
- Healthcare professionals credentialing.
- Healthcare and life sciences supply chain management.

A distinction is made between four types of initiatives for the deployment of blockchain, these are:

- New disruptive initiatives, which are based on the application of blockchain within an existing business model.
- Initiatives to improve transactions of assets and interactions between organisations, leading to increased transparency and traceability.

- Initiatives that lead to the creation of new virtual and physical markets.
- Initiatives that can contribute to the safe storage of data within a community. (Pessin, Shanler, Cole, & Stevens, 2019).

Several Systematic Literature Reviews have been published with the topic of blockchain in healthcare. Using the Google Scholar database, the notation: "Systematic Review "AND "Blockchain in Healthcare" with a range between the years 2019-2020 yields a total of 322 cited publications. If the range is increased from 2016-2020, it turns out that 363 publications comply with the above notation. The conclusion is that there have been more publications in recent years, which provide a systematic review of blockchain in healthcare (Mayer, Costa, & Rosa Rhigi, 2020). Looking at the most cited articles, it is striking that they mostly deal with the adoption process, the advantages and disadvantages and possible applications of blockchain. Little is known about initiatives and applications within the healthcare sector that have led to concrete solutions using blockchain and the considerations for adoption.

METHODOLOGY

For this Systematic Literature Review, the research field is limited to the domain of care and cure. Below, the methodology used is defined, which helps to gain insight into the extent to which the use of blockchain within healthcare has already led to implementable solutions and which considerations are important in the adoption of blockchain as a technology.

Research Questions

This study intends to answer the following research questions:

1. What is the development of implementations of blockchain solutions in recent years within the healthcare sector?
2. What are the main trends of implementations of blockchain solutions within healthcare?
3. What distribution is visible within the phases of adoption regarding blockchain solutions in healthcare?
4. What factors are considered in the adoption of blockchain solutions.

Use of Databases

The Scopus database was used to conduct this systematic literature review. To clarify which articles are important for answering the research questions, an evaluation took place based on the following criteria:

1. Scope: A data range of 2010-2020 was chosen. Furthermore, only original studies were included in the selected data.
2. Data sources: Only cited journals are selected for the data research.
3. Language: Only sources in English are included in the Systematic Literature Review.
4. Relevance: The titles of the studies were scanned for relevance to the defined research field "Implementations of Blockchain in Healthcare".
5. Inclusion: Studies should meet the inclusion criteria as mentioned in point 2, 3 and 4. Studies that do not meet these criteria were not included in this further study.
6. Specificity: Studies that meet the topic "Implementations of Blockchain in Healthcare" will be read.
7. Data: Studies that are read in their entirety are analysed to help answer the research questions. To search for relevant publications, a query, as defined below, was used to answer the first three sub-questions. The query and related strings are based on the research field and the defined research questions. The following search terms were defined and used:

   (blockchain OR "block chain") AND
   (healthcare OR health OR medic* OR
   Medical OR medicine OR *health*) AND
   (implementations OR usage OR realization OR execution)
   The search in the scientific database Scopus took place in November 2020.

The query containing the related strings was kept as broad as possible to include as many results as possible in the in-depth study. The search of the query resulted in 383 publications. The initial selection was based on the search terms in title, keyword and abstract. To answer the research question 'what factors are considered in the adoption of blockchain solutions', we looked for a relevant framework. This framework should provide insights from different contexts into what considerations are important when adopting blockchain as a solution. This insight was gained from the TOE framework. The TOE framework is described in the book by Tornatzky and Fleisher, entitled "The processes of technological Innovation" (Tornatzky & Fleischer, 1990).

In this book, Tornatzky and Fleisher describe the innovation process from development, adoption to final implementation. The TOE framework states that three principal contexts - technological, organisational, and environmental - influence the process by which an organisation adopts and accepts a new technology (Lippert & Govindarajulu, 2006). The aim is to use the TOE framework in identifying and categorising the factors within the technological, organisational, and environmental contexts that are considered when adopting blockchain as a technology. Figure 1 visualises the TOE framework.

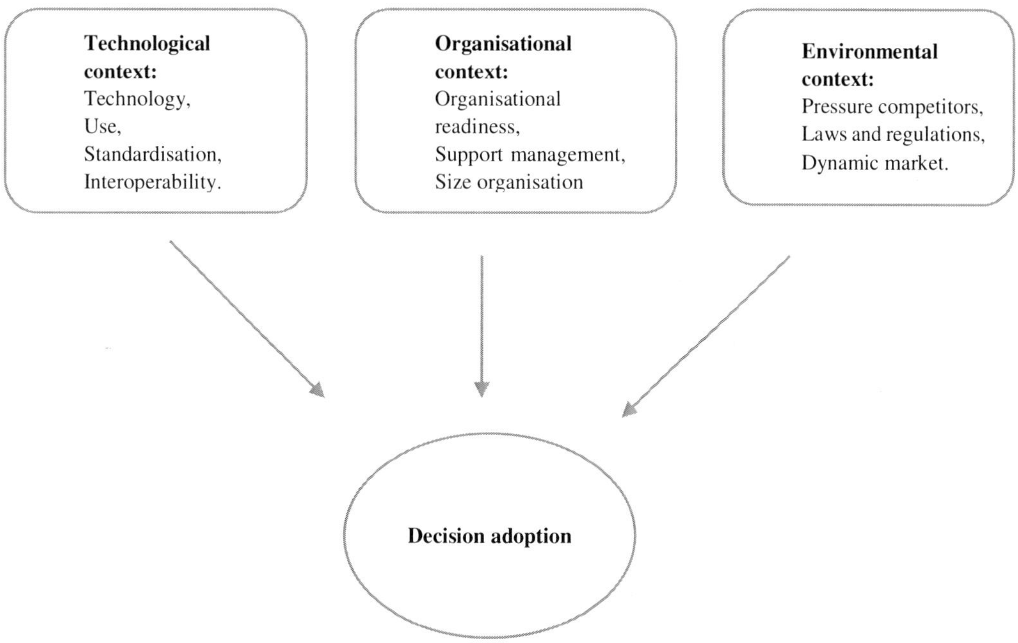

Figure 1. TOE-framework (Tornatzky & Fleischer, 1990).

To search for relevant publications, a new query was used, as defined below. The query and related strings are based on the research field and the defined research question. The search took place in March 2021. The following search terms were defined and used:

> ("factors" OR "restrictions" AND "Blockchain" AND "adoption");
> ("blockchain" AND "TOE" OR "toe-framework")

RESULTS

The selection from Scopus Database, based on the query mentioned on page 8, started with 383 publications for answering the first three sub questions. The further filtering and selection of the results can be divided into several phases. First, the filtering was based on the scope. The period 2010-2020 was taken as the scope. Based on this scope, 374 original publications remain. The choice to start with the year 2010 is related to the introduction of Bitcoin in 2008. After that, we filtered on data sources with the keywords "Blockchain" AND "Health Care". Only journals were included in the selection. Based on this selection, 120 publications remain. After that, we filtered on publications in English only. This resulted in 81 publications. Based on the 81 selected publications, a screening of the abstracts took place. We screened whether a publication says something about the implementation of a blockchain solution within healthcare. In the end, 38 publications were found to comply with this screening. These publications were included in the review. Figure 2 shows the entire selection process with the corresponding results once again.

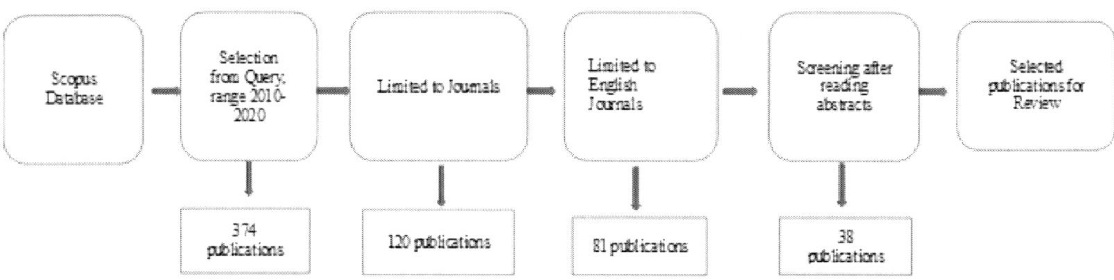

Figure 2. Examination of the selected journals.

About the scope, the choice was made to use the period 2010 to 2020 (present) for this purpose. If we look at the progression of the number of selected publications per year, it is striking that, based on the data from the Scopus database, publications on the application of blockchain in healthcare only started in 2017. Furthermore, it is noticeable that especially in 2019 and 2020, a lot has been published about blockchain applications in healthcare. Figure 3 shows the number of publications. The starting point is the publications described based on the keywords.

Looking at the research areas, Figure 4 shows that many publications about blockchain in healthcare have been published in "Computer Sciences" and "Engineering". This mainly indicates the focus on technology when it comes to blockchain.

In addition to the number of published articles and the research area, it is important to examine the development of the number of cited publications over the years.

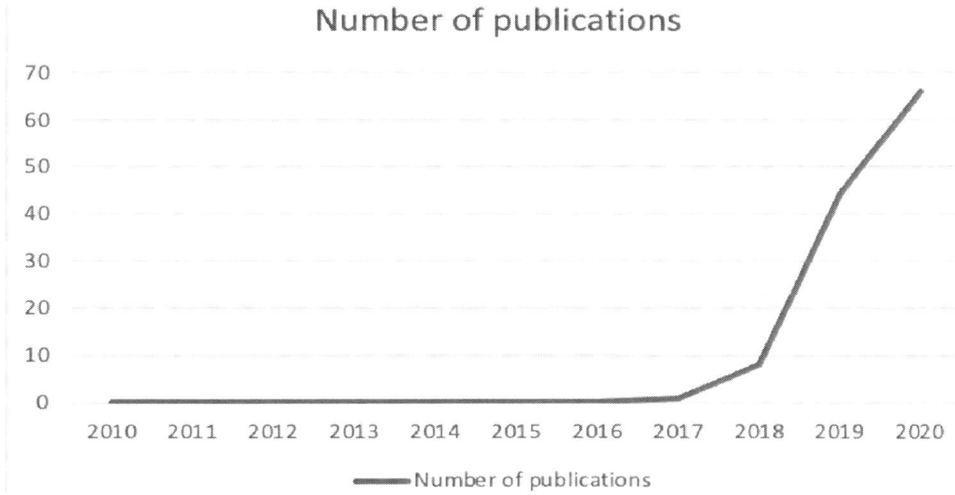

Figure 3. Development of the number of publications in relation to the scope used.

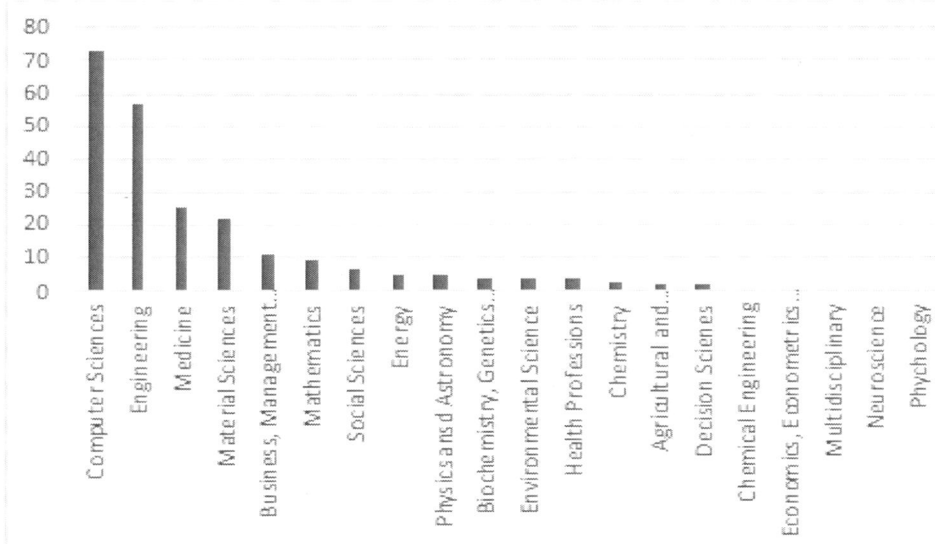

Figure 4. Research areas of selected publications.

Based on the results of this analysis, statements can be made about the importance of blockchain implementations in healthcare. For this analysis, the same scope was used as when determining the development of the number of publications. In addition, citations that are self-referring have not been included. Figure 4 shows the development of the number of citations in relation to the applied scope in years.

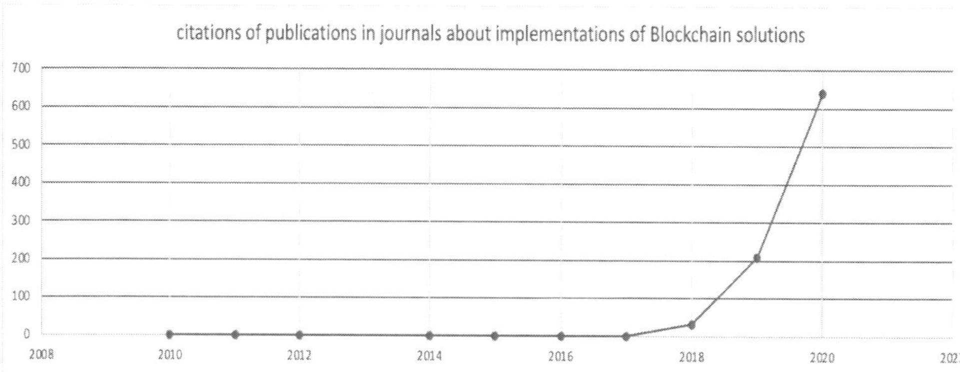

Figure 5. Development of the number of citations in relation to the scope used.

What stands out about Figures 3 and 5 is that both the course of the number and cited publications shows an upward trend from 2018. This trend can also be seen in the number of publications on the topic of "blockchain applications in healthcare" published in recent years. The importance of publishing on this topic is increasing. The same picture can also be observed in the research carried out by J. Veuger and published in the academic Journal of Property, Planning and Environmental Law (Veuger, Dutch Blockchain, real estate and land registration, 2020). It is also important to look at which countries are influential about publications that have an impact on the research area "implementations of blockchain in healthcare". To gain insight into this, a country analysis was carried out based on the 120 selected publications. The scope is based on the years 2010 to 2020 (present). The same scope has been used as when selecting the publications based on the defined query. Again, the Scopus database was used. The results are shown in Table 1 and Figure 6.

Table 1. Average number of citations by publications per country of origin based on scope used

Country	Number of publications	Numberr of citations	Citations by publications
Amerika	35	280	8,00
United Kingdom	19	205	10,79
China	18	243	13,50
India	16	134	8,38
Saudi Arabia	12	113	9,42
South Korea	10	11	1,10
Australia	9	112	12,44
Canada	6	113	18,83

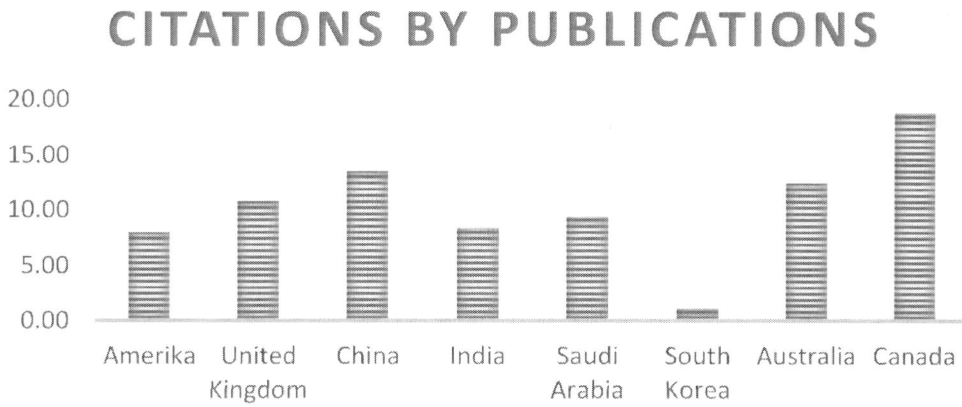

Figure 6. Average citations per article per country based on scope used.

Table 1 shows that the USA is the country where the frequency of the number of articles, which has as subject 'implementations of blockchain in healthcare', is the highest. This also applies to the number of citations. If we look at the number of citations per article, we see that Canada has the highest number of citations. This is related to the fact that two publications jointly have a score of 91 citations, which gives a distorted picture.

After screening the abstracts from the Scopus database, 38 publications were selected that say something about the implementation of a blockchain solution within healthcare. These publications were first screened for the purpose of the blockchain solution within healthcare. In addition, the phase in which the solution is situated was investigated. To determine the phases, we used the document 'Handreiking e-health implementatie' [E-health implementation guide] from the digital platform Zorg voor innoveren. This platform is a collaboration between five government organisations in the Netherlands. The following organisations are involved:

- Ministry of Health, Welfare and Sport
- Healthcare Institute Netherlands
- Dutch Health Care Authority
- Netherlands Enterprise Agency
- ZonMw

In this document, the following phases are identified for implementing e-health solutions:

1. Vision and strategy
2. Plan development
3. Development

4. Implementation and evaluation
5. Scaling up (Wolters & Hagen, 2019).

Below is a brief explanation of each phase of implementation.

Phase 1 This phase is about the forming of a vision and strategy.

Phase 2 This phase is about the introduction of a plan and investigate the impact of the solution.

Phase 3 This phase concerns the development of the solution and shaping the organisational change.

Phase 4 This phase putting the solution into practice and evaluating the quality of the solution. Putting into practice takes place through a pilot.

Phase 5 The final phase relates to scaling up the solution by standardising work processes, steering for structural use of the solution and re-evaluating the further development (Wolters & Hagen, 2019).

In Table 2, the 38 publications have been filtered according to the purpose of the study.

The result of the analysis of 38 publications held is that 20 of the 38 selected publications relate to the sharing of data between healthcare organisations using blockchain solutions. Furthermore, the analysis shows that 11 publications out of 38 relate to streamlining healthcare data using a blockchain solution. The number of cited publications per topic/research field was also examined. The result of this analysis is that 144 citations relate to publications with the topic/research field 'Data Sharing' There are 48 citations that relate to publications that have 'Healthcare Data' as their main topic/research field.

Table 2. Research field

Research area	Number of Publications	Number of citations	Number of citations in relation to number of publications
Sharing of Data	20	144	7,20
Electronic Health records	11	48	4,36
Access control	2	0	0,00
Logistic	1	1	1,00
Other	4	69	17,25
Total	38	262	

The subject/research field 'Other' shows a distorted picture. This distorted picture is caused by the fact that there is a publication in this domain with 61 citations. If the number of citations per subject/research field is set off against the number of publications per subject/research field, the result is that the subject/research field 'Data Sharing' has an average of 7.2 citations per publication. The subject/field of research 'Health care data' has an average of 4.36 citations per publication. Here too, a distorted picture arises because in the subject/field of research 'Other', one publication is categorised with 61 citations. Compared to the small number of publications in this category, this means an average of 17.25 citations per publication. In Table 3, the 38 publications have been selected according to the implementation phase. For this purpose, the five phases have been taken as the starting point.

The results are based on an analysis of the most important topics from the abstracts. These topics say something about the phase of implementation. Based on this, it was determined which phase is applicable to the publication. The result of this analysis is that sixteen of the selected publications are in the planning phase. In percentage terms, that is 42% of the total.

Table 3. Stage of implementation based on number of publications and citations

Phase of implementation	Number of Publications	Number of citations	Number of citations in relation to the number of publications
Vision and Strategy	6	28	4,67
Planning	16	153	9,56
Development	10	58	5,80
Execution and Evaluation	6	23	3,83
Scaling up	0	0	0,00
Total	38	262	

Also, of the 38 selected publications, 10 are in the development phase. Six publications were analysed in which the blockchain solution is in the implementation and evaluation phase. No publications were analysed that say anything about the scaling up of blockchain solutions within healthcare whereby processes are also standardised. To gain insight into the impact, the number of citations was determined for each phase of implementation. Based on this analysis, the result is that the 'Planning' phase, with 153 citations, has the largest share of the 262 citations. To obtain a relative picture, the number of citations has been set off against the number of publications per implementation phase. The result of this analysis is that the implementation phase

'Planning', with an average of 9.56 citations per publication, has the largest share as a phase, followed by the implementation phase 'Development' with 5.8 citations per phase.

To gain insight into the most important trends of Blockchain implementations within healthcare, the 38 selected publications were classified based on the type of initiative. In terms of methodology, a topic analysis by means of axial coding was used. A publication can have several initiatives. The initiatives used originate from the research of Pessin, Shanler, Cole & Stevens and can be found in chapter 5.

Table 4. Development of the number of initiatives for the implementation of blockchain as a solution

Initiatives of Blockchain as solution for implementation	Number of Initiatives identified	2018	2019	2020
Disruptive initiatives within existing business model	14		4	10
Initiatives that lead to improvement of transactions between organizations	21	2	5	14
Initiatives that lead to the creation of new virtual or physical markets	2		2	0
Initiatives that deal with secure storage of information.	16		6	10
Total	53	2	17	34

*Some initiatives occur more frequently in one publication

Table 4 shows that implementations, which lead to the improvement of transactions between organisations, with 21 initiatives (40%) have a large share compared to the total. Blockchain solutions with the initiative 'secure storage of information' also feature frequently (30%). To form a picture of the development of the initiatives studied, we looked at when the initiative was published in a Journal. Both initiatives in which the blockchain solution disrupts the existing business model and initiatives that lead to improved transactions between organisations show an increase between the publication years 2019 and 2020. Since the number of publications has also increased between 2019 and 2020, it is not yet possible to make a direct statement as to whether there is a trend.

The increase in the number of initiatives per initiative must be compared with the increase in the number of publications to establish whether there is an actual positive development. The results of this analysis are summarised in Table 5.

The result of this analysis is that initiatives concerning the improvement of transactions between organisations and initiatives that are disruptive to existing business models, show an increase. To determine whether there is a trend, more progressive insight is needed.

Table 6 shows, from three different contexts, the main considerations in adopting blockchain as a solution.

Table 5. Development of the number of initiatives between the years 2019 (index 100%) and 2020

Initiatives to implement blockchain as a solution	Increase in initiatives between the years 2020 and 2019	Increase in number of publications between the years 2020 and 2019	Difference
Disruptive initiatives within existing business model	150%	100%	50%
Initiatives that lead to improvement of transactions between organizations	180%	100%	80%
Initiatives that lead to the creation of new virtual or physical markets	-100%	100%	-200%
Initiatives that deal with secure storage of information.	67%	100%	-33%

Table 6. Adoption considerations from three different contexts

Important factors to take in consideration with the adoption of Blockchain					
Considerations at technology perspective	Number of mentioned in selected articles	Considerations at Organizational perspective	Number of mentioned in selected articles	Considerations at Environmental perspective	Number of mentioned in selected articles
Availability (technik)	6	Organizational readiness	6	Competive pressure	3
Complexity (technik)	3	Top Management support	5	Rules and regulations	3
Perceived use	3	Size organizations	3	Dynamic market	3

The considerations presented in Table 6 were obtained by applying the selection process and methodology presented in Figure 7 respectively.

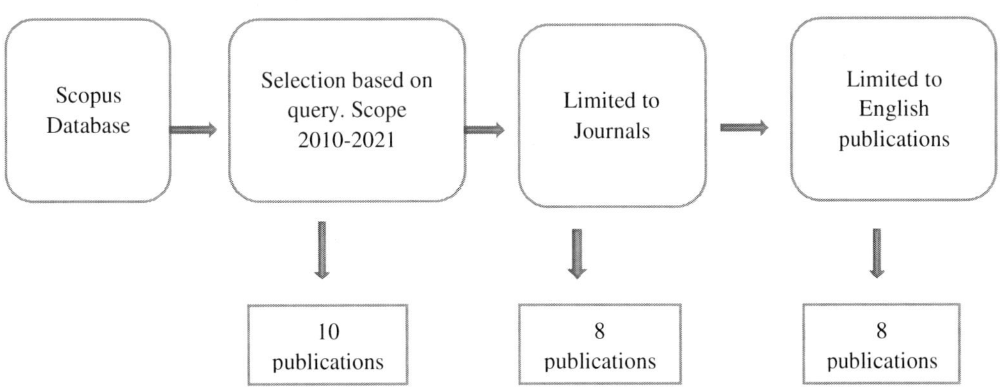

Figure 7. Selection process.

The selection resulted in 8 publications that were read in their entirety and coded for adoption considerations, which were described from the theory of Tornatzky and Fleisher (Tornatzky & Fleischer, 1990). Appendix 2 contains an overview of the selected publications with the mentioned adoption considerations. The result of Table 6 is that from the technological context, availability and complexity of technology are important considerations that influence the adoption of blockchain. Organisational readiness is an important consideration for adopting blockchain. Organisational readiness refers to the change readiness and efficiency of the members of the organisation to implement an organisational change. (Weiner, 2009) Important contextual factors from the organisational perspective are organisational culture, organisational structure, past experiences, and internal regulations. From an environmental context, pressure from competitors is especially seen as an important factor in the adoption of blockchain as a technology.

ANSWER TO THE RESEARCH QUESTIONS

In this section, the questions posed in Section 6.1 will be answered based on the data obtained and analyses made in the Systematic Literature Review.

The first research question concerns the development of implementations of blockchain solutions in recent years within the healthcare sector. Based on this systematic review, it can be stated that many implementations of blockchain in healthcare are still in the planning and development phase and have yet to be implemented and evaluated. However, the Systematic Literature Review does show that the number of publications dealing with the implementation of blockchain solutions has risen sharply. This means that the blockchain research field in healthcare remains interesting and is continuing to develop. This observation can be justified by the increase in the number of cited publications. As of 2019, a clear increase in the number of citations in relation to the number of publications can be observed. This means that the domain of blockchain in healthcare is gaining greater impact.

The second research question is about what the main trends of implementations of blockchain solutions within healthcare are. Important trends that emerge from this Systematic Literature Review relate to the sharing of data between organisations. This mainly concerns increasing interoperability. Another examined trend within the area of blockchain solution implementations concerns the sharing of healthcare data which is often linked to self-sovereign identification (SSI). Deloitte also outlines this trend in its report “five blockchain trends for 2020” (Deloitte, 2020).

Another important trend within healthcare is that many initiatives are being taken to disruptively adapt existing business models using a blockchain solution. Between the years 2019 and 2020, a clear growth can be observed in the number of publications that deal with initiatives to disruptively adapt existing business models using a blockchain solution. Of the selected publications, an increase of 50% can be observed on said initiative. This mainly concerns the disruptive adaptation of business models that deal with granting permission within the process of sharing medical data. In addition, there are initiatives about the implementation of blockchain solutions that improve the existing business model of transporting the blood supply from patient to blood test result. There is also a trend in publications leading to improved transactions between organisations. If the year 2020 is compared with the year 2019, an increase of 80% can be observed in the number of initiatives in which implementations of blockchain solutions lead to the improvement of transactions between organisations. However, the discussion is that the data collected relates to the years 2019 and 2020 and there is insufficient progressive insight as to whether these mentioned trends will continue.

The third research question concerns the division that is visible within the phases of adoption about Blockchain in healthcare. To answer the question properly, a connection was sought with the phases of adoption as defined by Rogers and Pierce & Delbecq (Pierce & Delbecq, 1977) (Rogers, 1995). The adoption process consists of three phases: Initiation, Adoption (decision-making) and Implementation.

The initiation phase relates to the need to identify a solution, for which awareness is created. This leads to identifying suitable innovations and proposing some innovations for adoption (decision making) (Duncan, 1976) (Rogers, 1995). The adoption (decision making) phase reflects the evaluation of innovations from technical, financial, and strategic perspectives, where the decision is made whether to accept an innovation (Meyer & Goes, 1988). The last phase concerns the phase of implementing the innovation. It involves actions related to adapting the innovation, preparing the organisation for use, trial use, acceptance of the innovation by users and scaling up the innovation (Rogers, 1995) (Meyer & Goes, 1988) (Duncan, 1976). By linking to Table 3, phases of implementation of blockchain in healthcare, a picture can be obtained of the adoption phase of blockchain in healthcare. The majority of the 38 selected publications are still in a plan or development phase. As described in chapter 7, the plan phase is about forming a plan and the impact of the solution offered on the organisation within the healthcare sector. The development phase is about developing the solution and shaping organisational change. This plan and development phase corresponds to the definition of the initiative phase from the adoption process, as defined by Rogers and Pierce and Delbecq (Rogers, 1995).

The fourth research question concerns the factors that are considered when adopting blockchain as a solution. To this end, a connection was sought with the theory of Tornatzky and Fleischer, in which insight was gained into the considerations relating to the adoption of technology from various contexts (Tornatzky & Fleischer, 1990). For this purpose, the TOE framework was taken as the starting point. Selection from the Scopus Database resulted in 8 publications, which were coded according to the different considerations, reasoned from three different contexts. The main factors considered are the availability of blockchain as a technology, organisational readiness, and competitive pressure. An interesting area of research within the adoption considerations is organisational readiness. Where, in terms of organisational readiness and organisational capacity, do barriers arise that prevent the adoption of new technologies such as blockchain?

Conclusion and Discussion

In this chapter, I present the results of a Systematic Literature Review of the development, trends, and impact of blockchain solution implementations in healthcare and the considerations for adoption. The findings show that the interest and impact in the field of implementations of blockchain solutions in healthcare is growing. The conclusions of the selected 38 publications, which were analysed using axial coding, show that many studies are still in the planning and development phase. The studies studied mostly present a framework for implementing blockchain solutions in healthcare. This finding is in line with phases 1and 2 and partly phase 3 from the 'Handreiking e-health implementatie' (e-health implementation guide) published by the digital platform Zorg voor innoveren (Wolters & Hagen, 2019). None of the publications contains a study on the evaluation of an implemented blockchain solution. The findings from the Systematic Literature Review show that blockchain is seen as a solution to promote data sharing within healthcare. This finding aligns with the main initiative to initiate a blockchain solution, which is to improve transactions between healthcare organisations. From the study of the selected publications, it appears that the adoption of blockchain is largely rooted in the technological aspects such as security, scalability, and flexibility. From an organisational perspective, there is a need for research into the acceptability of blockchain as a technology. This need is in line with the results obtained from the TOE framework of Tornatzky and Fleischer (Tornatzky & Fleischer, 1990). Holotiuk and Moormann describe that organisational adoption of blockchain is an important factor because organisations must be able to assess the use of a technology, such as blockchain, based on need (Holotiuk & Moormann, 2018). Organisational adoption is an ongoing, multifaceted process of technological innovation and organisational change management (Markus & Tanis, 2000). This Systematic Literature Review is limited because relevant data was collected only from the Scopus Database. A broader scope of relevant literature would have provided more in-depth information, thereby increasing the reliability and validity of this systematic literature review. This systematic literature review did provide sufficient insights into where there are gaps in the scientific literature. The insights obtained from this systematic literature review help to connect the research stream on blockchain with established research areas such as organisational and change management.

Further Research and Limitations

The conclusion of the fourth sub-question forms the starting point for conducting further research. This question focuses on the factors that are considered when adopting new technologies. In the introduction to this publication, it was described that there is a gap in the literature regarding the barriers to the adoption of blockchain by users (patients), but also service providers such as doctors and hospital administrators (Jaoude & Saade, 2019). Tandon et al and Holotiuk and Moormann confirm this gap (Tandon, Amandeep, Najmul Islam, & Mantymaki, 2020) (Holotiuk & Moormann, 2018). Further research is needed to gain insights into how healthcare organisations respond to changes caused using new technology, such as blockchain. Specifically, research is conducted on organizational readiness for change and organizational capacity. Organizational readiness for change focuses on the willingness and ability to change within an organization (Weiner, 2009). Organizational capacity refers to the competence, motivation, and support present within organizations to enable change because of new technologies (Bailey, 1993). On this basis, a research agenda was drawn up in which four studies take centre stage. In Figure 8, the different studies are visualised and brought into coherence with each other. Due to the rapid developments occurring within a disruptive technology such as blockchain, an additional Systematic Literature Review is necessary. This research will, given the strong development of the research area, take place with different terms. Relevant scientific literature published in the year 2021 will be included in this Systematic Literature Review.

In this way, a series of Systematic Literature Surveys will be created, forming a longitudinal picture. As recommended by Briner, Denyer, and Rousseau, to have sufficient evidence on objects (including a technology such as blockchain) that are constantly evolving, the collected literature from the first Systematic Literature Review would help to establish a preliminary theoretical framework. Literature data from the 2nd Systematic Literature Review serves to justify, supplement and/or extend the constructed theoretical framework (Briner, Denyer, & Rousseau, 2009). This means that a more sophisticated approach to a Systematic Literature Review is necessary. According to Greenhalgh & Peacock, no matter how many databases are searched, a Systematic Review of complex evidence cannot rely solely on predefined, protocolised search strategies. Strategies that may seem less efficient, (asking colleagues, following references that look interesting, and just being alert to chance discoveries) may have a better payoff and are likely to identify important sources that would otherwise be missed. Citation tracking is an important search method for identifying systematic reviews (Greenhalgh & Peacock, 2009)

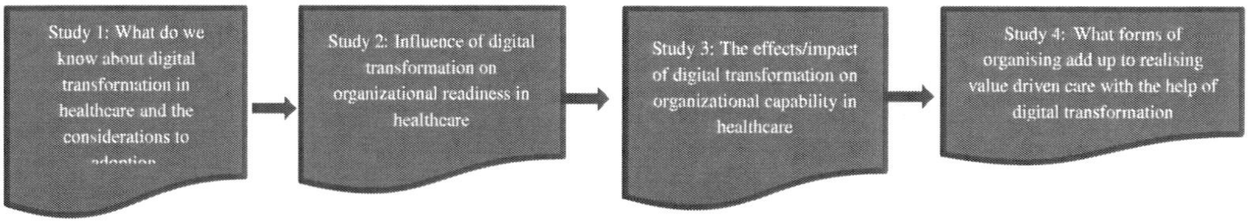

Figure 8. Research agenda in a coherent perspective.

- Theoretical background: Digital transformation (Blockchain)
- Field of research: Organisational readiness, organisational capability, forms of organising
- Level of analysis: Organisational level and between organisations.
- Unit of analysis: Healthcare organisations.

REFERENCES

Abou-Nassar, E., Ilyasu, A., El-Kafrawy, P., Song, O.-Y., Bashir, A., & El latif, A. (2020). DITrust Chain: Towards Blockchain-Based Trust Models for Sustainable Healthcare IoT Systems. *IEEE Access*, vol.8, 111223-111238.

Adrian, Husain, F., Willyanto, Wang, G., & Sfenrianto. (2020). Applying smart contract in E-logistics for monitoring and control. *International Journal of Emerging Trends in Engineering Research,* vol.8, 247-250.

Akkaoui, R., Hei, X., & Cheng, W. (2020). EdgeMediChain: A Hybrid Edge Blockchain-Based Framework for Health Data Exchange. *IEEE Access,* vol.8, 113467-113486.

Aste, T., Tasca, P., & Di Matteo, T. (2017). Blockchain Technologies: The Foreseeable Impact on Society and Industry. *Computer,* 18-28.

Bailey, T. (1993). D*iscretionary Effort and the Organization of Work: Employee Participation and Work Reform Since Hawthorne.* Columbia: Teachers College and Conservation of Human Resources Columbia University.

Beijen, M. (2020). *Succesvol Digitaal Transformeren.* 's-Hertogenbosch: van Haren Publishing. [*Successful Digital Transformation.*]

Berns, S., de Jong, J., Oosterkamp, H., Stolk, R., Wesseling, H., & Wieringa, W. (2019). *Naar werkende governance op blockchain in de zorg.* Den Haag: Berenschot. [*Towards working governance on blockchain in healthcare*]

Boulos, M., Wilson, J., & Clauson, K. (2018). Geospatial blockchain: Promises, challenges and scenarios in health and healthcare. *International Journal Health Geogr.*, 17-25.

Briner, B., Denyer, D., & Rousseau, M. (2009). Evidence-Based Management: Concept Cleanup Time? *Exchange; Academy of Management Perspectives*, 19-32.

Chukwu, E., & Garg, L. (2020). A systematic review of blockchain in healthcare: Frameworks, prototypes, and implementations. *IEEE Access,* vol.8, 21196-21214.

Cieplak, J., & Leefatt, S. (2017). Smart Contracts: A smart way to automate performance. *Georgetown Law Technology Review,* vol 1:2, 417-427.

Clohessy, T., & Acton, T. (2020). Investigating the influence of organizational factors on blockchain adoption: An innovation theory perspective. *Industrial Management and Data Systems,* vol 188.

Cubera, F., Dias, D., Simonyan, V., Yoon, W., & Casella, A. (2019). Blockchain: An enabler for healthcare and life sciences transformation. *IBM Journal of Research and Development,* vol 63.

Dai, J., & Vasarhelyi, M. (2017). "Toward blockchain-based accounting and assurance". *Journal of Information Systems,* Vol.31 No.3, 5-21.

Deloitte. (2020). C-Suite Briefing: 5 blockchain trends voor 2020. *Deloite*, 14.

Duncan, R. (1976). The Ambidextrous Organization: Designing Dual Structures for Innovation. Dans R. Kilmann, L. Pondy, & D. Slevin, *The Management of Organizational Design: Strategy Implementation 1* (pp. 167-188). New York: North-Holland.

Erokhin, A., Koshechkin, K., & Ryabkov, L. (2020). The distributed ledger technology as a measure to minimize risks of poor-quality pharmaceuticals circulation. *PeerJ Computer Science,* vol.6.

Fernando, Y., Rozauar, N., & Mergeresa, F. (2021). The blockchain-enabled technology and carbon performance: Insights from early adopters. *Technology in Society,* vol 64.

Gokalp, E., Coban, S., & Gokalp, M. (2020). Acceptance of Blockchain Based Supply Chain Management System: Research Model Proposal [Blokzincir Tabanli Tedarik Zinciri Yönetimi Sistemi Kabulü: Arastirma Modeli Önerisi]. *1st International Informatics and Software Engineering Conference: Innovative Technologies for Digital Transformation, IISEC 2019 - Proceedings,* vol 173.

Goossens, J., & Verslype, K. (2019). Blockchain en smart contracts;Het einde van de vertrouwde tussenpersoon? *Eerste hulpHulp bij rechtszaken: Blockchain in de juridische wereld: Enkele toepassingen* , 5-10. [Blockchain and smart contracts; The end of the trusted middleman? *First AidLegal Aid: Blockchain in the Legal World: Some Applications*]

Gopalakrishnan, S., & Ganeshkumar, P. (2013). Systematic Reviews and meta-analysis: understanding the best evidence in primary healthcare. *Journal Family Med. Prim. Care 2*, 9-14.

Gourisetti, S. N., Mylrea, M., & Patangia, H. (2020). Evaluation and Demonstration of Blockchain Applicability Framework. *IEEE Transactions on Engineering Management* (Volume: 67, Issue: 4, Nov. 2020), 1142-1156.

Greenhalgh, T., & Peacock, R. (2009). Effectiveness and efficiency of search methods in systematic reviews of complex evidence: audit of primary sources. *BMJ,* vol 331, 1064-1065.

Griggs, K., Ossipova, O., Kohlios, C., Baccarini, A., Howson E.A., & Hayajneh, T. (2018). Healthcare Blockchain System Using Smart Contracts for Secure Automated Remote Patient Monitoring. *Journal of Med. Syst.*

Hölbl, M., Kompara, M., Kamišalić, A., & Zlatolas, L. (2018). A systematic review of the use of blockchain in healthcare vol 10. *Symmetry.*

Hölbl, M., Kompara, M., Kamišalić, A., & Zlatolas, L. N. (2018). A Systematic Review of the Use of Blockchain in Healthcare. *Symmetry 2018, 10.*

Hanelt, A., Bohnsack, R., Marz, D., & Marante, C. (2020). A Systematic Review of the Literature on Digital Transformation: Insights and Implications for Strategy and Organizational Change. *Journal of Management Studies*, 1-39.

He, Q., Guan, N., Lv, M., & Yi, W. (2018). On the Consensus Mechanisms of Blockchain/DLT for Internet of Things. *2018 IEEE 13th International Symposium on Industrial Embedded Systems (SIES) 6-8 June 2018.* Graz: IEEE.

Hewavitharana, T., Nanayakkara, S., & Perera, S. (2019). Blockchain as a project management platform. Blockchain as a project management platform (pp. 137-146). *Proceedings of the 8th World Construction Symposium*, Colombo, Sri Lanka, 8-10 November 2019: https://2019.ciobwcs.com/papers.

Holotiuk, F., & Moormann, J. (2018). *Organizational adoption of Digital Innovation: The case of blockchain technology.* Portsmouth UK: Association for Information Systems.

Islam, A., & Young Shin, S. (2020). A blockchain-based secure healthcare scheme with the assistance of unmanned aerial vehicle in Internet of Things. *Computers and Electrical Engineering* vol 84.

Janse, A., & Lin Lim, C. (2020). *Basisboek Blockchain.* Amsterdam : De boekdrukker.

Jaoude, J., & Saade, R. (2019). Blockchain Applications-Usage in different domains. *IEEE Acess 7*, 45360-45381.

Kamble, S., Gunasekaran, A., Kumar, V., Belhadi, A., & Foropon, C. (2021). A machine learning based approach for predicting blockchain adoption in supply Chain. *Technological Forecasting and Social Change,* vol 163.

Kamel Boulos, M., Wilson, J., & Clauson, K. (2018). Geospatial blockchain: Promises, challenges, and scenarios in health and healthcare. *International Journal of Health Geographics,* vol 17.

Kim, S., Kim, J., & Kim, D. (2020). Implementation of a blood cold chain system using blockchain technology. *Applied Sciences (Switzerland)*, vol 10.

Kulkarni, M., & Patil K. (2020). Block chain technology adoption using toe framework. *International Journal of Scientific and Technology Research* vol 9.

Kumar, A., Krishnamurthi, R., Nayyar, A., Sharma, K., Grover, V., & Hossain, E. (2020). A Novel Smart Healthcare Design, Simulation, and Implementation Using Healthcare 4.0 Processes. *IEEE Access* vol. 8, 118433-118471.

Kuo, T.-T., Kim, J., & Gabriel, R. (2020). Privacy-preserving model learning on a blockchain network-of-networks. *Journal of the American Medical Informatics Association* vol.27, 343-354.

Lemieux, V., Rowell, C., Seidel, M.-D., & Woo, C. (2020). Caught in the middle?: Strategic information governance disruptions in the era of blockchain and distributed trust. *Records Management Journal.*

Liang, X., Zhao, J., Shetty, S., Liu, J., & Li, D. (2017). Integrating blockchain for data sharing and collaboration in mobile healthcare applications. *Proceedings of the 2017 IEEE 28th Anual International Symposium on Personal, Indoor, and Mobile Radio Communcations*, (pp. 1-5). Montreal QC, Canada.

Lippert, S., & Govindarajulu, C. (2006). Technological, Organizational, and Environmental Antecedents to Web Services Adoption. *Antecedents to Web Services Adoption,* 147.

Luijs, J., Bergen, M. v., & Engelen, L. (2020). *De gezondheids (zorg) toekomst van Nederland.* Deloitte. [*The health (care) future of the Netherlands.*]

Mackey, T., Miyachi, K., Fung, D., Qian, S., & Short, J. (2020). Combating health care fraud and abuse: Conceptualization and prototyping study of a blockchain antifraud framework. *Journal of Medical Internet Research* vol 22.

Madine, M., Battah, A., Yaqoob, I., Salah, K., Jayaraman, R., Al Hammadi, Y.,... Ellahham, S. (2020). Blockchain for Giving Patients Control over Their Medical Records. *IEEE Access,* vol 8, 193102-193115.

Malamas, V., Kotzanikolaou, P., Dasaklis, T., & Burmester, M. (2020). A Hierarchical Multi Blockchain for Fine Grained Access to Medical Data. *IEEE Access,* vol.8, 134393-134412.

Margheri, A., Masi, M., Miladi, A., Sassone, V., & Rosenzwieger, J. (2020). Decentralised provenance for healthcare data. *International Journal of Medical Informatics,* vol. 141.

Markus, M., & Tanis, C. (2000). *Framing the Domains of IT Management: Projecting the Future through the Pas*". Cincinnati: Pinnaflex Educational Resources Inc.

Mayer, A., Costa, C. d., & Rosa Rhigi, R. d. (2020). Electronic health records in a Blockchain: A systematic review. *Health Informatics Journal*, 1273-1288.

Mazlan, A., Daud, S., Abas, H., Rashid, S., & Yusof, M. (2020). Scalability Challenges in Healthcare Blockchain System-A Systematic Review. *IEEE Access,* vol 8, 23663-23673.

McBee, M., & Wilcox, C. (2020). Blockchain Technology: Principles and Applications in Medical Imaging. *Journal of Digital Imaging,* vol.33, 726-734.

Meinert E., A. A., Meindert, E., Alturkistani, A., Foley, K., Osama, T., Car, J., ... Brindley, D. (2019). Blockchain implementation in health care: Protocol for a systematic review. *Journal of Medical Internet Research,* vol. 21.

Menshikov, V., & Volkova, O. (2019). Digitalization for increased access security to healthcare services in Latvia. *Journal of Security and Sustainability Issues,* vol. 1, 171-183.

Meyer, A., & Goes, J. (1988). Organizational Assimilation of Innovation: A multilevel Contextual Analysis. *Academy of Management Journal 31*, 897-923.

Moon, J., & Kim, D. (2020). Design and implementation of distributed ledger based health data management system. *International Journal of Innovative Computing, Information and Control*, vol.16, 1117-1124.

Muzammalab, M., Qu, Q., & Nasrulin, B. (2019). Renovating blockchain with distributed databases: An open source system. *Future Generation Computer Systems,* vol. 90, 105-117.

Nakamoto, S. (2008). *Bitcoin a peer to peer electronic cash system.* Récupéré sur https://bitcoin.org/bitcoin.pdf

Nordrum, A. (2017). "Govern by blockchain Dubai wants one platform to rule them all, while Illnois will try anything". *IEEE Spectrum,* vol. 54. No.10, 54-55.

Omar, I., Jayaraman, R., Salah, K., Yaqoob, I., & Ellahham, S. (2020). Applications of Blockchain Technology in Clinical Trials: Review and Open Challenges. *Arabian Journal for Science and Engineering.*

O'Reilly, K. (2012). *Ethnographic methods,* second edition. New York: Routledge.

Orji, I., Kusi-Sarpong, S., Huang, S., & Vasquez-Brust, D. (2020). Evaluating the factors that influence blockchain adoption in the freight logistics industry. *Transportation Research Part E: Logistics and Transportation Review,* vol 141.

Orlikowski, W. (1992). The Duality of Technology: Rethinking the Concept of Technology in Organizations. *Organization Science,* vol. 3, No. 3, 398-427.

Pandey, P., & Litoriya, R. (2020). Implementing healthcare services on a large scale: Challenges and remedies based on blockchain technology. *Health Policy and Technology*, vol. 6, 69-78.

Pandey, P., & Litoriya, R. (2020). Promoting Trustless Computation Through Blockchain Technology. *National Academy Science Letters.*

Park, K. (2020). A study on sustainable usage intention of blockchain in the big data era: Logistics and supply chain management companies. *Sustainability (Switzerland)* vol 12.

Pawczuk, L., Massey, R., & Holdowsky, J. (2019). *Deloitte 2019 Global Blockchain survey-Blockchain gets down to business In: Deloitte Insights.* Récupéré sur https://www2.deloitte.com: https://www2.deloitte.com/content/dam/Deloitte/se/Documents/risk/DI_2019-global-blockchain-survey.pdf

Peral, J., Gallego, E., Gil, D., Tanniru, M., & Khambekar, P. (2020). Using visualization to build transparency in a healthcare blockchain application. *Sustainability (Switzerland),* vol. 12.

Pessin, G., Shanler, M., Cole, B., & Stevens, A. (2019). *Healthcare and Life Science Digital Transformation and Innovation.* Gartner.

Pierce, J., & Delbecq, A. (1977). Organization Structure, Indivdual Attitudes and Innovation. *Academy of Management Review 2*, 27-37.

Rahman, M., Rashid, M., Kernec, J., Philippe, B., Barnes, S., Fioranelli, F., ... Imran, M. (2019). A secure occupational therapy framework for monitoring cancer patients' quality of life. *Sensors (Switzerland),* vol 19.

Raval, S. (2016). *Decentralized Applications: Harnessing Bitcoin's Blockchain Technology*. Sebastapol CA, USA: O'Reilly Media.

Roehrs, A., Costa, C. d., Rosa Righi, R. d., Silva, V. d., Goldlim, J., & Schmidt, D. (2019). Analyzing the performance of a blockchain-based personal health record implementation. *Journal of Biomedical Informatics* vol.92.

Rogers, E. (1995). Diffusion of Innovation. Dans *Diffusion of Innovation.* New York: Free Press.

Sgantzos, K., & Grigg, I. (2019). Artificial intelligence implementations on the blockchain. Use cases and future applications. *Future Internet,* vol 11.

Shahnaz, A., Qamar, U., & Khalid, A. (2019). Using Blockchain for Electronic Health Records. *IEEE Access,* vol 7, 147782-147795.

Sharma, N., & Joshi, R. (2019). Enhancing the health care data security through blockchain. *International Journal of Engineering and Advanced Technology,* vol 8, 549-554.

Sung, M., Park, S., Jung, S., Lee, E., Lee, J., & Park, Y. (2020). Developing a mobile app for monitoring medical record changes using blockchain: Development and usability study. *Journal of Medical Internet Research,* vol. 22.

Swan, M. (2015). *Blockchain: Blueprint for an New Economy.* Newton, MA, USA: O'Reilly Media.

Tandon, A., Amandeep, D., Najmul Islam, A., & Mantymaki, M. (2020). Blockchain in healthcare: A systematic literature review, synthesizing framework and future research agenda. *Computers in Industry,* vol. 122.

Tornatzky, L., & Fleischer, M. (1990). *The processes of technological innovation.* Lexington, MA: Lexington Books.

Vazirani, A., O'Donoghue, O., Brindeley, D., & Meinert, E. (2019). Design choices and trade-offs in health care blockchain implementations: Systematic review. *Journal of Medical Internet Research,* vol 21.

Veuger, J. (2020). Dutch Blockchain, real estate and land registration. *Journal of Property, Planning and Environmental Law,* Vol 12, No2, 93-108.

Veuger, J., & Woldendorp, H. (2021). Blockchain in de zorg. *Dans Blockchain in de zorg.* Assen: Koninklijke Van Gorcum BV. [Blockchain in healthcare. *Dance Blockchain in healthcare.*]

Wang, Z., Luo, N., & Zhou, P. (2020). GuardHealth: Blockchain empowered secure data management and Graph Convolutional Network enabled anomaly detection in smart healthcare. *Journal of Parallel and Distributed Computing,* vol 142, 1-12.

Weiner, B. (2009, oktober 19). A theory of organizational readiness for change. *Implementation Science,* vol. 4.

Wolters, W., & Hagen, S. v. (2019). https://www.zorgvoorinnoveren.nl/. Récupéré sur https://www.zorgvoorinnoveren.nl/implementatie/ handreiking-e-health-implementatie: https://www.zorgvoorinnoveren.nl/implementatie/handreiking-e-health-implementatie

Wong, L., Leong, L., Hew, J., Tan, G., & Ooi, K. (2020). Time to seize the digital evolution: Adoption of blockchain in operations and supply chain management among Malaysian SMEs. *International Journal of Information Management,* vol 52.

Xie, J., Tang, H., Huang, T., Yu, F., Xie, R., Liu, J., & Liu, Y. (2019). A Survey of Blockchain Technology Applied to Smart Cities: Research Issues and Challenges. *IEEE Communications Surveys and Tutorials,* vol 21, 2794-2830.

Yanez, W., Mahmud, R., Bahsoon, R., Zhang, Y., & Buyya, R. (2020). Data Allocation Mechanism for Internet-of-Things Systems With Blockchain. *IEEE Internet of Things Journal*, vol.7, 3509-3522.

Yu, H., Sun, H., Wu, D., & Kuo, T.-T. (2019). Comparison of Smart Contract Blockchains for Healthcare Applications. *AMIA ... Annual Symposium proceedings. AMIA Symposium*, 1266-1275.

Zheng, Z., Xie, S., Dai, H., Chen, X., & Wang, H. (2017). An Overview of Blockchain Technology: Architecture, Consensus, and Future Trends. *IEEE International Congress on Big Data (BigData Congress)* 11-14 December 2017, (pp. 557-564). Boston, MA USA.

Zubaydi, H., Chong, Y.-W., Ko, K., Hanshi, S., & Karuppayah, S. (2019). A review on the role of blockchain technology in the healthcare domain. *Electronics (Switzerland),* vol 8.

APPENDIX 1: SELECTED AND CONSULTED ARTICLES

1. (Kamel Boulos, Wilson, & Clauson, 2018)	Geospatial blockchain: Promises, challenges, and scenarios in health and healthcare
2. (Hölbl M., Kompara, Kamišalić, & Zlatolas, 2018)	A systematic review of the use of blockchain in healthcare
3. (Vazirani, O'Donoghue, Brindeley, & Meinert, 2019)	Design choices and trade-offs in health care blockchain implementations: Systematic review
4. (Meinert E., et al., 2019)	Blockchain implementation in health care: Protocol for a systematic review
5. (Rahman, et al., 2019)	A secure occupational therapy framework for monitoring cancer patients' quality of life
6. (Cubera, Dias, Simonyan, Yoon, & Casella, 2019)	Blockchain: An enabler for healthcare and life sciences transformation
7. (Shahnaz, Qamar, & Khalid, 2019)	Using Blockchain for Electronic Health Records
8. (Yu, Sun, Wu, & Kuo, 2019)	Comparison of Smart Contract Blockchains for Healthcare Applications
9. (Sgantzos & Grigg, 2019)	Artificial intelligence implementations on the blockchain. Use cases and future applications
10. (Xie, et al., 2019)	A Survey of Blockchain Technology Applied to Smart Cities: Research Issues and Challenges
11. (Menshikov & Volkova, 2019)	Digitalization for increased access security to healthcare services in Latvia
12. (Sharma & Joshi, 2019)	Enhancing the health care data security through blockchain
13 (Roehrs, et al., 2019)	Analyzing the performance of a blockchain-based personal health record implementation
14 (Zubaydi, Chong, Ko, Hanshi, & Karuppayah, 2019)	A review on the role of blockchain technology in the healthcare domain
15 (Lemieux, Rowell, Seidel, & Woo, 2020)	Caught in the middle? Strategic information governance disruptions in the era of blockchain and distributed trust
16 (Kim, Kim, & Kim, 2020)	Implementation of a blood cold chain system using blockchain technology
17 (Malamas, Kotzanikolaou, Dasaklis, & Burmester , 2020)	A Hierarchical Multi Blockchain for Fine Grained Access to Medical Data
18 (Adrian, Husain, Willyanto, Wang, & Sfenrianto, 2020)	Applying smart contract in E-logistics for monitoring and control
19 (Islam & Young Shin, 2020)	A blockchain-based secure healthcare scheme with the assistance of unmanned aerial vehicle in Internet of Things
20 (Erokhin , Koshechkin, & Ryabkov, 2020)	The distributed ledger technology as a measure to minimize risks of poor-quality pharmaceuticals circulation
21 (Mackey , Miyachi, Fung, Qian, & Short, 2020)	Combating health care fraud and abuse: Conceptualization and prototyping study of a blockchain antifraud framework
22 (Omar , Jayaraman, Salah, Yaqoob, & Ellahham, 2020)	Applications of Blockchain Technology in Clinical Trials: Review and Open Challenges

Appendix 1. (Continued)

23 (Kuo, Kim , & Gabriel , 2020)	Privacy-preserving model learning on a blockchain network-of-networks
24 (Mazlan, Daud, Abas, Rashid, & Yusof, 2020)	Scalability Challenges in Healthcare Blockchain System-A Systematic Review
25 (Wang, Luo, & Zhou, 2020)	GuardHealth: Blockchain empowered secure data management and Graph Convolutional Network enabled anomaly detection in smart healthcare
26 (Litoriya & Pandey, 2020)	Promoting Trustless Computation Through Blockchain Technology
27 (Yanez, Mahmud, Bahsoon, Zhang, & Buyya, 2020)	Data Allocation Mechanism for Internet-of-Things Systems with Blockchain
28 (Abou-Nassar, et al., 2020)	DITrust Chain: Towards Blockchain-Based Trust Models for Sustainable Healthcare IoT Systems
29 (Moon & Kim , 2020)	Design and implementation of distributed ledger-based health data management system
30 (Akkaoui, Hei, & Cheng, 2020)	EdgeMediChain: A Hybrid Edge Blockchain-Based Framework for Health Data Exchange
31 (Pandey & Litoriya, 2020)	Implementing healthcare services on a large scale: Challenges and remedies based on blockchain technology
32 (McBee & Wilcox, 2020)	Blockchain Technology: Principles and Applications in Medical Imaging
33 (Chukwu & Garg, 2020)	A systematic review of blockchain in healthcare: Frameworks, prototypes, and implementations
34 (Peral, Gallego, Gil, Tanniru, & Khambekar, 2020)	Using visualization to build transparency in a healthcare blockchain application
35 (Margheri, Masi, Miladi, Sassone, & Rosenzwieger, 2020)	Decentralised provenance for healthcare data
36 (Madine , et al., 2020)	Blockchain for Giving Patients Control over Their Medical Records
37 (Kumar, et al., 2020)	A Novel Smart Healthcare Design, Simulation, and Implementation Using Healthcare 4.0 Processes
38 (Sung, et al., 2020)	Developing a mobile app for monitoring medical record changes using blockchain: Development and usability study

APPENDIX 2: OVERVIEW OF SELECTED PUBLICATIONS WITH ADOPTION CONSIDERATIONS

Auteur	Titel	Vaktijdschrift	Volume	Issue	Citatie	Document type	Jaartal	Construct	TOE-factor
Kamble S.S., Gunasekaran A., Kumar V., Belhadi A., Foropon C.	A machine learning based approach for predicting blockchain adoption in supply Chain	Technological Forecasting and Social Change	163		2	Article	2021	Druk van concurrenten	Omgeving
								Organisatorische bereidheid	Organisatie
								Waargenomen bruikbaarheid	technologie
								Waargenomen gemak	technologie
Fernando Y., Rozuar N.H.M., Mergeresa F.	The blockchain-enabled technology and carbon performance: Insights from early adopters	Technology in Society	64		0	Article	2021	Support top management	Organisatie
								Bekwaamheid	Organisatie
								Druk van concurrenten	Omgeving
Park K.O.	A study on sustainable usage intention of blockchain in the big data era: Logistics and supply chain management companies	Sustainability (Switzerland)	12	24	0	Article	2020	Technologische bekwaamhei	Technologie
								Support top management	Organisatie
								Organisatorische bereidheid	Organisatie
Orji I.J., Kusi-Sarpong S., Huang S., Vazquez-Brust D.	Evaluating the factors that influence blockchain adoption in the freight logistics industry	Transportation Research Part E: Logistics and Transportation Review	141		4	Article	2020	Infrastructuur	Omgeving
								Wet en regelgeving	Omgeving
								Beschikbaarheid techniek	technologie
Wong L.-W., Leong L.-Y., Hew J.-J., Tan G.W.-H., Ooi K.-B.	Time to seize the digital evolution: Adoption of blockchain in operations and supply chain management among Malaysian SMEs	International Journal of Information Management	52		36	Article	2020	Druk van concurrenten	Omgeving
								Complexiteit	Technologie
								Dynamiek markt	Omgeving
								Support top management	Organisatie
Kulkarni M., Patil K.	Block chain technology adoption using toe framework	International Journal of Scientific and Technology Research	9	2	1	Article	2020	Infrastructuur	Technologie
								Kennis/Leren vermogen	Organisatie
								Organisatorische bereidheid	Organisatie
								Druk van concurrenten	Omgeving
								Wet en regelgeving	Omgeving
								Dynamiek markt	Omgeving
								Beschikbaarheid techniek	Technologie
Gokalp E., Coban S., Gokalp M.O.	Acceptance of Blockchain Based Supply Chain Management System: Research Model Proposal [Blokzincir Tabanli Tedarik Zinciri Yönetimi Sistemi Kabulü: Arastirma Modeli Önerisi]	1st International Informatics and Software Engineering Conference: Innovative Technologies for Digital Transformation, IISEC 2019 - Proceedings	173		1	Article	2019	Complexiteit	Technologie
								Comptabiliteit	Technologie
								Interoperabiliteit	Technologie
								Schaalbaarheid	Technologie
								Support top management	Organisatie
								Organisatorische bereidheid	Organisatie
								Organisatie grootte.	Organisatie
								Wet en regelgeving	Omgeving
								Vertrouwen tussen organisat	Organisatie
								Druk van concurrenten	Omgeving
Clohessy T., Acton T.	Investigating the influence of organizational factors on blockchain adoption: An innovation theory perspective	Industrial Management and Data Systems	188		24	Article	2019	Support top management	Organisatie
								Organisatorische bereidheid	Organisatie
								Grootte organisatie	Organisatie
								Gebrek aan informatie	Organisatie

(Kamble, Gunasekaran, Kumar, Belhadi, & Foropon, 2021) (Fernando, Rozauar, & Mergeresa, 2021) (Park, 2020) (Orji, Kusi-Sarpong, Huang, & Vasquez-Brust, 2020) (Wong, Leong, Hew, Tan, & Ooi, 2020) (Kulkarni & Patil K., 2020) (Gokalp , Coban , & Gokalp, 2020) (Clohessy & Acton, 2020)

In: Blockchain and Health
Editor: Jan Veuger
ISBN: 978-1-68507-232-2

Chapter 2

Blockchain in Health Care

Jan Veuger[1,*], PhD and Harry Woldendorp[2]

[1] Saxion University of Applied Sciences,
School of Finance and Accounting, School of Creative Technology, School of Governance, Law and Urban Development,
Hospitality Business School,
School of Commerce and Entrepeneurship,
School of People and Society, The Netherlands
[2]PlatformVmz and Curaevitel Balie, Expert Partner
Research Group Blockchain Saxion UAS, The Netherlands

Abstract

In this chapter, we have demonstrated how Blockchain can contribute to addressing the major healthcare issues. These include recording medical data (security, interoperability, accessibility), recording the results of medical research, setting up care chains and ensuring the quality of the medicines. In current healthcare practice, avoidable errors are still made as a result of the lack of information. In addition, time is wasted on double healthcare activities. Therefore, the electronic exchange of healthcare information between healthcare professionals and healthcare institutions should become the standard. Electronic data exchange takes place in a very complex environment. Important developments for the implementation of Blockchain include: increasing the agility of organisations and professionals (including due to COVID-19), a sense of urgency to continue digitisation, artificial intelligence focused on early diagnosis and self-diagnosis, standardisation of healthcare activities, and lifestyle interventions. Among other things, COVID-19 needs to accelerate the provision of good information. Blockchain contributes

* Corresponding Author's E-mail: j.veuger@saxion.nl.

to clear, validated and reliable recording. So while Blockchain is at an early stage, we believe it will converge with Artificial Intelligence and the Internet of Things. This makes a fundamentally different way of organising care processes possible.

Keywords: blockchain, health care, organization, innovation

Preface

It is evident that the current Dutch health system is changing. Developments in data science and the associated technical and organisational infrastructure play a significant role in this, as do the 'contextual factors' including European and national policies. An unexpected contextual factor has become COVID 19, which has demonstrably influenced the healthcare system nationally and internationally. In addition to all the known problems caused by COVID 19, the pandemic has also contributed to the 'digital literacy' of the healthcare sector, especially in the Netherlands.

Now that existing eHealth solutions appear to be entering daily healthcare practice, there is a need for more effective and efficient management of the healthcare system and thus for more applied knowledge in areas such as Blockchain. Blockchain, which is the subject of this book, is one of the emerging technologies in the Dutch healthcare landscape. Several studies show that Blockchain can make a relevant contribution to improving our healthcare system in several ways. Examples of this are discussed extensively in this publication. This involves increasing the efficiency and effectiveness of the healthcare system by, among other things, increasing the safety, consistency and transparency of the multitude of information exchanges circulating in the healthcare system.

This book discusses examples where Blockchain technology has already left its mark in the Dutch healthcare landscape, such as applications and apps for structured notifications of what the healthcare provider has done to the healthcare recipient, which allows the administrative and financial process to be completed more quickly for the various parties. This has not only to do with networks around the client but also with cooperation between healthcare professionals, both inside and outside the walls of the institution.

In addition to this undeniable added value for the healthcare system, in my view the most important contribution of Blockchain is the potential to promote the autonomy and control of healthcare users by bringing their ownership and control over their own medical records closer. Whereas less than 10% of the data in healthcare worldwide was stored electronically in 2008, the electronic health record has become an established concept in 2020. According to the WHO (2016), the adoption and deployment of national electronic health care systems (EHR) has increased by no less than 50 percent worldwide in five years. It appears that these electronic healthcare systems are integrated into more than two thirds of the laboratories and pharmacies.

Nevertheless, that does not tell the whole story, and there are still many challenges to be overcome before there is a global adoption and integration of data technology in healthcare. The most frequently cited obstacles to the implementation of EHRs are, on the basis of a World Health Organisation report, the lack of funding, infrastructure, capacity and in particular legislation. Care and privacy can be considered synonymous. In this digital age, it is essential that information is recorded reliably in methods and systems such as Blockchain.

This chapter, like other studies, also stresses the importance of what is called interoperability, which can be defined as applying the same definitions and data standards.

You often hear that 'data' is the 'new money' or the 'new oil' in the fourth industrial revolution we are now experiencing. This is changing the meaning of communication and also of economy and services. For years, we have been sharing information with each other via the internet, social media, etc. Often we use 'free applications'; in other words, we exchange our data for a service. As a result, our digital currency has become data, and we pay with our data.

Services within the healthcare sector naturally rise above monetary value. Nevertheless, one of the major challenges within the current healthcare system is its financing system. Technology has made it possible with virtual money and digital infrastructure, i.e., cryptocurrency, with Bitcoins as the best known, and Blockchains, to exchange services with each other without thinking in euros. This makes it seem that we are returning to the primary objective of money: a means by which we can exchange our services and products with each other. Can these technological solutions develop new possibilities for exchanging services and completing 'payments' only once the intended 'value' has been achieved?

It is a perspective to which this book aspires and which, given the pace at which technology is developing, seems feasible in the foreseeable future. (Preface by Prof. Dr MSc Engineering Masi Mohammadi, Eindhoven University, The Netherlands).

INTRODUCTION

Storing medical records in a safe manner is vital for any healthcare system. Sole reliance on centralized servers increases the likelihood of sensitive information being leaked. Transparency and increased security of Blockchain technology make this an ideal platform for storing medical records. Patients can store their privacy-sensitive information securely by securing their data on a Blockchain by means of cryptography. This enables them to share their medical information with each healthcare institution with their approvals. The healthcare system is currently very fragmented, but if all users used a secure global database, the flow of information between those users would be much faster. A great advantage of a global database is that clients do not have to tell their story every time. For example, a medical specialist can see exactly what a patient has been through and what treatments and examinations have taken place. The information is also available in *real time* to that care professional whose client has indicated that the professional may access the file.

Digitisation in Healthcare

A new revolution is underway which is clearly different from the third industrial revolution (internet, communication and globalisation). This fourth industrial revolution is about a fusion of technologies such as biotechnology, nanotechnology, artificial intelligence, robotics, the Internet of Things, *cloud computing* and Blockchain. Our healthcare society is also fundamentally changing, also under the influence of COVID-19.

These fundamental changes require an integrated and comprehensive response, involving stakeholders in public and private society. The challenge is how to take healthcare to a new level with innovations from the fourth industrial revolution and at least solve the most urgent problems in care and society. Blockchain will play a major role in this. This is a core technology that has the potential to combine digital data with physical systems.

The starting point of our care is that patients can choose the care that suits them. But how can a patient do this in a field where complexity is only increasing?

In addition, ageing will increase the demand for care. Rising medical costs and an increase in chronic diseases also require a new approach. And more and more often, treatment takes place in a home environment instead of a hospital or healthcare institution. There is therefore a great need for innovation in healthcare.

Healthcare is a high-tech and information-intensive environment. Partly because of this and because of the importance of good communication for the client, you would expect the exchange of information in healthcare to be well regulated. However, care is organised in such a complex way that there is insufficient oversight and insight for both professionals and clients. For example, healthcare professionals describe diseases and treatments in a variety of ways, making it difficult to interpret information from different healthcare records unambiguously. In addition, care parties use a variety of information systems, which makes the information difficult to connect. Of course, security of information is an important issue, which also contributes to the complexity of data exchange.

Digitalisation makes it possible to implement fundamental changes in business operations (Brynjofsson and McAfee 2014). The art for administrators is to securely and intelligently connect all applications and information systems that care parties use. In this book, we elaborate how Blockchain will contribute to overcoming these challenges. Blockchain is a decentralized data storage network. It is designed to achieve integrity, transparency, efficiency and accuracy of data.

Blockchain technology distributes data and decentralizes management, which means that data are stored across multiple servers and managed by the members of the network. PharmaLedger – the European Centre for the Blockchain Consortium in healthcare - aims to bring Blockchain technology to healthcare. Figure 1 shows the relationships between multiple servers.

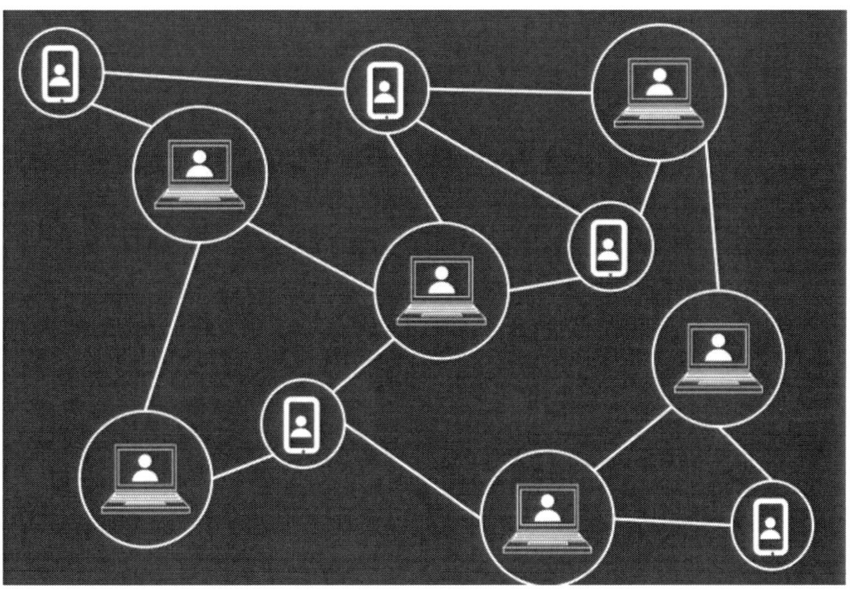

Source: Pixabay.

Figure 1. Distribution and management in Blockchain technology.

Despite the convincing possibilities, there have only been a few large-scale implementations of B*lockchain* technology (Veuger 2020b: 22). In the book, we discuss a case about an application after each chapter:

1. All the parties responsible for Mijn Zorg Log
2. Case: How Microbiome Centre closes the knowledge gap
3. Case: Health information exchange at MedFAbric4Me
4. Case: The VGZ innovation team develops an app for maternity care
5. Case: Deventer GROZzerdam innovates with an app

However, there are also some alternatives in development to creating a decentralised platform for exchanging medical data. The Swiss Medicalchain and the Austrian Grapevine World have solutions that are under development. Another example is the submission of initiatives around Blockchain Enabled Healthcare with the Innovative Medicines Initiative (IMI), a partnership between the European Union and the European pharmaceutical industry.

Blockchain monitors real-time transactions, simplifies regulatory compliance, promises efficiency gains by reducing intermediaries and reduces the risk of fraud and cybercrime (Veuger 2020b). Blockchain thus has an opportunity to address the challenges in the areas of trust, transparency and bureaucracy that various (government) bodies are confronted with and offers new opportunities for collaboration between different profit and non-profit actors.

METHODS

Not everyone needs to become a Blockchain expert, just as you don't have to be a qualified automotive engineer to drive a car. However, with this book we want to achieve that you can 'drive' your organisation with Blockchain, so that goals can be achieved effectively and efficiently on the basis of recorded unchangeable data.

We'll start with a general chapter to guide you in how Blockchain works, such as accessing a Blockchain platform, data storage, and what types of applications there are for Blockchain in healthcare. The subject area contains many unfamiliar terms, but we use as many common terms as possible so that you are familiar with them more quickly.

In Chapter 2, we delve deeper into the characteristics of Blockchain and thus this chapter forms a deepening of Chapter 1. We explain the types of Blockchain applications in healthcare in Chapter 3, and of course we give many examples of applications and experiments. We pay special attention to making patient information accessible and the security of drug production and distribution. We will also discuss the possibilities of Blockchain with *artificial intelligence* and the *Internet of Things*.

In Chapter 4, we elaborate the four basic principles of Blockchain in healthcare. Nictiz's five-layer model plays an important role in this. Chapter 5 is about designing applications. We provide a *roadmap* for interoperability and discuss the role of Blockchain for the Electronic Health Record. In the last chapter, we give advice on how to use and implement Blockchain in healthcare. This chapter therefore has a different character and does not end with a case.

Incidentally, we have opted for the male form for readability, with the exception of the case on maternity care, since virtually all maternity care providers are women. First of all, a chapter to introduce you to the world of Blockchain.

INTRODUCTION TO BLOCKCHAIN

Within healthcare, complexity is caused, among other things, by regulations, funding, organisation, coordination between domains and interaction between clients and professionals. Blockchain enables a fundamental recalibration of the position of clients: complete control of your own data. In this chapter, we expose the complexity of care and tell you how Blockchain is a solution for this.

How Blockchain Works

The name *Blockchain* comes from the way data is stored within the chain. Network users can allow transactions to take place, share information and exchange documents. Each transaction or set of transactions - called a *block* - refers to the previous transaction or set of transactions.

This is because data are stored in blocks. These blocks are connected to each other, creating a chain: the Blockchain. When a transaction has been created, signed, sent and checked within the network, the *blocks* are linked to each other. After the transactions are written and the user has signed them, the blocks are linked to each other.

Each block contains coded data and can be included in the chain if these data refer to the previous data. A block is thus linked by means of a reference to a previous block and thus the blocks form a chain. Figure 2 shows an illustration of this.

A Blockchain, a chain of blocks, is a system that can be used to record data. Examples of this are banking matters, title deeds and product data. What is unique about Blockchain is that it legitimately exists without there being a single central point and without a trusted intermediary.

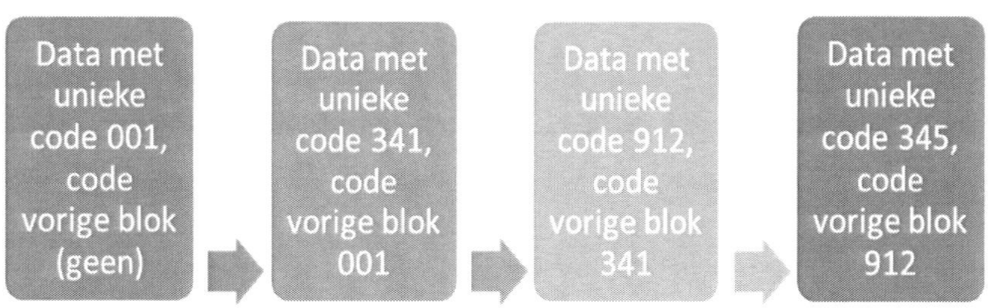

Source: Veuger 2020b.

Figure 2. Chain of blocks.

Blockchain can be used in any domain where information is transferred:

- Currency: electronic financial systems without intermediaries

- Payment infrastructure: transferring payments
- Digital assets: exchanging information
- Digital identity: Digitally sign IDs to combat fraud
- Verifiable data: verify the authenticity of information
- Smart contracts: software programs that perform actions without trusted third parties (Nichol 2017)

Blockchain has four basic principles that distinguish Blockchain from other automation technologies.

1. Growing chain: a chain of data blocks that builds up over time and cannot be unilaterally changed.
2. Distributed network: the chain is distributed to all participating parties and is a shared truth.
3. Consensus: Parties involved must agree on the data stored in the last block.
4. Data storage in the form of cryptography for the data in a Blockchain.

These four basic principles form the character of Blockchain. For all applications and every use, you will see these basic principles applied.

Blockchain as an index

In order to benefit from Blockchain in healthcare, it is mainly about controlling access to medical data. One perspective is to see a healthcare blockchain as an *index*, a list of all healthcare records and medical data of a client. The index is equal to a catalogue in a library. The catalogue contains metadata about a book and the place where the book can be found.

This also applies to healthcare: transactions within the blocks contain a unique opportunity to identify the user, a secure link to the healthcare file and a time marker of when the transaction was created. The healthcare Blockchain thus contains a complete indexed history of all healthcare data (individual history of a patient). The patient determines who gains access to the information, which gives the user full influence on what data is collected and how his data can be shared (Linn and Koo 2016). For example, a GP can view all the data of his own patients, but the patient ultimately determines which data he wants to show to third parties.

Ledger

The Blockchain is therefore a distributed database (the library from the framework text) where data in each instance of this database are stored, comparable to a *ledger*. Everyone connected to the network on which the Blockchain runs has the same copy of the ledger. Before data are permanently stored, there must be *consensus* within a majority of the parties who received these data on the accuracy, origin and completeness of these data.

Where we are familiar with the exchange of information via the internet, Blockchain is about transferring value, as we know it from banks or the notary, but digitally. Key concepts for Blockchain are:

- Ledger: a list of information about all blocks.
- Stored: All the desired information is stored in each block.
- Distributed and decentralised: in the Blockchain, there are many parties - so it is not centralised - and all these parties are connected with each other. All these parties also have the same ledger. Everyone gets a copy of the full ledger and receives an update when something is added.

Peer-to-peer ledger

Blockchain can be seen as a decentralized, distributed ledger or log. This is also called a *peer-to-peer ledger*, in which all participants keep the ledger together. After all, there is no central authority for determining the identity of users, storing files or opening sources. The digital ledger (the Blockchain) is distributed over different *nodes* (network of computers), which check the changes for accuracy. Each node in the Blockchain has a copy of the ledger. There is no centralised official copy and there are no users more trusted than others. Everyone is equal. Transactions are sent to the Blockchain network using applications such as Mijn Zorg Log. This application is central to the case after this chapter.

The most widely known is the application of Blockchain for Bitcoin. In principle, a Blockchain is a database in which different data can be stored. In the case of the Bitcoin Blockchain, the entire transaction history of all Bitcoins is kept and the Blockchain therefore knows exactly how many Bitcoins everyone has.

What makes the Bitcoin Blockchain unique is that this Blockchain (or database) is maintained by a network of servers that basically all have an exact copy of the Blockchain.

Decentralised

A server can be a computer but is in principle a device on which data can be stored. This could therefore also be a mobile phone or a smart TV. The servers check the Blockchain data for accuracy and synchronize the content of their Blockchain with the databases of all other servers on the network. As a result, the servers connected to the

Blockchain network, in the best case scenario, always share the same copy of the Blockchain (Lim and Janse 2020).

> In principle, a Blockchain is: a database comparable to a ledger, that is copied and distributed across different computers and reliable.

Each action of each participant is recorded in a database, which is not only in one place (decentralised). Partly because the database is stored decentrally on thousands of servers around the world, the information remains securely stored and the system is fraud-proof. Every user has an up-to-date copy of the database with all transactions at all times. Data is never lost as a result. Figure 3 shows the difference between a central and decentralised database.

A Blockchain can be explained at different levels. At the simplest level, a simple analogy is often made with a database or ledger that keeps track of all transactions. An exact copy of this ledger is distributed across different computers that are connected to the network. To hack the ledger, you need to hack a majority of these different computers at the same time and change the same data at the same time to the same results. The probability of such a large-scale hack taking place is very small and depends of course on the number of connected computers. This is what makes the Blockchain so reliable.

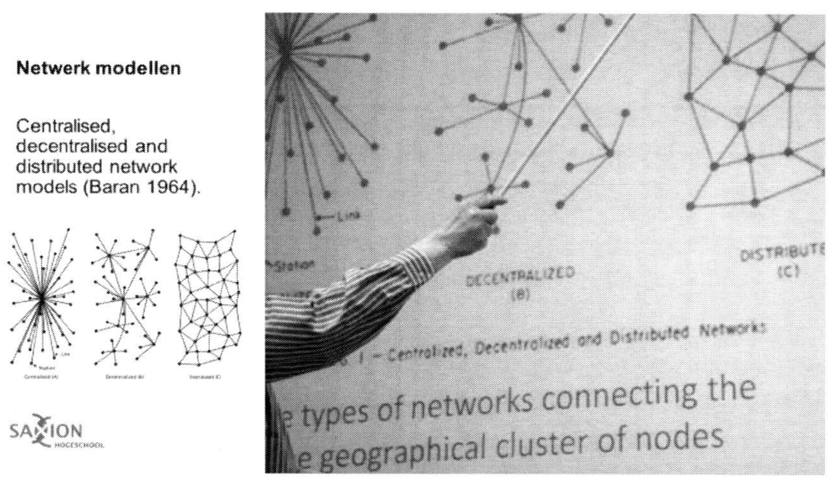

Source: Veuger 2020b.

Figure 3. Network models according to Baran (1964).

Characteristics

Because the Blockchain is a database distributed across different servers, this technology is also seen as a form of *distributed ledger* technology. When a distributed network is used, this leads to the following interesting consequences:

1. There is no single point of failure.
2. New data must be confirmed by other nodes (see box).
3. A form of consensus is required.
4. A Blockchain is difficult to hack.
5. Censoring or changing the data on the Blockchain is difficult.
6. It is a peer-to-peer network that does not require trust in a central party.

These consequences can be regarded as emergent characteristics of the Blockchain.

From the perspective that Blockchain is considered a database that records information, Blockchain has the following characteristics:

- data are arranged in data blocks
- incremental
- reliable because the data are cryptographically verifiable
- digital

Companies, governments and individuals can use a Blockchain among themselves or with each other together form a Blockchain network. A Blockchain has four characteristics:

1. Data - with the exception of private data - are public and accessible to everyone.
2. Information is stored on a decentralised basis.
3. All data are stored in combination with corresponding times.
4. The code is open source, which means that everyone can view it.

Nodes

Transactions on the blockchain take place peer-to-peer without an intermediary, also called trusted third party, which has interesting consequences for users. A peer-to-peer network is a network of computers, also called nodes, which are equivalent to each other and can provide services to each other. A node is a device that is connected to and participates in the blockchain network. This can be a computer, telephone, television or even a printer as long as it is connected to the network via the internet. They can have a variety of tasks, such as distributing data across the network, validating and confirming transactions and helping to secure the network.

The 'full nodes' download each block of the blockchain and also verify transactions. Their main task is to ensure consensus on the blockchain and to ensure that it remains secure. Full nodes also send blocks and transactions to the network for others to download. They also make decisions about the future of the network. They do this by voting on improvement proposals for the network such as the Bitcoin Improvement Proposals (BIPs) (Lim and Janse 2020).

In summary, blockchain technology has the potential to:

- facilitate registration and validation
- eliminate copies
- save on costs
- authenticate transactions
- record data permanently
- make transactions possible without an intermediary
- realize self-executing contracts
- shorten transaction times
- make more automation possible

With this in mind, we will look at care and what complex problems are involved here.

Increasing Complexity in Healthcare

Although the basic principle is that the (vulnerable) elderly citizen can continue to live in his own living environment for as long as possible, care in the Netherlands is designed in such a way that it is sometimes difficult to find the right (and financially viable) care. We mention four reasons that healthcare in the Netherlands is so complex.

Methods of Financing

Healthcare is divided into three funding regimes: the Social Support Act (Wmo), the Healthcare Insurance Act (Zvw) and the Long-Term Care Act (Wlz). The Zvw requires an indication from a district nurse, the Wmo usually runs via a kitchen table conversation, and the Wlz requires an indication from the Central Indication Body for Care (CIZ). For requesting a personal budget, access is often even more difficult.

Fragmented First Line

What further increases the complexity is that primary care is traditionally organized and financed in a fragmented fashion. All this applies while care needs to be increasingly integrated and personalised. As far as ICT is concerned, much more is possible than is currently customary in healthcare, and here too, there is enormous fragmentation that reinforces complexity. ICT has been set up per subsector.

Everyone Has Their Own Policy

The complexity of care is great, as well as the coordination with the social domain in terms of funding and organisation. The coordination mechanisms make the complexity structural. Within the Zvw, a limited number of health insurers conclude health contracts with a large number of integrated, small-scale organisations and professionals in elderly care and the social domain. Often, these organisations are also regionally or locally oriented. In addition, there are 355 municipalities that have their own policy in the area of the social domain. Clients and patients have the option of choosing, but they often do not have the information required to make a considered choice. These different ordering systems lead to suboptimization in the relationship between client and healthcare professional. Clients thus have a navigation problem.

New Transactions

Interaction takes place between healthcare professionals and clients. This interaction takes place in the form of a transaction: there is a (care) agreement, there is a consideration (payment via Wmo, Zvw or Wlz), and a delivery (care deployment) takes place. The arrival of digital platforms such as Platformvmz.nl and Curaevitelbalie.nl creates new interactions and transactions between professionals and clients.

Blockchain enables a new model for the exchange of care information. This reduces the current fragmentation in the various care systems and enables a better view of the results of care interventions.

Blockchain as a Solution for Verified Data

The Blockchain can respond to the challenges currently confronting healthcare. These challenges include medical data (security, interoperability, accessibility), medical research, clinical trials, the medical supply chain and the quality of the medicines. Blockchain in healthcare is mainly about data from and about people.

Standardising information strengthens communication between professionals and between clients and professionals. The client determines which information is available to which healthcare professional. A different design for making data accessible and information provision based on that can reduce complexity. Digitisation of care leads to clients and patients managing their own information in a Personal Health Environment (PHE).

In this book, we want to show that it is necessary to make shifts in the way we think and how we manage. This concerns the formation of decentralised structures where the interaction between client and healthcare professional is central. That means exploring network control and self-control (Topol 2015) with Blockchain.

Benefits and Opportunities

What are the benefits and opportunities of Blockchain in healthcare? Healthcare professionals can be active in multiple networks such as the patient file, interest organisation and the like. A network determines and justifies its own area of responsibility. The starting point for improvement of data management is the complexity and reality of the specific needs and questions of the target group within this area of responsibility.

Complexity requires innovative solutions. This in turn follows from data, information and knowledge that lead to common understanding and joint action (Wallin 2018). Digitalisation increasingly enables virtual integration of business processes between organisations.

The advantages of working with Blockchain are an effective organisation of care information that is easily interchangeable, data security and user control of the care data. Blockchain enables a fundamental recalibration of the position of clients: complete control of your own data. In this way, Blockchain shifts the control that institutions exercise to control exercised by the individual himself (Huizinga 2018). Standardising information strengthens communication between professionals and between clients and professionals. The client determines which information is available to which healthcare professional. Digitisation therefore leads to clients and patients managing their own information in a Personal Health Environment (PHE) or Electronic Health Record (EHR).

Blockchain also offers new opportunities to shape collaboration between healthcare organisations and healthcare professionals. *Real-time* available information can thus be made safely accessible. Because no intermediaries are required, cost savings can be realized. Blockchain provides a decentralised healthcare structure and thus strengthens the position of professionals and clients. Blockchain technology also allows citizens and professionals to exchange and share data directly, resulting in benefits such as greater transparency in the care process of patients and professionals.

App

The use of Blockchain technology is often supported by a user-friendly application, such as a website, database or app. Such an application layer facilitates use. A user can thus see in an app where he can enter data, which then becomes visible to others who have reading rights. The Mijn Zorg Log app from Zorginstituut Nederland works like this. This app is illustrated in Figure 4.

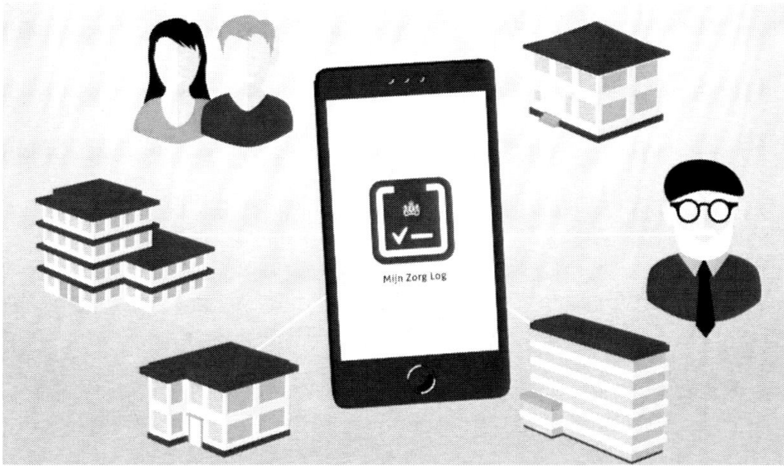

Source: Blockchain: Mijn Zorg Log - iStandaarden.nl.

Figure 4. Mijn Zorg Log.

Other sources of information can also be connected to the application and made visible to the users. The Blockchain itself can be linked to information from external sources. In principle, Blockchain enables the following developments:

- an effective health information management system that is interoperable
- data security
- control by users over care data (Lim 2020).

However, Blockchain applications are not yet being developed on a large scale in the Dutch healthcare sector. Important reasons for this limited development are that several parties in the chain must simultaneously agree on the added value that can be achieved, on how risks can be mitigated and on how a specific Blockchain is created. This requires knowledge, mutual trust and a shared sense of urgency. Like other digital transformations, the introduction of Blockchain applications is also hampered by outdated IT systems used by healthcare parties and suppliers. The expectation is that this will change in the long term (Veuger 2020a and b), and we would like to contribute to this with this book.

Three Forms of Access

A common way to make it clear who is allowed to join is to see if everyone is allowed to join in principle. Or are there conditions that you must meet imposed by the network? Either permissionless or permissioned entry. A healthcare blockchain infrastructure can take three forms: a public, private or hybrid system. The aim is to clarify which roles are needed to manage the network, as well as what role the entrants ('participants') can receive. We briefly explain the three forms of access.

Public System

Anyone can join a public system; there is permissionless entry. Everyone has the right to use and view the ledger. Everyone is free to assume any role they want within the system, even that of validating transactions. This system, where everyone is treated equally, is mainly used if a group of 'like-minded people' want to work together, such as Bitcoin or the internet. The like-minded can join the decentralised network themselves. The user group determines the content or operation of the blockchain in line with group motives such as openness, neutrality and freedom in line with decentralised cooperation.

If it is decided that everyone is allowed to join, the option can be offered to give everyone anonymity, of course within the blockchain rules. Trust about the shared 'truth' is very high, because it is enforced by the blockchain rules, not by knowing who the entrants are. The users determine the function of the blockchain.

This public model is not always desirable for organisations in a more regulated environment such as healthcare. After all, care is a highly regulated system.

Private System

If it is decided that only a limited group may join, a *private system* is created. The blockchain rules do not impose enough trust, which means that the activities of the entrants must be controlled. This is done by drawing up rules that an entrant must comply with, by a kind of separation of responsibilities, by checking transactions and possibly reversing them: permissioned entry.

A private system is often an organisation where a central body has control options with regard to, for example, the establishment of an intranet facility. For example, a director or management team starts a blockchain system and invites participants to participate within a certain role. A comparison in a private system is an intranet in which the nodes, data and the program code are checked.

A private system empowers the organization, where a public system empowers the individual (Lim and Janse 2020). The three most relevant roles within a management control system are initiating, verifying and viewing a transaction. Other questions you want to ask yourself here are:

- Who owns the data?
- Who ensures that data are not tampered with?
- Who is allowed to change or delete data?
- Who creates and maintains the software? (Consensys 2018)

Healthcare institutions that use a Blockchain with each other together form a Blockchain network. This Blockchain has four characteristics:

- Data - with the exception of private data - are public and accessible to everyone.
- Information is stored decentralised, distributed between different computers.
- All data are stored in combination with the corresponding time of those data.
- The code is open source, which means that everyone can view it.

Smart contracts exist to fulfil agreements between the parties within the Blockchain. These are not contracts in the legal sense, but software that automatically executes those rules between parties within a Blockchain (Zorginstituut 2018). In Chapter 2, we go deeper into this.

Hybrid System

A hybrid system has characteristics of both the public and private system. An example of a hybrid system is using existing systems with sources on which a Blockchain is built. This can be done, for example, with the delivery of medication in which not all sources of the manufacturer are visible, but the qualification of the product medication that is delivered is visible. Figure 5 is an illustration of the public, private and hybrid system by Lim and Janse (2020).

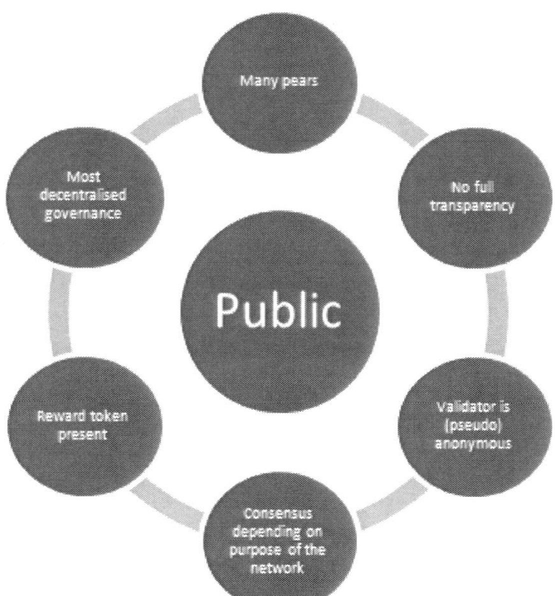
Many pears
No full transparency
Validator is (pseudo) anonymous
Consensus depending on purpose of the network
Reward token present
Most decentralised governance
Public

Many unknown pears

Figure 5. (Continued)

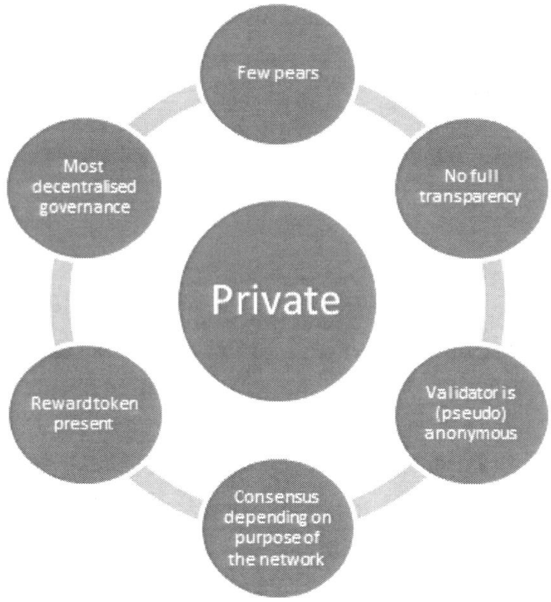

Known users

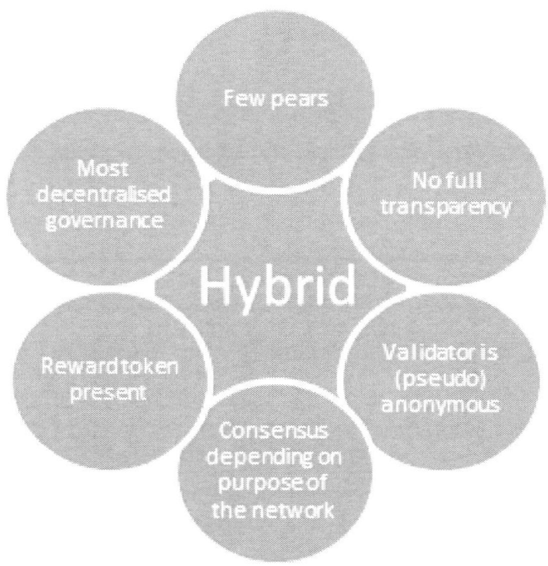

Known users from multiple organizations

Figure 5. A public, private and hybrid system.

Healthcare has specific substantive values for healthcare governance (healthcare-wide governance). These also apply to blockchain. According to Berenschot (2019), the combination of decentralised hardware and personal data (especially the special, medical personal data) means that public blockchain is now not a possibility for care. The risks are still too great. However, nothing stands in the way of care using private blockchain platforms, i.e., a private system. For blockchain to be used responsibly in healthcare, it is necessary to optimise blockchain's possible contribution to safe, accessible and affordable healthcare and to manage the risks thereof. Good cooperation is crucial for development.

The design of healthcare logistics can therefore be supported efficiently via blockchain technology. The interoperability of secure data significantly simplifies access to healthcare information for organisations, professionals and clients. Blockchain makes it possible to share client data in a uniform manner.

Storing Data

The blockchain is therefore technology that is used to store data. And the blockchain does not exist as a storage medium. Not singularly, anyway. Several blockchains will be created that can have very different characteristics and that are tailored to the application built on them. The best-known blockchain application is Bitcoin, a digital currency that cannot be copied due to the characteristics of the technology. blockchain also stands for supply chain optimization and control tools to work together more efficiently.

A blockchain platform can be operational on four types of infrastructure.

1. A blockchain platform can be installed as a blockchain node on a local computer. This is common for private development or testing environments.
2. One or more blockchain nodes are installed on servers within the ICT infrastructure of a healthcare institution (*on-site*), to which different computers or devices can connect.
3. Nodes can 'host' on one or more remote servers, such as cloud servers.
4. A blockchain platform may use the global infrastructure of a public blockchain platform (VNG 2019).

With blockchain, a safe digital infrastructure can be built within the healthcare system. In this book, we show what this infrastructure can look like.

Generic Benefits

Edriouch et al. (2018: 26-27) assert that the characteristics of blockchain are: no central storage, not changeable, impossibility of error correction, energy consumption (*proof of work*), circulation speed, scalability, privacy and semi-democratic nature. Blockchain at its core is therefore an intelligent way to combine cryptographic techniques in a public, distributed database. The *Basisboek Blockchain* (a blockchain primer) by Chhay Lin Lim and Arthur Janse from 2019 gives the most complete picture possible of blockchain philosophy, technology and many other related issues around blockchain.

As far as the storage of data is concerned, blockchain has the following generic advantages:

Irrefutable

Because stamps are placed in the blockchain, which meet certain agreements and are checked by all members of the network, these data are in fact irrefutable. Irrefutable here means that you cannot simply delete data. This ensures that it can be trusted that one party cannot make changes or delete data without the others being aware of this.

Control over Your Own Data

By means of the *wallet* (see box), the user has control over who is allowed to do what and when with his data. Within the framework of a blockchain, it is irrefutably recorded who has done what and when with the data.

Intelligent Layer

It is still difficult to connect different data silos. Think, for example, of hospitals that all have their own data islands, which has been set up over time. In this context, blockchain forms an intelligent layer that connects these sources, so that patients can follow the reliable 'stamps' path.

Administrative Optimization

When you look at data within an administrative process, the administrative process follows the operational and financial processes and is therefore set up reactively.

Wallet

With a *wallet*, a user sends and receives blockchain transactions. The wallet signs transactions with a digital signature (*public key*). The secret piece of the digital signature (*private key*) keeps a user secret. The private key is used as mathematical proof that the transactions originate from the owner of a particular wallet. The private key also prevents the transaction from being changed by someone once it has been issued by the user. All transactions are exchanged between users and are confirmed within minutes by a process called *mining*.

The user's wallet is the personal environment or the user-friendly application with which the user can access the blockchain. Personal data about the user (such as the private key of the user) can be stored in the wallet. The personal data stored in the wallet are considered *off-chain* personal data (Zorginstituut 2019).

Security

The importance of blockchain ensuring the reliability and accuracy of data. This is an essential development for healthcare. So you can see that security is crucial in the design and application of this technique. For example, all transactions require a digital signature that confirms the reliability of the transaction. Unauthorised transactions are detected on time and not processed. All data are also encrypted by *cryptography* (see box).

Guarantees for the correct handling of personal data are necessary when sharing information, because (encrypted) information ends up on hardware of parties who may not have the right to view this information.

Personal data can be processed in different ways. They are processed *off-chain* when the personal data are not processed in the transactions included on the blockchain. Personal data are processed *on-chain* when the personal data are processed in the transactions included on the blockchain.

When the blocks are linked to each other, they use a reference to the previous block. This reference is a *hash*, an encrypted and calculated numeric code. A hash cannot be used to derive what the actual data looks like. Also, a hash is meant to be unique. If a bit or character changes in a piece of code or a document, the hash will change completely. Any change in the blockchain can thus be seen immediately.

Cryptography

Cryptography deals with techniques for hiding or encrypting information to be transmitted. A cryptoanalyst is the person who has access to the channel between transmitter and receiver and can therefore 'listen in' as it were. It must be impossible for him to deduce from the transported data, with an acceptable effort, which information was transmitted by the sender and which parties were involved. The term Proxy encryption network fits here, about which we will say more in the case MedFAbric4Me after Chapter 3.

Security is also created by control by the users. Users can make the computing capacity of their computer available. This makes them a mining node. The mining nodes ensure consensus between all copies of the ledger. Mining nodes check all transactions - and the order of those transactions - before they are added to the blockchain. Each new transaction is encrypted with the entire history of all previous transactions like a kind of DNA.

During the mining process, the mining nodes solve a cryptographic puzzle. This determines whether the transactions offered are valid and may become part of the blockchain. In the case of tampering with one copy of the ledger, no consensus is reached in the network and all other participants refuse the faulty transaction. This will then not be added to the blockchain.

Conditions for the Application

With blockchain, trust lies in the system itself and not so much between parties (Lim and Janse 2020: 488). Data standards can play an important role in this. With blockchain technology, a more sustainable, safer and reliable digital infrastructure (Veuger 2018b and 2019d) can be built. That makes this technology potentially revolutionary.

Because blockchain technology is also very complex and still developing, it can only be realized if open cooperation takes place. On the one hand, because bundling knowledge is necessary due to the complexity. On the other hand, because the decentralized nature of blockchain requires new, decentralized forms of governance (Veuger 2020b: 8).

Criteria

Blockchain is useful if the following criteria are met (Lim and Janse 2020: 490):

- Digital innovation is part of the strategy.
- Different parties share data.
- These data relate to monetary value.
- The data are confidential.
- Several parties process data.
- Data must be verified.
- A clear *return on investment* can be calculated.
- Verification is complex and costly.
- The solution of choosing blockchain is the simplest to solve the problem.
- The solution affects the organisational form.
- The solution affects the existing work processes.
- The solution affects the existing ecosystem.
- The technical solution is close to existing systems.
- The solution is data-intensive but scalable.

Future

Blockchain is a *disruptive technology* that gives industries and sectors a *wake-up call* through a totally new and secure method of data file management: the 21st century operating system. Blockchain cannot solve all social, economic, cultural and technological problems. It does have the potential to greatly improve trust issues in our society and in particular the economy. Uncertainties can be removed by blockchain in the (financial) world through new forms of chain cooperation(s) (Veuger 2020b: 18).

It is important to note that blockchain technology is complex and still at a development stage for healthcare. Blockchain applications are not yet being developed on a large scale in the Dutch healthcare sector. Despite the potential benefits, large-scale applications, for example, have not yet been developed in care chains.

The research firm Gartner predicts that blockchain will converge with other complementary technologies such as the Internet of Things and artificial intelligence in 2025. As a result of these developments, there is increasing interest in decentralised solutions (Lim and Janse 2020: 520). Blockchain offers a lot of potential advantages, 'potential' because application possibilities have not yet been used in a combined way on a large scale and have not been proven until then. One reason for this is that not everything is technically possible yet. Experiments are therefore needed to make this technology more stable. Before we delve deeper into the characteristics of blockchain, we would like to tell you about the application Mijn Zorg Log in maternity care.

Case 1: All the Parties Responsible for Mijn Zorg Log

An important example of Blockchain's application in the Netherlands is Mijn Zorg Log in maternity care. This application has been tested as a practical trial and has demonstrated secure information exchange of personal data via a blockchain application with different players: the client, healthcare provider, insurer and supervisor.

Zorginstituut Nederland has investigated whether Blockchain is applicable in healthcare. This has led to the first working Blockchain in healthcare: Mijn Zorg Log. The Dutch blockchain specialist Ledger Leopard built Mijn Zorg Log on an Ethereum blockchain platform. Mijn Zorg Log uses this blockchain technology and is therefore one of the innovations in the exchange of digital information in healthcare.

Mijn Zorg Log is a tool that provides insight into how Blockchain technology can contribute to the exchange of information in healthcare. It works on the basis of a closed blockchain with permissions, what is called a permissioned blockchain. In 2017, Mijn Zorg Log was awarded a legal certificate that indicates that the application complies with laws and regulations relating to care and privacy in the Netherlands (Zorginstituut 2018).

Development

During the development of Mijn Zorg Log, it was taken as a starting point that parties who exchange personal data with each other in the blockchain all have the role of 'controller', to use the language from the General Data Protection Regulation. Parties that only run a node and cannot add transactions themselves or cannot see certain transactions are 'processors'. They process personal data exclusively for the benefit of controllers. A processor agreement has been concluded with the processors by all controllers. In the practical trial, the maternity care providers and the insurer were controllers.

The insurer, Zorginstituut Nederland and Ledger Leopard played the role of processor. In the practical trial, a processor agreement was concluded between the three maternity care providers, health insurer VGZ and Zorginstituut Nederland. A sub-processor agreement was concluded with blockchain builder Ledger Leopard. Nodes were set up at VGZ, Zorginstituut Nederland and Ledger Leopard.

In the practical trial, there was a ledger - the blockchain - located in a limited number of places (nodes). The choice was made for a limited number of participants in the practical trial, namely 33, which enabled good control. Because a permissioned blockchain was the starting point, it was possible to reach unambiguous agreements and to comply with the laws and regulations regarding privacy.

How It Works

A maternity care provider provides home care, documents what she has done and sends this information to the office. The office takes over this in a system and forwards it to the paying agency. What is sent is therefore not also checked by the client (the mother), the source. The paying agent takes over the information in its own system and makes payment after 30 days or more. This takes a long time, is inefficient and expensive because the financial process follows the labour-intensive administrative process.

By means of blockchain technology, the maternity care provider sends a structured notification of what she has done for the client with an app. The client can reject this notification, then there is a discussion at the source as to why a particular service has not been provided or has been experienced as such. If the client accepts the notification, both the administrative and the financial process will be completed within a few seconds for the different parties; this has already been checked by the client at the start, so no further questions or discussions should arise when the client actually has to pay. Here, the process is much shorter, more reliable, more efficient and cheaper, because the administrative and financial processes run in parallel. Figure 6 shows the functioning of Mijn Zorg Log. The choice for a permissioned blockchain for the practical trial was made because work had to be (and could be) done in a protected environment with a number of known parties involved in the care of the insured person (client/mother). In addition, the transaction speed of a public Blockchain was not (yet) suitable for the requested functionality in the practical trial.

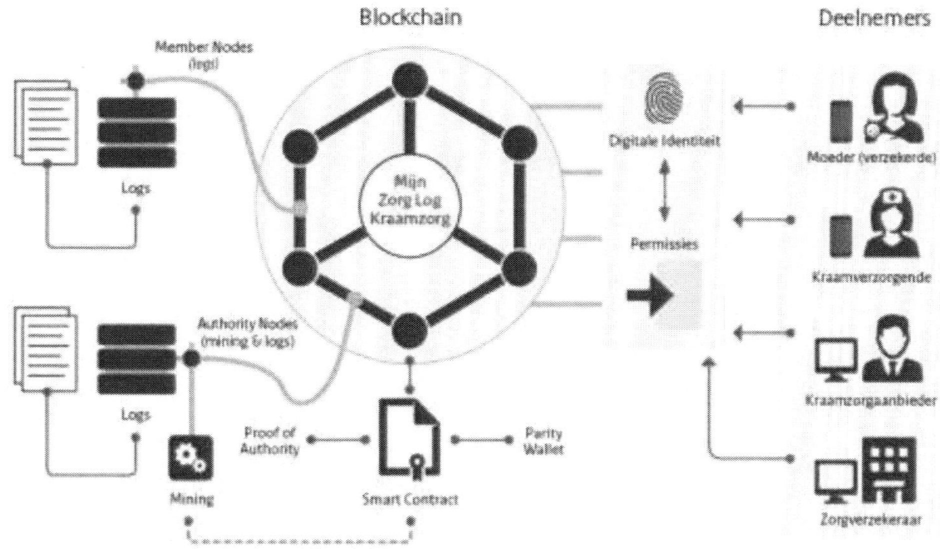

Source: Blockchain: Mijn Zorg Log - iStandaarden.nl (Zorginstituut Nederland and VGZ (2018)).

Figure 6. The function of Mijn Zorg Log.

The generic advantages of Blockchain are elaborated as follows in 'Mijn Zorg Log'.

Irrefutable

The blockchain irrefutably records that concrete services have actually been provided by the maternity care provider and that these have been approved by the parents, the source.

Control Over Your Own Data

The parents were able to determine which parties could access the data themselves via the app, and this was also recorded irrefutably.

Intelligent Layer

The blockchain connects the systems of the maternity care organisations, authorities and the insurer with respect to the mother and baby. This creates the same source that the different parties were authorised to access.

Administrative Optimization

The maternity care provider sent a notification to the parents about the actual work performed via the Mijn Zorg Log app.

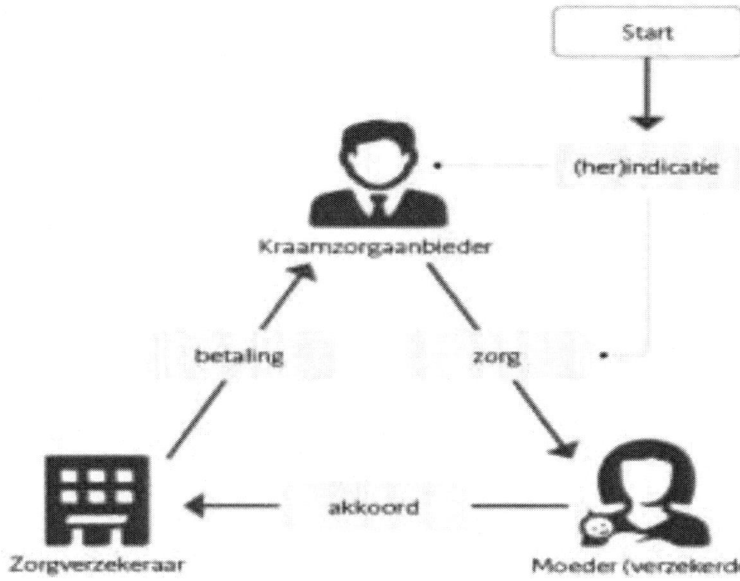

Source: Blockchain: Mijn Zorg Log - iStandaarden.nl (Zorginstituut Nederland and VGZ (2018)).

Figure 7. The adapted maternity care process as the bases for Mijn Zorg Log.

Here, the financial and administrative processes run in parallel and are therefore much more efficient and cheaper, see also Figure 7.

'Mijn Zorg Log' is a Blockchain application, which has been successfully tested in and by practice to organise maternity care more efficiently (Megchelen 2020).

Two Characteristics of Blockchain

A blockchain, a chain of blocks, is a system that can be used to record data. Each block contains coded data and can be included in the chain if these data refer to the previous data and thus form a chain. The most unique thing about the blockchain is that no *trusted third party* is needed to store, monitor or control the data. The function of, for example, a notary will therefore be abolished.

In this chapter, we delve deeper into the characteristics of blockchain and how they form a trilemma. We discuss solutions for this blockchain trilemma and show how different infrastructures use the features. We will also focus on the transfer of information, smart contracts and cybersecurity. Blockchain has four basic principles that distinguish blockchain from other automation technologies. We will repeat them briefly and explain them further.

- Basic principle 1 Growing chain. A blockchain offers a new method of data storage by a chain of data blocks that builds up over time and cannot be unilaterally changed.
- Basic principle 2 Distributed network. The chain is distributed to all participating parties and is a shared truth. The growing chain (basic principle 1) can always be stored and used by one party. Blockchains are extra reliable because the entire chain can be shared and distributed to other parties.
- Basic principle 3 Consensus. Parties involved must agree on the data stored in the last block (consensus). When working in a distributed network (basic principle 2), the biggest challenge is reaching agreement on the content of the last data block. No consensus is possible if the parties do not agree on the data in the last block.
- Basic principle 4 Data storage. The programming code with cryptography can be stored and executed in Blockchains. The data in a Blockchain can contain logic, procedures and a programming code. These data are securely synchronised between all parties and can be executed decentrally (VNG 2019).

The distribution and decentralisation level of the blockchain plays a major role in scalability. When introducing blockchain, the blockchain trilemma plays a role: scalability, security and decentralisation. A highly decentralised blockchain is better secured, but at the expense of scalability. If it is scalable and centralized, it is then less secure.

The Blockchain Trilemma

Blockchain was first developed in 2008 for Bitcoin. Interest in blockchain technology has increased since the idea of blockchain was introduced in a 2008 white paper by Satoshi Nakamoto. He argues for an electronic payment system in which unknown parties can realize transactions directly and without the intervention of a third party such as a bank. The payment method of this system is the Bitcoin. Nakamoto improved his system on a number of points, such as the prevention of *double spending* and the introduction of a *timestamp*. He thereby created a system in which trust - the keyword for blockchain - is embedded in the blockchain technology. Nakamoto thus ensured that a *trusted third party* (TTP), to which he objected in principle, was no longer necessary. This created the certainty that the recipient could be sure that the previous owner had not executed a previous transaction and that the first (money) transaction is the only valid one. The main reasons for the interest in blockchain are security, anonymity and data integrity without an external organization controlling the transactions.

Research into Blockchain

The characteristics of blockchain create interesting research areas, especially from the perspective of technical challenges and limitations. The study by Yli-Huumo Ko, Choi, Park and Smolander (2016) is a systematic study to collect all relevant research into Blockchain technology. The aim of the research was to understand the current research themes, challenges and future directions with regard to blockchain technology from 41 primary *papers* from scientific databases.

The results show that the focus in more than eighty percent of the papers is on the Bitcoin system and less than twenty percent on other blockchain applications such as smart contracts and licences. The majority of the research focuses on revealing and improving limitations of blockchain from a privacy and security perspective. In many of the proposed solutions, a concrete evaluation of their effectiveness is lacking. Many other scalability-related challenges such as transit and response times have not yet been studied.

Trilemma

Blockchain can have a huge impact on the value chain in our society. After all, it can play a role in efficiency, transparency, ownership, value (transfer), automation and services.

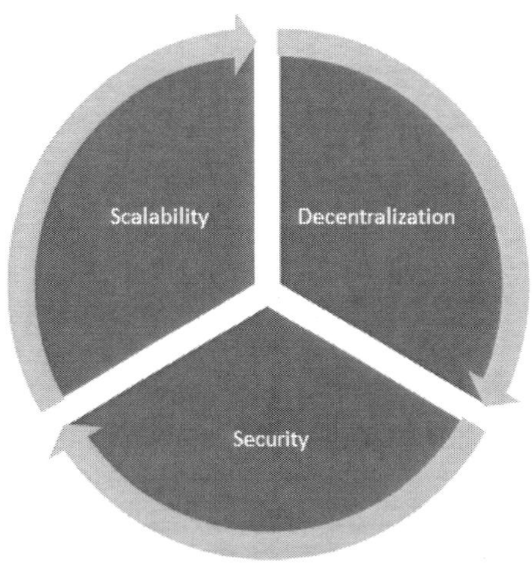

Figure 8. The Blockchain trilemma.

When introducing Blockchain, the Blockchain trilemma always plays a role:

- scalability
- security
- decentralization

A highly decentralised blockchain is better secured but at the expense of scalability. If it is scalable and centralized, it is then less secure (Lim and Janse 2020: 188). This is shown in Figure 8.

Scalability

Scalability is an important challenge for the application of Blockchain. Scalability refers to the number of transactions that the Blockchain network can process. Scalability can be increased by adjusting the way blocks are produced and transactions are verified (Lim and Janse 2020).

The block time is the average time in which a block is produced. For Bitcoin, the block time is 10 minutes. If your transaction is not included in the current block, then you will have to wait 10 minutes to be included in the next block. A faster block time can be achieved by reducing the difficulty for *miners* to find valid hashes and be able to produce blocks. This is described in detail in *Basisboek Blockchain* by Chhay Lin Lim and Arthur Janse.

In addition to block time, block size plays an important role in scalability. The discussion about increasing the block size has led to disagreement within the Bitcoin community. In 2017, a group of developers wanted to increase the block size of Bitcoin from 1MB to 2MB so that more transactions can be processed per block. With the same block time, doubling the block size would mean that twice as many transactions can be processed every 10 minutes.

The distribution and decentralisation level of the Blockchain plays a major role in scalability. This is because there is a strong correlation between the centralization and the processing speed of the Blockchain. As mentioned earlier, BitShares can process significantly more transactions per second than Bitcoin by using delegated Proof-of-Stake. The idea behind this is that a Blockchain is considerably more scalable with a select group of nineteen witnesses, where it is pre-determined who can produce the next block and validate those transactions.

Security

The security of the Blockchain takes place in all kinds of ways, through the nodes, smart contracts, and the hashes to link blocks. Any form of security entails limitations in scalability and decentralisation.

Decentralization

The most unique thing about the Blockchain is that no *trusted third party* is needed to store, monitor and control the data, as we are familiar with at banks or a notary. Blockchain is therefore a *type* of distributed ledger technology. A *distributed ledger* is a database that exists in multiple locations or between multiple users. Organizations often use a centralized database that is at a fixed location, and this centralized database therefore has one failure point. However, a distributed ledger is decentralized to avoid a third-party trusted agent or authority from having to process, validate, or authenticate transactions. Blockchain is therefore a *type* of distributed ledger technology.

Figure 9 shows the differences between a centralised network, decentralised network and a distributed network according to Baran (1964).

Arguments for decentralisation are:

- resistant to one or more parts of the network
- no sensitive central points that can be manipulated
- resistant to collusion of participants acting at the expense of others (Lim and Janse 2020: 199)

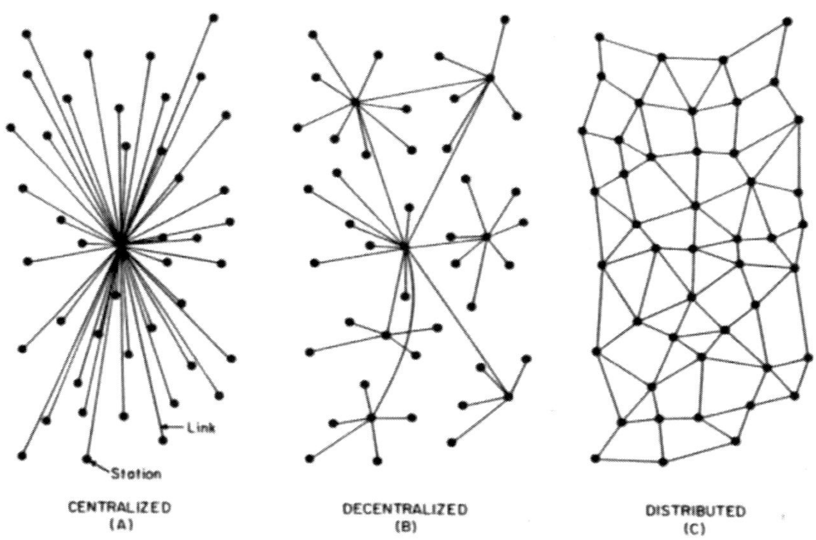

Source: Baran 1964.

Figure 9. Network models.

The Solution to the Trilemma by Bitcoin

If we want to understand the world of Blockchain, we need to understand the innovation of the currency of Bitcoin in 2009 terms, which is based on the underlying technology of Blockchain.

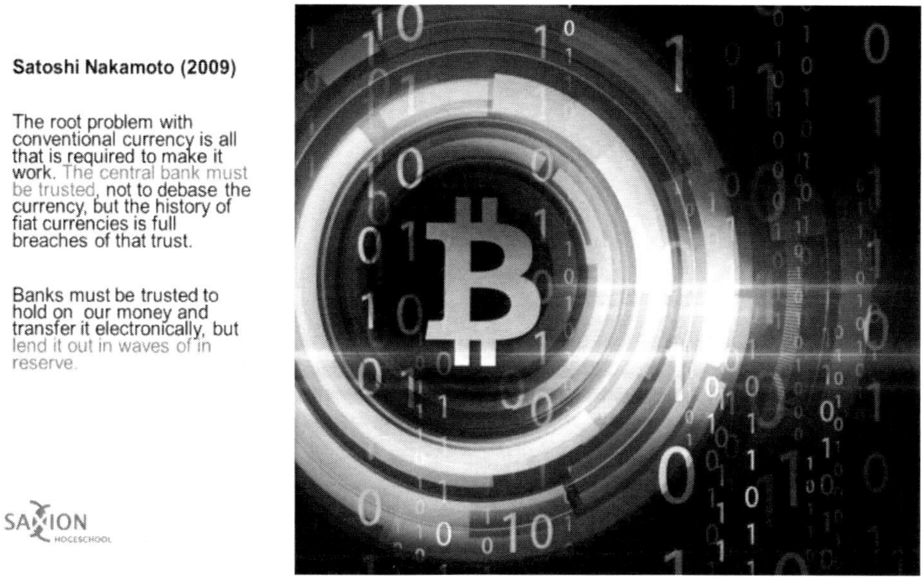
Satoshi Nakamoto (2009)
The root problem with conventional currency is all that is required to make it work. The central bank must be trusted, not to debase the currency, but the history of fiat currencies is full breaches of that trust.
Banks must be trusted to hold on our money and transfer it electronically, but lend it out in waves of in reserve.
SAXION

Source: Veuger, 'Belastingdienst, Blockchain, Finance, Taks & Advice', August 27, 2019; 'ABN AMRO & Blockchain ontwikkelingen', September 19, 2019 and 'Themadag Politie & Blockchain', October 10, 2019.

Figure 10. Statement by Satoshi Nakamoto (2009).

Bitcoin is a combination of four individual elements: cryptography, a peer-to-peer network, an open-source protocol and a shared ledger. This makes it a phenomenon about which people are enthusiastic.

When talking about Bitcoin, it is essential to distinguish between the Bitcoin currency and the Bitcoin network (Lim and Janse 2019):

- bitcoin is the digital currency
- the Bitcoin network is the underlying infrastructure consisting of the nodes that help track all bitcoin transactions by means of the Blockchain.

Bitcoin as a digital currency is written with a small b; the Bitcoin network with a capital B (Veuger 2020b). This is illustrated in Figure 10. The Bitcoin phenomenon therefore includes both the virtual money and the infrastructure. It is therefore a sophisticated and revolutionary way to store data in a certain way without the intervention of a third party.

The Creation of Bitcoin

Chaum (1982) is seen as the godfather of the bitcoin. He now lives in California and is one of the best cryptography experts in the world. Already in the eighties and nineties, he was working on systems to enable digital transactions without the intervention of a bank or credit card company. Chaum (1982) described the necessary blockchain technology with which he laid more than a foundation for bitcoin. Then the well-known Satoshi Nakamoto document appeared on the internet about blockchain. He solved the remaining problem of double payments and came up with the solution that the payments are stored everywhere in the network.

At the Science Park Centre for Mathematics & Information in Amsterdam, there came the headquarters of the Digicash company, which Chaum founded in 1990 and which presented eCash three years later. This made safe and anonymous payments possible. The research by Sherman, Javani, Zhang and Golaszewski (2018) provides an interesting historical exploration of the work of Chaum, whose vault systems embody many of the elements of blockchains. Figure 11 provides an overview of some important cryptographic discoveries that underlie Blockchain technologies (according to Veuger 2020a: 36).

Only needed a money system

Nobel Prize winner in economic sciences in 1976 Milton Friedman, saw back in 1999 (Gobry 2014) that the internet would play a major role in reducing the role of government in our economic and social life. According to Friedman (Gobry 2014), only a reliable electronic money system was lacking that allows people to make money mutations without knowing the fellow operators. Such a system then resembles cash transactions with anonymity. According to many, Bitcoin has delivered on this promise. The internet already makes it possible to transfer information quickly and cheaply without paper and without intermediaries. Blockchain offers the same benefits for transferring values. The internet is used to transfer word and image; Blockchain, transactions.

Year	Discoveries
1970	James Ellis, public-key cryptography discovered at Government Communications Headquarters (GCHQ) in secret
1973	Clifford Cocks, RSA cryptosystem discovered at (GCHQ) in secret
1974	Ralph Merkle, cryptographic puzzles (paper published in 1978)
1976	Diffie and Hellman, public-key cryptography discovered at Stanford
1977	Rivest, Shamir, Adleman, RSA cryptosystem invented at MIT 1979
1979	David Chaum, vaults and secret sharing (dissertation 1982)
1982	Lamport, Shostak, Pease, Byzantine Generals Problem
2002	Adam Bach, Hashcash
1992	Dwork and Naor, combating junk mail
2008	Satoshi Nakamoto, Bitcoin
2017	Wright and Savanah, nChain European patent application (issued in 2018)

Figure 11. Timeline of discoveries in cryptography and Blockchain technology.

Bitcoin as a Decentralised System

Bitcoin as a digital currency for transactions – who transfers how much money to whom? - is registered in blocks, similar to journal entries in a ledger. A transaction is therefore a *record* with different fields and thus blocks. The account numbers are unique public keys, and every transaction also has a fee for the miners. Blocks (data or text) form a chain because each piece of data refers to the previous piece of data. This creates a chain (Veuger 2020b) as in Figure 12.

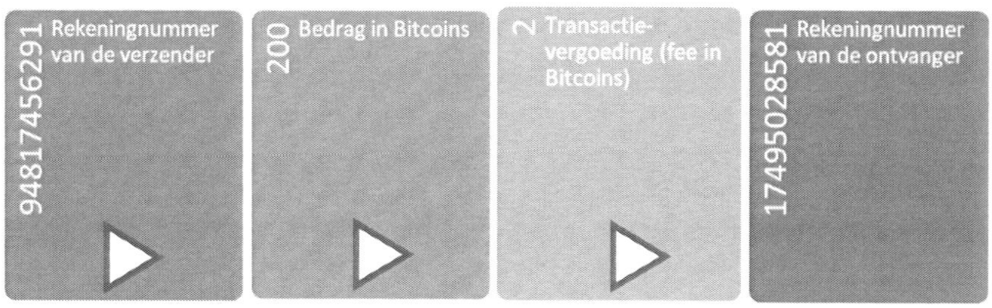

Figure 12. Transaction in Bitcoin.

Everyone can participate in this system and add new transactions (blocks) to the chain. These blocks are stored *decentrally*, and no one monitors the reliability of the transaction, where the immediate challenge is to design the system in such a way that only valid transactions are added without the person behind the transaction being known and without a central control.

The challenge is therefore to keep Blockchain's ledger up to date, with consensus on its content. This is known as the *Byzantine Generals Problem*[1]: the problem of a number of generals who jointly coordinated an attack on an enemy.[2] The problem consists of:

- Completeness: a message from one general to the others may not arrive because, for example, the messenger is attacked. In terms of Blockchain: a valid transaction does not reach the others and is not included in the ledger.
- Authentication: an untrustworthy general can represent himself as another general. In terms of Blockchain: C wants to give money from A to B.
- Integrity: the message from the reliable general can be falsified, for example by the messenger. In terms of Blockchain: A makes a valid transaction but the content thereof is changed.
- Consistency: an untrustworthy general can send different and conflicting messages to different generals. In terms of Blockchain: A may have 10 euros but gives it to both B and C, also known as double spending.

Blockchain essentially solves the Byzantine Generals Problem because all participants agree on the content of this ledger, a technique that has been around for centuries. Namely by using different cryptographic techniques:

---

[1] Satoshi Nakamoto wrote about the Byzantine generals in https://satoshi.nakamotoinstitute.org/emails/cryptography/11/.

[2] The original article can be found at: https://people.eecs. berkeley.edu/~luca/cs174/byzantine.pdf.

- Public-private key encryption: this is an encryption that requires a public key and private key, which together form a pair and are each other's counterpart. What is unique about this is that the decryption is only possible with the use of both keys.
- Cryptographic hash functions: converting a (large) piece of text into a fixed-length text. This is applied as a guarantee of the integrity of the data.
- Hashcashing: the reverse process of cryptographic hashing. This is a labour-intensive process, also called the proof of work, where there is a lot of calculation work for a computer.

Examples of Infrastructures

Various Blockchain systems are being developed in the world, and they work in different ways - publicly or privately. Differences in the infrastructures are also determined, among other things, by the way in which consensus has been reached to arrive at that infrastructure. There are currently three different structures that are widely used: Hyperledger Fabric, Ethereum and Corda. We explain them briefly.

Hyperledger Fabric

Hyperledger Fabric has a refined consensus model that is not only dependent on proof-based mining. After all, a check has already been done for the transaction data and the authorizations therein. Nodes – which validate the reliability and integrity of transactions – have a different role and tasks within Hyperledger Fabric to reach consensus than for Ethereum.

Hyperledger Fabric is very suitable for streamlining the supply chain. This infrastructure focuses on the chain management of a sector. Information is only shared with stakeholders who are not visible to all (involved) parties in the entire chain, so it is a private system (see Chapter 1.4). An example of this are material certificates, the processing of the material and the final assembly of these steel elements. This application is described in Jansen's research (2018).

Medicalchain is one of the first healthcare organizations to use Blockchain within the Hyperledger community. Medicalchain is focused on ensuring that clients have access to their medical records.

Ethereum

Within Ethereum, all users must reach consensus on all transactions within the network, the order of transactions being essential for consistency within this network. As a result, duplications and fraud can be prevented. Consensus is reached on the basis of mining, a proof of work mechanism, whereby common agreement is reached in the ledger and all users give permission for all transaction data in this Blockchain. With

Ethereum, the nodes for all functions are identical, do exactly the same thing and fulfil the role of client, peer or orderer.

Ethereum aims to innovate globally in several sectors with decentralized distributed systems. Governments can function on this, but also the financial sector, logistics systems and the (supply) chain, the energy market, music and gaming industry, healthcare (Hölbl, Kompara, Kamišalićand Zlatalas 2018) including the pharmaceutical market et cetera. Ethereum is a platform for the development of decentralized applications for different industries. It lends itself well to decentralized applications, smart contracts and digital payment units. Ethereum, with a more transparent character, could be at the expense of privacy and scalability.

Corda

With Corda and Hyperledger, a check has already been done for the transaction data and the authorizations therein. With Corda, consensus is achieved in a similar way to that with Hyperledger Fabric, because for both the consensus is determined by transaction validity and transaction individuality through an automatic check that all signatures are correct.

The Corda Blockchain has been created through intensive cooperation between banks and has therefore been developed especially for this sector. This collaboration in a hybrid system is known as R3CEV, and its main purpose is the management, synchronization and distribution of financial applications. The consortium is convinced that not all Blockchain data are suitable for publicly accessible Blockchain infrastructure with regard to financial transactions. Privacy and scalability are the most important principles for the consortium for the development of an infrastructure like Corda.

A critical comment and therefore also an opportunity is whether Corda is still a Blockchain, or whether future use lies precisely in sector-specific distributed networks such as insurance policies; see Figure 14 With this, it can act in isolation as well as forming a worldwide Blockchain that is compatible with other distributed networks. For example, the coincidence of different networks can occur with each other, from which an interaction arises.

Reaching consensus is an important factor in ensuring that a distributed network can function optimally, and that can be done in a permissionless way – where everyone can use it – or a permissioned – limited access – way. Ethereum is permissionless; Hyperledger and Corda are a permissioned Blockchain. Corda and Hyperledger Fabric do not have a necessary built-in cryptocurrency. Fabric does offer this option. Hyperledger Fabric does not have these problems, due to the use of an algorithm for the Byzantine Generals Problem and the limited accessibility, and it is therefore suitable for various applications.

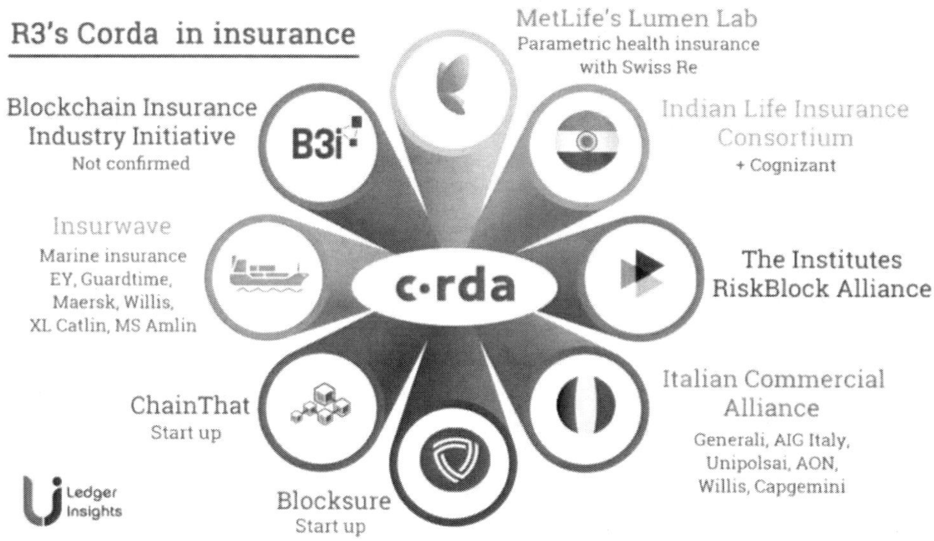

Source: Ledger Insights 2018.

Figure 14. Corda in insurance.

Infromation Transfer with Tokens

Blockchain has the potential to make and keep digital data safe and private with the help of a database and cryptography. Tokens provide a flexible and varied form to transfer or capture value, information, ideas, rights and obligations quickly, transparently and securely between multiple parties through self-executing smart contracts and using sensors based on the *Internet of Things*. *Tokenization* is a central method in which tokens are programmed in a Blockchain.

A token is a stand-alone value system outside the network, where the user must rely on the central methodology, also in terms of the liability and obligations of the central publisher. A token is independent of the data and contains authorisation keys as shown in Figure 15.

With tokens, the peer-to-peer capability of the Blockchain can be used whereby the value of the tokens depends on, for example, a non-digital system: a bank account. The value is also determined, checked and managed by a *trusted third party*. As a methodology, it is already being used for the Facebook Credit, which can be exchanged for regular money. Of course, this is also possible with other centrally issued virtual currencies.

The cryptocoin or the digital coin is therefore not dependent on a central publisher. It is a digital *asset* within a decentralized network and is given a value as a result of market forces, has an independent value and is an independent digital coin unit. Incidentally, other centrally-managed cryptocoins are coming onto the market, such as Utility Settlement Coin. This is a project by a number of major banks such as UBS, BNY

Mellon, Deutsche Bank and Santander. A critical question that can be asked here is whether the cryptocoin is a centrally controlled cryptocurrency or a complex tokenization. Ethereum is now the foundation of many Initial Coin Offers: offering a first token that is outside the influence of the Financial Markets Authority. Ethereum will be used for the launch of Security Token Offerings by Polymath, which represents a share in an organization or right to a profit distribution.

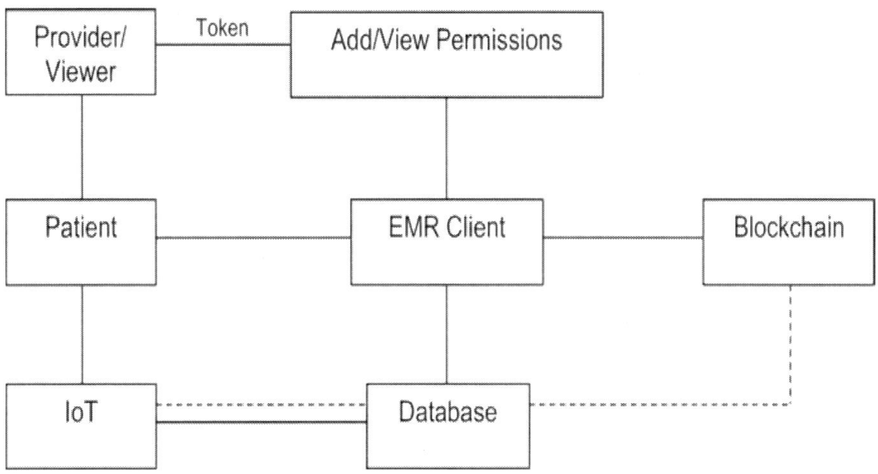

Source: Vazirani et al. npj Digital Medicine 3, 2020.

Figure 15. Authorisation keys.

Automatic Processing with Smart Contracts

Recorded agreements are used to perform actions in the blockchain quickly and safely. These can be done automatically if all the conditions are met. A *smart contract* is software that can carry out pre-programmed actions if certain conditions and agreements are met. In this way, obligations (claims) can be recorded in healthcare.

Smart contracts manage all the agreed commitments decentrally in a Blockchain network. This method is very efficient because manual verification or (bank) transfers are no longer necessary, it is safe, and conflicts are prevented.

When participating in a smart contract, the conditions are known and coded in advance, so that the conditions cannot be changed after the contract has been placed in the Blockchain. At the time of the transaction, it is already known that and how the conditions have been met.

Smart contracts can run on a Blockchain and are therefore compliance with a standard. Due to this compliance with applicable laws and regulations, the Blockchain can therefore enforce this compliance through legal enforceability.

For speed and costs, it is desirable that participants can register in a Blockchain platform and the Blockchain can function independently without the intervention of people. At the moment, however, it is not (yet) profitable to autonomously run registrations on smart contracts and Blockchain, as Herian (2018) asserts. The technological ambitions, legal norms and cultural differences could crystalize how a hybrid construction can work at a higher level. Smart contracts can then work in a combination of online and offline and on-chain and off-chain in different modalities. New legislation should also be in line with this, and/or new rules and principles should provide robust and equitable support for the legislation.

In automated processing with smart contracts, a DAO can be an appropriate infrastructure. A *decentralized autonomous organization* (DAO) consists of a number of connected smart contracts and thus forms an autonomous organization. Looking at the design of the digital environment and forms of independent future entities, then the DAO is one development. It is a business model with no central decision point or employees in an organization. An example of this is, for example, an autonomous car or taxi that is managed by a group of people, whereby revenues and expenses are automatically settled through a smart contract. Or tools that are managed by a group of people whereby revenues and expenses are automatically settled through a smart contract.

Recommendations for Cybersecurity

With every new technology, security risks are increased or reduced, depending on the characteristics thereof. Recommendations for organizations that want to adopt existing Blockchain applications or want to design existing processes with Blockchain can be found in the report *Blockchain Security: A Framework for Trust and Adoption.* The Dutch Blockchain Coalition makes 24 recommendations in this regard.

This report offers a framework for the most important security considerations that should be taken into account when applying Blockchain technologies. The framework is written for decision makers who are planning to use Blockchain technology. In addition, it is a practical, high-level guide to the most important security issues that an organization should consider when starting its own Blockchain application or transferring from a current application to this new environment.

The top 18 safety risks to be taken into account when using the technology are:

1. Security of smart contracts
2. Forks
3. Crypto algorithms
4. Cryptographic key management
5. Access control
6. Scalability
7. Intrusion detection

8. Targeted attach resistance
9. Data propagation attach resistance
10. Operations & communications security
11. System acquisition, development, and maintenance
12. Asset management
13. Human resource security
14. Supplier relationships
15. Incident management
16. Organization of information security
17. Information security policies
18. External/internal compliance

The following are the top 6 security risks when migrating a current application to this new environment:

1. Choosing the right Blockchain
2. Special considerations for testing
3. Awareness and training
4. Contingency planning
5. Simplicity as a security measure
6. Privacy

In addition to identifying safety risks, it is especially important to eliminate these risks or to bring them to an acceptable level. The following case is a good example of this in which different intermediate layers of data exchanges disappear and fewer risks are involved.

CASE 2: HOW MICROBIOME CENTRE CLOSES THE KNOWLEDGE GAP

The health of your intestines largely determines how you feel. If the bacterial collection in the intestines (the micro-organism) is not balanced, this may lead to various medical complaints. Nevertheless, the knowledge about this was limited until a few years ago and was anything but useful. 'Doctors simply did not know what to do with it and patients also knew nothing about it', says Henk Duinkerken, CEO of Microbiome Centre (Ledger Leopard 2019).

Network Organization

The Microbiome Centre is not a traditional clinic for intestinal complaints. This knowledge gap around the microorganism of intestines gave the founders the idea to set up a network between patients, general practitioners, pharmacists, laboratories and scientists: a Blockchain network in which medical and personal data are recorded securely and irrefutably. Microbiome treatments are always performed by physicians who have their own treatment location. In 2017, this network organisation started on Blockchain. A large number of parties are connected to this Blockchain: doctors, a laboratory, pharmacist, three universities and the AMC to improve intestinal health by making personalised microbiome treatment possible.

The Blockchain always makes it clear which party has access to which data and gives the patient an explicit role in granting consent. Dunkirk states: 'Medical doctors can request faecal analyses based on this if a patient has complaints; the laboratory then carries out the requested analysis. Based on the analysis, the doctor writes out a prescription, and the patient can determine whether he agrees with the proposed treatment. Finally, the pharmacist looks at the prescription and sends the requested medicine to the patient. With a smooth integration of payment.'

Medicines Act

The Microbiome Centre's network environment eliminates the need for signed agreements. These have been replaced by smart contracts, which automatically trigger actions when the conditions are met. 'The agreement between doctor and pharmacist is very important according to the Medicines Act, so we have anchored it in a Blockchain. Just like the data traffic between the doctor and the laboratory. That must be absolutely safe, and nothing must go wrong. The client is in charge', Dunkirk explains (Rabobank).

Correspondences and research data are all stored watertight on the Blockchain. Dunkirk: 'The doctors who use our system can view results in our network. The pharmacist sees which probiotics to mix. Checks by parties are stored in the system, as well as confirmation that the patient has received his medication.'

Five Principles to Get Started

As an experience expert Dunkirk provides a number of basic principles for organisations (Rabobank).

Does Blockchain Fit Your Company?

Take a good look at whether Blockchain fits your business. Whether it is a suitable solution depends on the problem. If you use a lot of files as an entrepreneur, archive a lot of documents, put ten damage forms in a system every day, as it were: you can then see whether a blockchain will save a great deal of time and money.

Choose a Platform

Do not wait until there is one final Blockchain platform; that will never happen. Dunkirk does, however, expect connections to be established between different platforms at some point.

Dare to Ask

You don't have to re-invent the wheel. There are plenty of parties that can help you fulfil your wishes in a blockchain application. Microbiome Centre ended up at Ledger Leopard with their work process, which they had neatly incorporated into a table. Ledger Leopard has developed the network environment.

An Open Mind

In the beginning, people also had doubts about email. Then you were asked questions like: 'Where do you buy a mail account?' Today, emailing has become very common, and that's how blockchain will work. A number of things can be done very well with blockchain. For example, to irrevocably record mutual agreement without having to involve a central authority. If you look at business processes with those eyes, there are many places where Blockchain is useful.

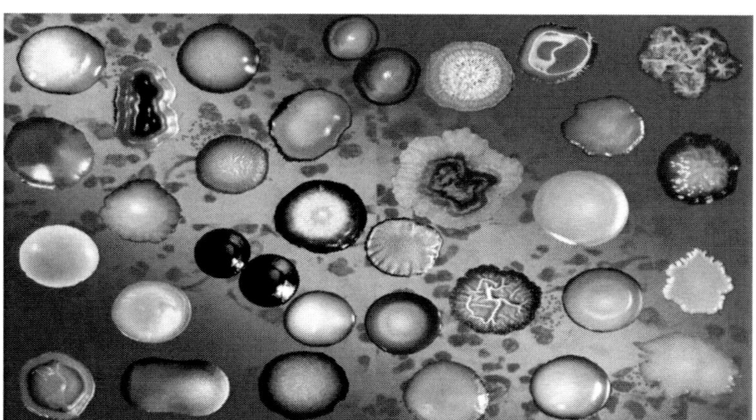

Source: Pixabay.

Figure 16. On Thursday January 16, 2020, the Blockchain lectorate, together with Health Valley, Zorginstituut Nederland and Novel-T, organised an afternoon on Blockchain & Health with the cooperation of Microbiome Centre: https://novelt.com/nl/events/blockchain-health/.

Three Applications in Healthcare

The Blockchain can respond to the challenges currently confronting healthcare. These challenges include medical data (security, interoperability, accessibility), medical research, clinical trials, the medical supply chain and the quality of the medicines. Many healthcare organizations do not use efficient and ineffective methods to deal with medical data. Failure to properly manage data affects patient care. In addition, the problem arises that many health services each use their own methodology for medical data and access to such data.

The Blockchain can shape data efficiency in healthcare. It can ensure flexibility, interconnection, accountability and protection in accessing those data that are necessary for the provision of good care. In this chapter, we mainly talk about how Blockchain can be applied in healthcare in practice.

Transparency of Information

Medical data on patients are spread across many organisations, insurance companies, doctors and the like. As a result, the medical file appears to be a complex of information that is incoherent, and it is a question whether all very important information is available. Currently, there is (not yet) a universal data storage system and the associated standards, both medical and ethical. This is therefore the crossroads between the medical sector and Blockchain to develop healthcare applications.

The use of Blockchain technology in healthcare makes a difference in data management. The technology will make sharing medical data more effective, efficient, secure and transparent for all healthcare stakeholders. A network for healthcare institutions can exist without having a patient's personal data. The details are all part of the Blockchain.

Patients are identified in this network by means of their hash identification which is a unique identification. A *hash* is an encrypted and calculated numeric code (see Chapter 1). The hash identification makes the ID unique and protects the privacy of the user. As a result, the Blockchain can also form a platform for exchanging patient data. In this way, you can prevent information from being blocked, as it is possible to keep the exchange of information between the various stakeholders active. When the data changes within one of the blocks, a chain reaction is set up that can freeze the entire Blockchain. Because this is theoretically impossible, the data contained in the Blockchain cannot be tampered with.

But what if non-stakeholders want to *hack* information and/or influence it incorrectly? This is solved by Blockchain technology: it is a transparent tool in which everyone who is part of this network will look at the Blockchain to see how each transaction takes place and whether or not relevant information is passed on. In addition, data cannot be fraudulent; if a non-interested party wishes to block the data, this will drastically change the hash due to the snowball effect. Each block in the Blockchain stores the data hash stored in the previous block (see Chapter 4.4). Blockchain thus ensures enormous transparency of patient information so that patients can be better helped.

Accessibility of Patient Information

Although it is considered an unethical activity, blocking information in healthcare has been a problem. In the medical sector, for example, blocking patients' data can be recognised by a doctor as the result of unreasonable restrictions on the exchange of patient data or electronic health information. There are three reasons for blocking information, the US Office of the National Coordinator for Health Information Technology states:

- interference
- knowledge
- there is no justification for inaccessibility of data

It goes without saying that blocking information is a huge disadvantage for efficient and effective practice in healthcare. The explanation for this seems very clear: hospitals do not want to miss patients and want to make it as difficult as possible for them to go to another hospital or claims behaviour produces undesirable effects. This actually should already have been the practice in the current digital age.

Research shows that blocking information is very widespread and that the various steps taken to curb this remain extremely inefficient. In fact, 50% of respondents have been involved in blocking information from health IT companies, says Adler-Milstein, associate professor and director of the Centre for Clinical Informatics and Improvement Research at Harvard University (Adler-Milstein and Pfeifer 2017). A quarter of these respondents say that this practice is due to hospitals and health systems. According to the researchers, the following methods can prevent blocking information:

1. Greater clarity so that any action taken by members can be justified.
2. Good financial rewards so that the participants want to exchange data.
3. A partnership between healthcare IT companies, hospitals and the Healthcare Information Exchange can prevent information from being blocked.

Blockchain technology can help set up medical records in Blockchain. This reduces unnecessary administrative costs and also allows better use of health data. In addition, its application may reduce the need to contact different intermediaries to supervise the exchange of essential health information.

Complete Information

A single patient's medical records can now be split across different facilities, doctors and insurance companies. This means that the entire medical history of a patient is always distorted or incomplete. Virtual medical records stored on a Blockchain can help healthcare stakeholders bring all parts of the health data complexity together. Therefore, the patient records, medicines received, completed procedures, facilities used and other details will also be up-to-date and usable for everyone involved.

Accessible and complete information will greatly simplify the key role of healthcare professionals. After all, this role consists of providing patients with reliable, timely and good treatment. By using Blockchain technology in the field of healthcare, service providers will always have a clear picture of the patient's medical record. It is crucial to note and acknowledge that all past health data are unchangeable in a Blockchain and healthcare environment and that any improvements to that data are obvious.

Guarantee of Information Storage

Medical information in a Blockchain can be processed from various sources such as:

- patient records
- *wearables* such as smartwatches
- mobile devices
- laboratories

Effective and efficient control over medical data is one of the most important advantages of Blockchain and healthcare. Many health-related problems can be avoided: interoperability, completion of data, misuse and even loss of data during a disaster. It is also worth noting that Blockchain technology can provide solutions to complex issues following a crisis like a pandemic.

To help organizations improve preparation for a future pandemic and to support, accelerate and safeguard an economic recovery after the COVID-19, the World Economic Forum has released the Blockchain Deployment Toolkit available on Weforum.org.

Critical to the provision of adequate medical services is the ability to ensure that the health data are correct. It must be avoided that junk becomes automated junk. Exposure to appropriate medical records means that healthcare professionals can make an accurate diagnosis. In addition, any adjustments are almost impossible until the data reaches a Blockchain.

Care Is (Still) Lagging Behind Blockchain

Pharmaceutical companies of medical equipment are enthusiastic about the Blockchain, but this technology is still being introduced slowly, GlobalData observed in 2020. However, they expect Blockchain's role in healthcare to grow rapidly. According to GlobalData, the main reason that this rapid growth is not yet achieved is the high start-up costs to get started. After all, many healthcare organizations have outdated legacy systems that are not adapted. There are also concerns about scalability, government regulation and privacy. Blockchain will certainly play a major role in future care, especially in the flow and exchange of information between stakeholders such as pharmaceutical companies, doctors, insurers and patients.

Data can be exchanged quickly, easily and securely with Blockchain, with a high degree of interoperability and the assurance that everyone has the latest data. Privacy legislation and the US Health Insurance Portability and Accountability Act play a role in this development, while one can also wonder whether it is not too leading. Laws and regulations always follow social developments and not the other way around.

Another application is to better safeguard data integrity by using Blockchain. Within clinical trials, it is of great importance that data and research results are not manipulated. Blockchain could at least theoretically offer a solution for this (Nictiz 2017).

Experiments in healthcare with Blockchain are already taking place in various countries. Estonia has set an example internationally in the field of digital services for years. Estonia uses Blockchain in the national database with patient files and medication regulations. At the beginning of 2016, the company Guardtime announced that together with the government they would secure the data of a million patients with the help of Blockchain. This concerns ensuring data integrity and making all operations performed on the data transparent. So it is not about putting medical data on Blockchain.

Blockchain pilots are also used in healthcare in the US. The US Food and Drug Administration is working with IBM, KPMG, Merck and Walmart to improve the pharmaceutical supply chain with the Blockchain. This supply chain contains many intermediaries that become unnecessary with the arrival of a Blockchain. In 2019, companies completed the Interoperability Pilot as part of the FDA's DSCSA Pilot Project Program (DSCSA 2020). In addition to the big advantages of a Blockchain, it also poses challenges such as data integrity, data storage options and development costs. The challenge of data integrity is no different in today's traditional systems.

The main components of GlobalData's Blockchain in Health Care Thematic Research (2020) research include:

- Key Industry Players: the major players in the blockchain industry and where they are in the value chain.

- Trends in the Blockchain: the main trends that stimulate the introduction of the Blockchain, divided into four main categories: trends in the supply chain, technological themes, macroeconomic themes and regulatory themes.
- Industry analysis and the impact of the Blockchain in healthcare: the key applications of Blockchain in healthcare, including case studies that demonstrate how the healthcare industry uses Blockchain for better results.
- Value chain: Blockchain implementation and integration in the healthcare industry, highlighting market drivers and barriers.

GlobalData provides a good overview of how investments in Blockchain relate to other trends in pharmaceutical and medical companies. For example, 71% of the pharmaceutical companies spend money on Blockchain. Around 55% of companies involved in medical equipment also invest in technology (GlobalData 2020). This puts investments in Blockchain in the middle bracket of the topics surveyed, including big data, artificial intelligence and cybersecurity, for example.

Security of Medicine Production and Distribution

Blockchain can be used for traceability of medicines and not only for traceability of the recipe but even counterfeit medicines. Counterfeiting medicines or imitation medicines is a major problem in the pharmaceutical industry and a social problem. As early as 2017, the Health Research Funding Organisation found that:

- 10 to 30% of medicines sold in developing countries are falsified;
- the market for counterfeit medicines is worth two hundred billion dollars per year;
- the sale of counterfeit products on the internet represents a value of USD 75 billion from the global market;
- the majority of counterfeit medicines are produced in India and China;
- in 2014, approximately sixty different Pfizer medicines and products were counterfeit worldwide. (World Health Organization 2017)

Incidentally, the WHO estimates that sixteen percent of counterfeit medicines contain the wrong ingredients, while seventeen percent contain the wrong levels of necessary ingredients. From a financial point of view, counterfeiting causes an annual loss for the European pharmaceutical industry of 10.2 billion euros.

Using Blockchain not only reduces the possibility of placing incorrect prescription products on the black market, but also reduces the chance of counterfeit products entering the black market. Regardless of the type of product, pharmaceutical companies must have incredibly safe chain cooperation. Pharmaceutical products are regularly stolen from the supply chain to be illegally marketed to various customers.

Blockchain for a Secure Supply Chain

Chain management is a field in which the blockchain is developing very strongly. Efficient supply chains form the core of many successful companies and deal with the transit of goods from the supplier to the consumer. Where there are several stakeholders in a particular sector, coordination is usually rather difficult. However, blockchain technology can enable new levels of transparency in many industries. An *interoperable supply chain* ecosystem that revolves around an unchangeable database is exactly what many industries can use to become more future-proof and effective.

Companies that register a product on a blockchain must be reliable to guarantee the validity and traceability of the products. Because of this reliability, it is therefore not unusual that private blockades operated by a central authority ensure that no counterfeit medicines are registered.

The companies determine which actors in the chain are active as *miners* and these can be suppliers, distributors or retailers. Depending on their role, each individual will have different rights: a laboratory technician can register medicines, while a wholesaler can only confirm transactions.

Tracking Down Medicines

When a medicine is registered for the blockchain, a hash is created that contains all relevant product data. The information is stored on the blockchain when the medicinal product goes from the manufacturer to the distributor, which makes traceability clear. A pilot shows that the use of blockchain technology can drastically reduce the time required to track down a prescription drug: from up to 16 weeks to 2 seconds. We already mentioned the US Food and Drug Administration's DSCSA Pilot Project Program. In addition to the visibility of the supply chain, this pilot uses the blockchain to improve patient protection and patient safety. The application helps users to locate, investigate and handle a particular criminal or illegal drug easily and efficiently.

When a drug needs to be withdrawn from the market, blockchain makes it easy to remove it from the market and thus prevent complications. *Blockade technologies* therefore help with two important issues when it comes to the traceability of drugs.

- They support companies to track down their medication in the supply chain, creating a closed network that is impenetrable to counterfeit medication.
- They help stakeholders to take action with knowledge from experience in the event of a problem by recognizing the exact position of their medication.

Collaboration with Artificial Intelligence and the Internet of Things

Because blockchain, *artificial intelligence (AI)* and the *Internet of Things (IoT)* connect perfectly, care processes can be fundamentally redesigned. This inevitable convergence of Blockchain, AI and the IoT will form an impactful combination of security, interconnectivity and autonomy to bring about a revolution in the way processes run. This is illustrated in Figure 17.

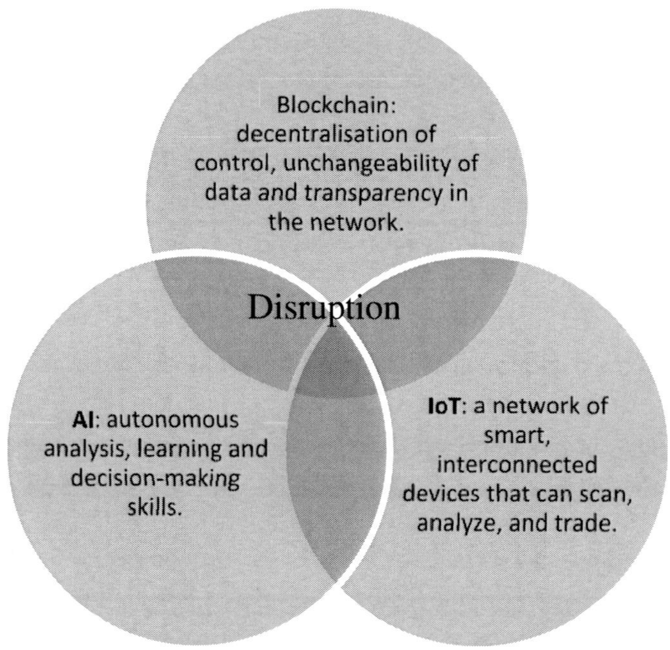

Source: Veuger 2020b and ICT Magazine, "Transparency in the medicines supply chain."

Figure 17. The individuals and disruption between Blockchain, AI and the IoT.

A combination of blockchain, AI and the IoT technologies that influence the potential of how companies, industries and even economies function will redefine these three more than they do now. Some applications and concepts have already shown an overlap between these technologies with promising results. The use of Blockchain makes it possible to securely record personalised data, so that these data can be used for diagnostics and treatment. We will first explain the operation and possibilities of AI and IoT.

Artificial Intelligence

Artificial intelligence gives complete autonomy when analysing data, making decisions and taking action on computers or other smart devices. AI can be replicated under certain circumstances and can even surpass human math and cognitive capabilities.

Organizations use AI to automate mainly repetitive, routine processes that may require large amounts of data processing and fast decision making based on pure logic.

Blockchain also strengthens the autonomy of the users. Blockchain strengthens the integrity and quality of firstly the exchange of information and secondly (the preparation for) automated decision-making in chains (Berenschot 2019) in a (semi-)autonomous way.

Internet of Things

The IoT is about familiar devices such as televisions, garage doors, refrigerators, coffee machines, lighting, speakers, heating etc. that are given an IP address, with which they have digital accessibility. The IoT offers seamless interconnectivity between different everyday objects that are equipped with sensors, microprocessors and transducers. This creates a network that can independently perceive and collect data, continuously analyse it and perform programmed tasks.

This infrastructure of devices, machines, homes, business premises, institutions, vehicles and people offers the possibility to share and process information with each other. More than 50 billion devices will be connected in the near future. In principle, the IoT consists of three elements:

- sensors
- communication
- processes

Sensors consist of data with regard to, for example, electricity, payment units or traffic information, or everything that can be measured. These data can then be recorded in a network, of blockchain for example. Within the IoT, blockchain technology is perfectly designed to communicate small objects with each other, the second element. IoT is going to have a huge impact on our economy and society. High-tech products and forms of service are expected to develop rapidly in the coming years, with blockchain technology playing a very important role.

Example of Heat Stress Levels

A proven convergence of blockchain, AI and the IoT is, for example, Fujitsu's algorithm to measure the heat stress levels of employees (Petitjean 2019; Fujitsu 2019). The algorithm constantly monitors the physiological data of employees (temperature, humidity, activity levels, pulse etc.) using portable In-vitro Diagnostic Devices (IDA) and sensors to track the correlation between various factors related to employee health. The analysis can help the organization to improve working conditions and prevent employee health problems.

Applying blockchain in this system can help to keep more personalized data by safeguarding privacy or can help pay out health insurance amounts through Smart contracts. Legal investigations in this area are being researched and can be found in an article by Automatie pma[3].

Smartly Combining Blockchain with AI and the IoT

The convergence of blockchain, AI and the IoT can enable organizations to maximize the benefits of each of these technologies while at the same time minimizing the risks and limitations associated with them. Given that the IoT networks include a large number of connected devices, there are numerous vulnerabilities, making the network susceptible to hacker attacks, fraud and theft. To prevent security issues, AI powered by *machine learning* can proactively defend itself against *malware* and hacker attacks. The security of the network and the data can be further improved by means of a Blockchain that can minimize illegal access to and alteration of the data on the network. AI can also improve the functional capacity of the IoT network by making it more autonomous and smarter.

A combination of Blockchain, AI and the IoT technologies that influence the potential of how companies, industries and even economies function will redefine these three more than they do now. Some applications and concepts have already shown an overlap between these technologies with promising results (Odyssey 2020). An example of this is the combination of AI and Blockchain to manage the unmanned air traffic, making mass autonomous flying safer. This application alone will redefine the aviation and logistics business.

The expected impact of the convergence of Blockchain, AI and the IoT is not (yet) foreseeable, and existing applications are not (yet) perfect. Many organizations, especially the *early adopters*, have very high expectations for the value of cognitive technologies and therefore want to invest in them. Findings from applications are now (still) at an early stage and are not yet as advanced as necessary to achieve real transformation, nor are the business models that will be key in this. The same can be said of the IoT in combination with Blockchain. With increased interest, investment and innovation, the convergence of the Blockchain, AI and the IoT will become reality.

Blockchain and Health Information Exchange (HIE)

Blockchain enables a distributed and decentralised environment with each central authority. Healthcare is an industry in which Blockchain is expected to have significant consequences. In recent years, health information exchange (HIE) has shown that it benefits the health care system. Research (Vishnoi 2020) has shown that Blockchain can help to improve several aspects of the HIE system.

When Blockchain meets HIE, there are only two issues. Firstly, the existing systems are not patient-oriented in terms of data governance. Patients do not own their data and

---

[3] For the article, see: https://automatie-pma.com/files/b764795652df2cd2343d25c49488f 980.pdf.

have no direct control thereover. Secondly, there is no particular protocol between the different systems for sharing sensitive data. In order to refute the two issues, the Blockchain Lab of Arizona State University conducted a study and presented a MedFabric4Me. This is a system for HIE based on Blockchain. In this rather technical case about MedFAbric4Me, we delve deeper into this system.

Healthcare Information Exchange (HIE)

Healthcare Information Exchange (HIE) is the electronic transfer according to national standards of healthcare related data between medical facilities, public authorities and health information organisations - companies that supervise and regulate the exchange of these data.

The purpose of HIE is to promote proper and safe access and retrieve health information from a patient in order to improve the cost, quality, safety and speed of patient care. Although HIE usually refers to the act of exchanging information between two or more organisations or healthcare providers, it may also refer to an organisation responsible for facilitating the exchange.

Case 3: Health Information Exchange at MedFAbric4Me

MedFabric4Me is a patient-focused system where patients own and share their healthcare data based on necessity. Arizona State University with its Blockchain Lab is a knowledge partner of the Blockchain professorship and also conducts specific research into Blockchain and healthcare. This case MedFabric4Me is an example of how Blockchain can be used effectively in healthcare.

First, an analysis was performed of the requirements for a patient-oriented system that ensures fraud-proof sharing of the data among the participant. This system contains a mechanical system that ensures that data cannot be manipulated. A distributed Proxy encryption system has been used to securely encrypt data during storage and data sharing. In addition, the combination of on-chain storage and on-chain access management has been applied for authenticity and privacy.

On-Chain and Off-Chain

MedFabric4Me is a two-part solution platform consisting of on-chain and off-chain components. The on-chain solution is implemented on the secure network of Hyperledger

Fabric while the off-chain solution uses an Interplanetary File System to store data securely. An Ethereum-based Nucypher – a Proxy re-encryption network – provides cryptographic access control to actors for encrypted data sharing.

To demonstrate usability and scalability, a prototype solution from MedFabric4Me has been implemented and evaluated as the performance benchmark of the system against an already implemented HIE. The results show that decentralised technology such as Blockchain can help to reduce some of the problems HIE faces today, such as patient transparency, slow emergency response and better access control. The research (Vishnoi 2020) therefore concludes that MedFabric4Me benefits in terms of operation and performance.

Properties of MedFabric4Me

The experiment has demonstrated the potential in an interoperable network of a private and public blockchain. If we compare this application with the HIE, intervals of scalability and performance, we see the following:

Privacy

As previously indicated, data from healthcare and the electronic patient file are protected by laws and regulations. Therefore, each system must comply with the Health Insurance Portability and Accountability Act (HIPAA) privacy guidelines. HIPAA is the 1996 US healthcare legislation. MedFabric4Me meets all minimum requirements.

A patient can delete their account at any time on MedFabric4Me. So when you leave the network, MedFabric4Me immediately deletes all information for the participant. Although the exchange of information must be recorded as a transaction history, MedFabric4Me as a general ledger is unchangeable.

A patient manages data sharing in MedFabric4Me and can therefore unsubscribe from file sharing at any time. A patient therefore determines their own policy for sharing data. In addition, a patient may request the supplier to change incorrect health information. Although the patient cannot change his electronic patient record himself, any discrepancy can be changed by a next doctor.

Partial Sharing of Data

De-identification is required when the patient's data are shared for study purposes. To comply with the same, MedFabric4Me may partially share data, hide personal information, or may not be required to share data for structured data only. For unstructured data, it has not (yet) been implemented in the system, but can still take place at a later stage.

Scalability

For scalability of Hyperledger Fabric, we will need to compare it to the state of the art of the Arizona company Health Current. Health Current completes an average of 23.4 million HLF transactions, 1.2 million CCD transactions and 10.4 million warnings per month.

IPFS versus Cloud

Cloud services offer about 20MB per second of upload and download speed, while Interplanetary File System (IPFS) provides a constant upload time of 0.4 seconds for encrypted files. For unencrypted files, the speed decreases even more (Taylor 2020). This shows that IPFS performs better for most uploads than cloud services with unencrypted file sizes. In the case of downloading, IPFS offers a speed of about 7 MB per second and is lower than the download speed of cloud services. This can be improved by creating a private cloud service and duplicating data across multiple *peers*. The researchers (Vishnoi 2020: 80) therefore conclude that IPFS may not be the best database for applications, but that it works to store files with a hash and when access control via Hyperledger Fabric is regulated.

Nucypher

PRE is the most popular coding algorithm (Aminubaba et al. 2014) in the cloud and has a speed of about 55 MB per second for encryption, compared to Nucypher with 115 MB per second. PRE therefore offers better performance in terms of encryption time than existing cloud services.

Comparisons of Use between MedFabric4Me and HIE

Finally, we look at six scenarios in which HIE offers benefits to healthcare providers and participants and compare them with the implementation of MedFabric4Me.

ADT Messages

When patients are admitted, discharged or transferred to an emergency situation, the patient's caregivers receive a warning with the basic information (date of admissions, place of admissions, reason for admission, etc.) and can thus reach the patient and take care of follow-ups. This warning is an ADT message, where ADT stands for Admission, Discharge and Transfer.

However, MedFabric4Me does not (yet) have an implementation for emergency visits, although the most important functionality of the ADT messages are implemented in an unchangeable ledger. When a patient visits the emergency room and files are updated, Fabric4Me records the transaction of data unchangeably. Providers will then not receive ADT messages at the exact time of status change. But when patients visit providers, those providers get a general history of the updated files with the patient's visit to the emergency room for what reason.

Improvements in Pandemic Warnings

A pandemic is an epidemic of diseases that spreads across a large region. Very well-known examples of this are SARS and COVID-19. In general, test laboratories provide rapid results during a pandemic. HIE will have to adapt and create an infrastructure to adapt to a pandemic that initially slows down the response. Even once the infrastructure is there, HIE is vulnerable because warnings must always be in *real time* and generally on a certain scale. During COVID-19, for example, Health Current initially provided the alerts and data without the Secure File Transfer Protocol.

MedFabric4Me does not have to adapt to a pandemic every time. Although it does not provide emergency alerts, no new functionality or complete infrastructure needs to be created to support pandemic reporting. An institute or test laboratory that conducts mass tests can provide safe results for the specific patient and those data can be exchanged further.

Management of Medical Devices

HIE has a very specific functionality, namely to share medical records with providers' suppliers and with the participants. The medical industry is enormous, and there are several other industries involved. One of these are manufacturers of medical devices that supply medical devices to suppliers, research institutes and healthcare institutions. Manufacturers pass on the use of a device to providers or institutes. Currently, medical suppliers have a limited view of the use of the device, which results in careless service.

MedFabric4Me's policy on the partial sharing of data can help device manufacturers to have a good view of the use of the device with vendors and to trust the data. The manufacturer can determine which medical devices are required. For the rest, manufacturers can gain insight into the inventory of a particular location, which helps them make a well-considered decision as to whether they should move it within the providers at the location or call for a new machine.

With these experiments and comparisons, the researchers conclude that MedFabric4Me is a viable decentralized alternative to the current centralized alternative. Some outlined benefits of MedFabric4me are:

- MedFabric4Me has the capacity to perform better in the field of transit.
- Decentralisation ensures that there is no single point of failure.
- MedFabric4Me reduces the overhead costs of *cloud computing*, expensive encryption and helps to divide costs between insurers, healthcare providers and patients.

- MedFabric4Me provides data governance to patients, which leads to transparency, decreasing delay and improving the services.

Although MedFabric4Me showed potential in some areas, there are some areas where there was a lack of a centralized solution. We will review them briefly.

Ease of Setup

It is very easy to set up and scale a centralized system – much simpler than a decentralized system like MedFabric4Me. The centralized HIE is largely based on what is called *enterprise cloud computing*, which manages and scales multiple services to analyse system applications. For MedFabric4Me, it is complicated to develop a company-level system application with multiple independent components.

System Upgrade and Updates

It is easier to update a centralized system as all servers and application code bases are controlled from a single central location. Blockchain setups are difficult to upgrade as nodes are distributed and each node is updated at the same time to keep the network functional.

Easier Data Backup

In a centralized system, it is easier for the current HIE to back up health data. This can be complex for MedFabric4Me when patients own their data and are free to choose their own data storage service providers. It is possible that the patient may permanently lose data due to a lack of data backups.

The Basic Principles of Blockchain in Healthcare

Blockchain offers opportunities for healthcare, but there is also a need for knowledge and insight into how to use blockchain safely and responsibly in healthcare (Zorginstituut 2019). Blockchain is currently being implemented more theoretically than practically. The legal, organisational, social and technical preconditions under which blockchain can be of value to healthcare require clarification.

The four basic principles are central to this chapter; we already mentioned them in Chapter 1 and at the start of Chapter 2. In order to achieve a more effective realization of the care, we expand on the four basic principles for the use of Blockchain.

- Basic principle 1 Growing chain. In order to be able to work together, it is necessary that information can be shared. This is implemented through information standards and Nictiz's five-layer model.
- Basic principle 2 Distributed network. Blockchain acts as a digital infrastructure (a care information system). An example is the functioning of the IT platform within value-driven care to arrive at a record of outcomes of care.
- Basic principle 3 Consensus. Since there is no central party that steers, the parties involved must reach agreement.
- Basic principle 4 Data storage. The recording of the digital identity and the safeguarding of privacy results from working with Blockchain.

Basic Principle 1 - Growing Chain

Healthcare is a digital island empire. Data exchange between professionals does take place, but there are still major points for development. Blockchain can play an important role in a new relationship between the patient and his data, the fourth basic principle, for example through greater transparency and control over data exchange. This is already being used by various parties:

- Blockchain for repeat prescriptions: Prescrypt. This is considered one of the first applications of Blockchain in healthcare (Radboud UMC).
- The MIT MedRec project is addressing fragmented access to medical data, improving interoperability, safeguarding patient rights and taking the amount and quality of data to a higher level for scientific research. In Chapter 5.4 you can read more about MedRec.
- Google has made it possible with its artificial intelligence department 'DeepMind' for hospitals in England to put health records on the Blockchain.
- Guardtime has already successfully implemented the same solution for the governments of Estonia and the United Arab Emirates.
- Coralhealth uses Blockchain to make personalised medicines possible.
- EncrypGen has launched a platform that allows people to sell their DNA in exchange for cryptocurrency.
- Lancor has developed a tool to bring the reliability of cancer screenings from sixty percent (by people) to ninety percent, through a combination of artificial intelligence and Blockchain.

Blockchain ensures a secure transfer of data between different parties, who can use them for personalised medicines, for example.

A care process can be described in part in terms of *transactions*: a moment of communication during which care information is exchanged. A combination of regulatory space, focus on the wishes of clients and quality of care and a digital working environment ensures that teams or care organisations are *in control*. By placing responsibility with professionals, organizational forms can arise around work processes and chains that transcend the boundaries of one's own organization. Because information is available, professionals can independently realize:

- distribution of common resources
- accountability for own resources
- mapping effectiveness and efficiency
- development of operational plans

Information standards

The digital transmission and sending of patient data is now more or less solved technologically. Nictiz is a Dutch knowledge organization that is committed to digital information exchange in healthcare. This organisation has developed *information standards* that, together with care providers, now apply to virtually all sectors of care. Examples include nursing transfer, acute care, obstetric care, the exchange of data from laboratories, medication safety and care for people with chronic diseases.

The information standard describes why and how medical data are used in practice. Examples of this type of data include blood pressure, discharge date, diagnosis and weight but also civil status, gender and name. The information standard also describes the technical infrastructures and networks through which the data can be transmitted and the international standards and communication systems that can be used for this purpose. Because the healthcare field is complex to describe in a single information standard, information standards are always developed for specific and well-defined situations in which healthcare professionals exchange information, with each other and with their patients. The dataset is a crucial part of an information standard. The dataset describes which data are involved and also provides a description of technical details that are understandable to software programmers.

A dataset consists of *healthcare information building blocks* (zibs) such as body weight, medication and alcohol consumption. These are indispensable building blocks for a secure, reliable and unambiguous exchange of medical data in all healthcare sectors. Figure 4.1 shows the relationship between the information standard, dataset and zib. In the Dutch context, it has been agreed that the collection of zibs is a national standard, which we call the *Basic Care Data Set* (Basisgevensset Zorg; BgZ). Nictiz plays a central and facilitating role in the development of information standards and care information building blocks (zibs) in the Netherlands.

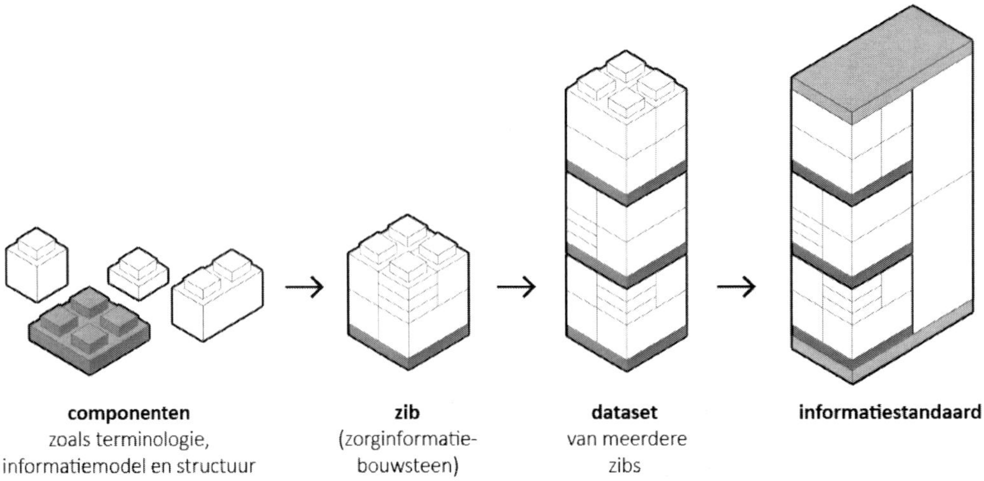

Source: Nictiz.

Figure 18. The dataset is a crucial part of an information standard.

For example, the *real-time* availability of data via mobile applications enables 24-hour monitoring of high-risk patients.

Care teams can remotely monitor and leverage treatment options for early intervention. The care professional and the client have access to the same information and can reach joint decisions (Linn and Koo 2016).

Five-Layer Model

Depending on what a blockchain implementation is used for, an information and data model will be required. In order to arrive at an effective network structure, it is important to record and share information unambiguously. This interoperability arises when healthcare parties can make agreements on the information architecture at five levels. Nictiz has developed the five-layer model for this, in which each level has its own parties, concepts and standards:

1. Organizational policy concerns the organizational side of the collaboration. An example of a standard is referring a patient.
2. The care process concerns the way in which healthcare processes work together, such as a guideline for the transfer of medication data in a network structure.
3. Information is about recording data used for transmission moments in the network. An example is a terminology standard.
4. Applications concern the information systems required to share process information. An example is a standardized domain data model.
5. The IT infrastructure concerns the technical infrastructure within which the information systems of the network partners operate. This concerns the technical set-up that enables the exchange of information.

For a good exchange of information, agreements must be made at all levels of the five-layer model. This is shown in Figure 19.

Network structures are a specific form of inter-organizational cooperation to connect actions of organizations. The aim is a coherent approach to actions that the client needs or wishes (Van der Aa 2001: 16). To arrive at chain agreements, it is necessary to have (Van der Aa 2001: 123):

- insight into and view of interdependencies
- trust between the chain partners
- a chain described in a process design
- clarity about everyone's contribution to the chain
- registration of key figures
- a quality system with regard to the chain
- forms of chain management
- chain automation

A major problem is that organizations make insufficient agreements at the highest level, the organizational policy. Care organisations tend to focus quickly on the lower layers of the model: the IT infrastructure. There is a key element for care: trust must exist between organisations before data exchange can begin. The more remote the party with whom data is to be exchanged, the lower the trust.

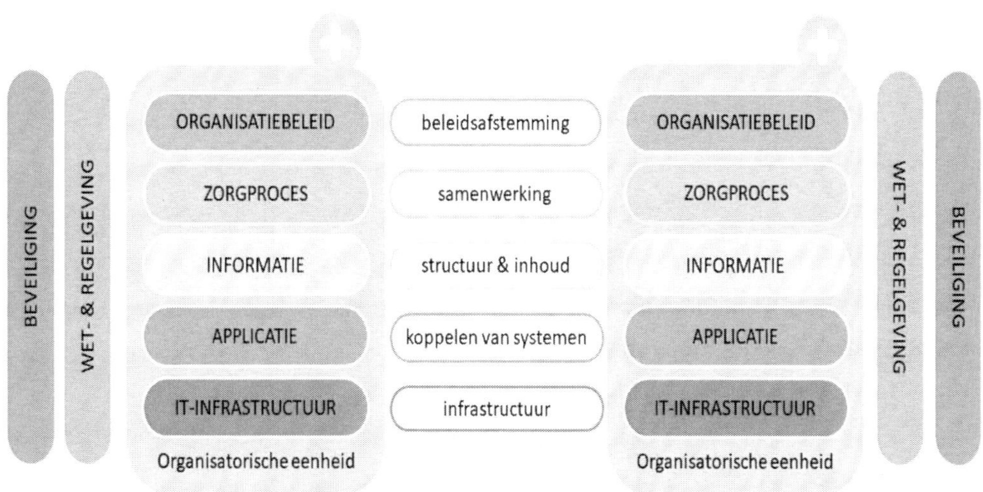

Figure 19. Nictiz's five-layer model.

For this purpose, the required standardisation is specified. The agreements are made by various parties:

- Policy coordination is usually an administrative process.
- Cooperation in the network takes place between the healthcare professionals and any supervisors.
- Structure and content require coordination between care and ICT professionals.
- Linking systems requires coordination between healthcare professionals and, for example, application administrators.
- The infrastructure requires coordination between ICT professionals.

Together, this is a complex agreement system. For good information exchange in healthcare, therefore, a number of facilities are always required. Together, they form the infrastructure on which information can be shared. This involves, for example, recording what is happening, ensuring secure communication such as encryption, authentication (verifying that someone is who they say they are) and being able to determine that the patient is giving permission for data exchange.

When and When Not to Use Blockchain

Decisions that require a decision-maker to fill in *discretionary space* (a large degree of regulatory freedom) with regard to the outcome and the process carried out with blockchain are not suitable for automated decision-making. Blockchain is therefore not suitable for less structured issues in which the process and the results can be the subject of interventions that have not been devised beforehand.

Blockchain can lend itself to (part of) the preparation of such decisions. Prescribing medications, for example, must remain the decision of the doctor and not be automatically decided by a blockchain. At the same time, the fact that the doctor prescribed the medicines and the pharmacist provided them (which is also not suitable for an automatic decision) can be used for an automated decision on the financing of care (Berenschot 2019).

Any type of information can be stored in a blockchain. The network that implements the blockchain determines the type of information that takes place in the transaction. It is essential that the information is correct and the system is well designed. By using blockchain, information (anonymised) can be shared irrefutably and in *real time* with different parties. Blockchain can thus support healthcare processes, make them faster and make them less sensitive to human errors. The technology can help to make healthcare safer, better, more accessible and cheaper. However, if blockchain is not well structured, the technology leads to risks, but that applies to every technology. As indicated earlier, blockchain does not have a central party: parties must make agreements at all levels of the five-layer model for a good exchange of information.

Basic Principle 2 - Distributed Network

The need of the patient is the starting point where different players in the network can add value to the patient at different times. *Network medicine* is care in which the patient is central and manages his health with the help of his relatives and healthcare professionals. The control is therefore increasingly placed with the client (Jeninga and Woldendorp 2019).

A properly functioning underlying digital infrastructure is a condition for effective and efficient collaboration in networks while maintaining the quality of care. In the future, digital and physical networks will be created at local, regional and (inter-)national levels. This is not only about networks around the patient but also about networks between healthcare professionals both inside and outside the walls of the hospital. As a result, bulkheads will disappear and specialisms will flow together (Porter and Teisberg 2006). What is needed for network care is:

- management of care (measurement, management and funding of care)
- fully integrated chain care
- notion of a system approach
- financing
- transparency with regard to costs and innovations

Blockchain contributes to this by effectively and efficiently setting up a healthcare information management system. This provides a basis to arrive at value-driven care.

The Outcomes of Care

Value-driven care is characterised by a focus on outcome indicators. The outcomes of care are broadly understood and seen in perspective with the costs of a treatment course. The outcomes of care are quality, costs and the appropriateness of care.

Appropriateness is understood to mean the extent to which care for a patient is actually indicated. Indicators are required to be able to measure results. The care process thus becomes a chain of care delivery, in which all activities are included that offer value to the patient, from prevention and diagnostics to treatment and aftercare. The results of quality and efficiency measurements are the basis for improving care. These outcomes are data, and a blockchain platform can be helpful in making good use of those data.

Facilitating IT Platform

In the thinking of Michael Porter (Porter and Teisberg 2006), an IT platform that facilitates the movement is of great importance. Despite much effort, there is still limited information exchange and limited availability of reliable outcome measures. In addition, exchanging or being able to exchange outcome information in order to learn from it is still very limited. Interoperability is of great importance: use the same definitions and set IT and data standards.

The design of an IT platform makes it possible to integrate (technological and digital) innovations intelligently into the delivery of care. An IT platform is needed to facilitate collaboration within integrated practice units and to enable comparison and reporting of results and costs. An IT platform has the following elements: it is designed around (the condition of) the patient, uses standardised terminology and data fields so that everyone speaks the same language and includes all different types of data so that all healthcare providers have the complete overview. It is therefore an IT platform:

- that makes it possible to communicate digitally with other professionals
- that makes it possible to exchange registered data, such as health records and care plans
- that makes it possible for the patient to have access throughout the entire care process
- that monitors performance to facilitate (integrated) care provision
- that offers digital tools for patients to be active in self-management

The healthcare organisations involved, whether or not collaborating in networks, need a data platform that supports primary and supporting processes in conjunction. Blockchain offers possibilities for exchanging data.

Basic Principle 3 - Consensus

One of the unique features of Blockchain is the absence of a central controlling party. This leads to basic principle 3, consensus. A form of consensus is needed to implement updates and agree on what the proper state of the Blockchain is. In Chapter 2.3, we already saw that different infrastructures have their own form of consensus: Hyperledger Fabric, Ethereum and Corda. The more parties involved, the stronger the consensus.

But Blockchain is not, of course, a neutral, impartial, non-political technology. Precisely because the use of Blockchain can mean that existing processes, data exchange and relationships can change, attention to control is important (Zorginstituut 2018). If no consensus is reached within a group, separate Blockchains may arise with their own rules and currencies, as was the case, for example, in 2017 with Bitcoin, resulting in the creation of Bitcoin Cash (Edriouch 2018).

Blockchain offers opportunities for healthcare, but there is a need for knowledge and insight into how to use Blockchain safely and responsibly. The challenge for the development of Blockchain lies in differences between knowledge levels and interdependencies between (chain) parties. Since Blockchain is about cooperation in a chain, the parties involved must agree on conditions before a Blockchain platform or application can be developed (Berenschot 2019). By means of a smart contract, it can be determined which users on the platform have access to which personal data.

The study by Berenschot (2019) shows that it is necessary to regulate governance at three levels:

1. Regular governance for optimizing and controlling working Blockchain applications in practice.
2. Development governance for the processes in which Blockchain applications are (further) developed.
3. System governance for the general management and supervision of Blockchain development and application in healthcare at system level.

The legal frameworks for governance on Blockchain depend on what the Blockchain application is used for. Blockchain requirements in healthcare can be divided into three groups:

- generally applicable requirements
- requirements for the use of personal data in the Blockchain
- requirements for automated decision-making

Blockchain is an automation technology that allows information to be shared and processes to be executed automatically without the intervention of a trusted third party.

Basic Principle 4 - Data Storage

Central to data storage is the ability to determine the identity of data subjects and safeguard privacy.

Digital Identity

With solutions based on *self-sovereign identity*, a citizen himself has a digital vault with information about his own identity. These data can then be used in situations where it is essential to confirm your own identity (care; buying a home). An infrastructure for the digital identity and a new agreement system will be built. This lays the foundation for the provision of services from government and business, in which people are central, instead of individual solutions devised by a single organisation. This still requires the necessary laws and regulations in the current context (Lizanova and Veuger 2019) and should be reviewed completely.

In practice, for example, everyone should first have a complete digital identity.

Events or achievements can always be added to this, such as a diploma and driving licence (Rathenau Institute 2018).

Nevertheless, Blockchain already offers possibilities. For example, Blockchain can be used for:

- the exchange of data (e.g., between healthcare provider and health insurer)
- giving the patient access to his data
- sending and paying expense claims
- recording evidence of, for example, medical operations that have taken place

Although these applications are of great added value to healthcare, there are also barriers to their implementation:

- complexity of Blockchain
- doubts about guaranteeing privacy (GDPR) when personal data are included in the Blockchain
- increasing energy costs due to additional transactions in the chain
- lack of uniform infrastructure and consensus on algorithms (smart contracts)
- long processing time (seconds) of transactions

In addition, failure to delete data reveals the limits of storage periods and storage capacity (Kennisgroep Keteninformatisering 2019). There are many Blockchain ideas and partly working initiatives in healthcare, but according to Nictiz (2017) they are not yet ready for large-scale use. The main objective is to experiment and become familiar with the capabilities and limitations of the technology. This means investing time and money in acquiring knowledge and experience.

Privacy

A key issue within healthcare is safeguarding the privacy of clients. It is extremely important that medical data is not disclosed. Only with the permission of the patient may the care information be disclosed to another person.

Current legislation does not allow medical data to simply be shared. One healthcare provider may therefore not provide data from the file to one of the other two healthcare providers. This professional secrecy of the healthcare provider expires if the patient has consented to this.

As a result, every healthcare professional who would process personal data in a Blockchain must check whether they are authorized to do so. To avoid errors, it is therefore wise to work within a *permissioned Blockchain* in a private system (see Chapter

1). Read and write rights can be granted to specific users. This can be done in various ways:

- In the smart contract, it can be regulated which users have access to which personal data.
- In a smart contract, it can be arranged that the sender of a transaction per transaction can determine which users within the Blockchain can read the transaction.
- The personal data for unauthorised users are hashed so that the impact of the processing is limited.
- The unauthorised users can act as processors and thus view personal data (Zorginstituut 2019).

In order to prevent data subjects from incorrectly viewing information, it is desirable to store personal data off-chain (outside the chain) and to include a link to the relevant information on-chain. In other words: the Blockchain is used as an *access control* ledger.

A good example from practice is the Microbiome Centre, which facilitates a chain via Blockchain for analysing human excrement for the development of personalised medication (see also the case after Chapter 2). The Blockchain connects the physician, the laboratory, the pharmacy and the patient within a certain process, domestically and abroad (Zorginstituut 2019).

The Impact

Blockchain can deliver value in the short term. Most Blockchain applications can have an effect on data recording and execution in the short term. For example by:

- improving effectiveness
- improving efficiency
- innovating products and services
- involving stakeholders
- develop the organisation (VNG 2019)

Blockchain can facilitate a reliable insight into a single shared data source for a chain or cluster. This means that the right people can have the right information at the right time. This facilitates, among other things, the faster and better handling of applications from citizens and thus the effectiveness. Reducing administrative effort and costs ensures that employees can be more involved in the primary process. Blockchain technology offers various opportunities to innovate applications. It offers additional transparency in a chain and can make ownership more flexible. Blockchain can engage clients and improve partnerships between stakeholders, such as in chains. Blockchain strengthens knowledge and experience and develops employee competencies (VNG 2019). In the next chapter, we delve deeper into the application possibilities.

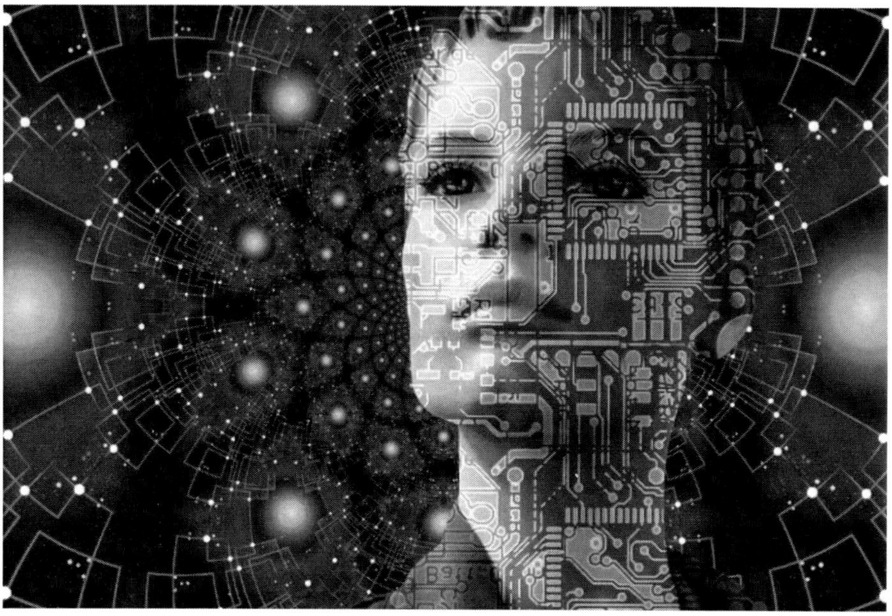

Source: Veuger 2020b: 17-32.

Figure 20. Blockchain convergence & competences.

Case 4: The VGZ Innovation Team Develops an App for Maternity Care

Health insurer VGZ is strongly focused on mapping innovation and technology for care. A lot of attention is paid to the practical implications of technological innovation (basic principle 2). There is an innovation team that is focused on the innovative application of relevant technology for the health insurer and healthcare. The I-Team Digital Innovation deals with:

- trend monitoring (e.g., digital humans and quantum computers)
- design of pilots (e.g., the Maternity Care practical trial and working with chatbots)
- advising on a digital care strategy for VGZ

Development

Blockchain is one of the topics proposed by the Board of Directors to move on to a deeper level. The first advice of the innovation team was to follow the development, but not yet to do any concrete experiments with it. At the request of the Supervisory Board, the Blockchain phenomenon was examined further. As a result, knowledge has been built up so that VGZ can take a good look at developments and any application for healthcare and the health insurer. Subsequently, the opportunity arose to run a practical trial in maternity care. Together with the Healthcare Institute, the I team developed a demo to test the added value of the growing Blockchain chain (basic principle 1). The Zorginstituut had developed a working app – called Geertje - which was converted together with VGZ for maternity care.

The maternity caregivers involved were very enthusiastic about the functionality of the app. This also applied to the three maternity care organisations involved. The app led to a clear reduction in the administrative burden. Nevertheless, it was decided not to continue. The reasons were:

- Blockchain works best when many parties are involved (the practical trial had a limited number of participating parties). Blockchain is about building consensus (basic principle 3). Consensus becomes stronger if more parties are involved. The number of parties in the various care chains is limited and the strength of the consensus is therefore also limited.
- Blockchain in healthcare is mainly about data around people. This puts the privacy issue at the centre. Although the personal data were encrypted, the process around logging in and retrieving encryption keys today requires a trusted third party. One of the most important advantages of Blockchain is that no dominant trusted third party is needed. But precisely because it is created for security purposes, this advantage is gone.
- Existing technology was able to deliver the same functionality via an app. This means that administrative burden reduction can also be achieved at lower costs at this stage.

Safeguarding privacy with data storage (basic principle 4) is an essential part of Blockchain's application in healthcare. There are developments around *self-sovereign identity* – validation by combining data from different parties – that will guarantee privacy in the long term. On the other hand, the best way to store data reliably is to disseminate it as little as possible. Data storage can take place on a private Blockchain. Important developments include:

- Increase agility of organizations and professionals
- A sense of urgency to continue digitisation (including due to COVID-19)
- Artificial intelligence focused on early diagnosis and self-diagnosis (e.g., SkinVision)
- Standardisation of healthcare operations (e.g., Bergman Clinics)
- Lifestyle interventions (e.g., GezondmetSalut)

DESIGN PRINCIPLES FOR INTRODUCING BLOCKCHAIN IN HEALTHCARE

The basic function of each Blockchain is to bring digital information together in a collection (a block) that cannot be changed. This is of great importance when designing an electronic client file (ECD) or electronic health record (EHR). For healthcare, Blockchain offers the opportunity to improve collaboration, safeguard trust and achieve interoperability.

In this chapter, we discuss developments in technology, the design principles for introducing Blockchain and the design of interoperability.

Different Way of Thinking

Blockchain leads to a different way of thinking by being able to capture transactions, creations and events. It is a *foundational technology*: it has the ability to create new foundations for our economic and social system (Harvard Business Review 2019: 7). There are five principles that determine this technology.

1. Distributed database: Each party on a Blockchain has access to the entire database and history.
2. Peer-to-peer transmission: horizontal communication.
3. Transparency and pseudonymity: Recording identity with the possibility of anonymity.
4. Irreversibility of files: Once a transaction has been recorded in the database, it can no longer be changed.
5. Computer logic: algorithms can be applied.

As a group, Blockchains are called *distributed ledger technologies* (Williams 2019: 60) or a distributed ledger. Blockchain is in fact a simple technology that works like a permanent, non-hackable ledger for virtually any type of information that someone wants to capture (Williams 2019). Anyone participating in a Blockchain is considered a ‘node’ in a network. When changes are made to a Blockchain, this is done in all nodes. Decentralised systems are non-hierarchical groups of interconnected nodes. Distributed systems are radically decentralized systems (Williams 2019: 47).

The IBM Institute for Business Value Blockchain Survey identifies nine areas of healthcare where disruption by Blockchain technology will take place (Nichol 2018): medical device data integration; asset management, client files, clinical trials, safety monitoring with regard to side effects, medication compliance, regulatory compliance, invoicing and claims and contract management.

In the area of COVID-19, Blockchain can capture an unchangeable trace of whether patients have developed antibodies. Access to information is significantly simplified through the use of technology. Clients can take better decisions if they have the right information. We therefore increase our *healthcare literacy*: the extent to which we have the ability to collect, record and understand healthcare information in order to arrive at better health decisions.

Technological Developments in Healthcare

Blockchain can play multiple roles in technological improvements (Williams 2019: 125):

1. Provide medical reports (ECD and EHR).
2. Agreement to share data in these files.
3. Payments to clients who promote health and thereby reduce healthcare costs.

Blockchain can bring an important innovation to the activities of health insurers. Blockchain technology applied to healthcare has the potential to reduce fraud and develop new business models (Nichol 2018). Medication policy is essential for effective healthcare (Czeschik and Stambolija 2018). When information about diagnoses and procedures is stored on Blockchain, there is virtually no room to manipulate this information to increase revenue. Medical devices are connected via Wi-Fi, Bluetooth and other interfaces. However, this leads to vulnerabilities caused by hackers.

How does Blockchain work within healthcare in practice:

- The client receives a code (hash) and an address that provides codes to unlock client data. If the client data are not stored in the Blockchain, the Blockchain provides authentication or the necessary hashes to access data.
- Care providers (care professionals) receive a separate universal signature (code or hash). When this hash is combined with the hash of a client, this ensures the authentication in order to be able to unlock data in a file.
- In his profile, the client defines the access rules required to access his file.
- When the client defines a 2-of-2 code via *eHerkenning*, two computers (hashes) are required to gain unauthorized access to data.

The advantages of this (Nichol 2018) are avoiding intermediaries, strengthening the management role of clients, integrity of data and reaching consensus.

Blockchain's application in healthcare can be distinguished in five separate fields (Czeschik and Stambolija 2018):

- ECD management
- medication management and planning
- invoicing and payment cycle
- logistics and chain management
- connected medical devices

What other application possibilities are there? This concerns the following areas:

- Chain management: monitoring and tracking of medicines; temperature determination for transport.
- Clinical *trials*: building consensus between different websites, systems and protocols and client data profiles.
- Online database of a provider: maintain worklists quickly and adequately.
- Client reports: bringing information from different data files together; translation into user-friendly development (diagnosis; medicines; consultations).

These applications greatly reduce costs:

- Costs for 'searching' for cases to almost zero (everything can be found quickly).
- Smart contracts replace current contracting and payment.
- Coordination costs of sources outside the organization are largely eliminated.
- Costs for trust largely expire.

Defibrillator with smart contracts

A practical example from healthcare. A patient with arrhythmias has an atrial defibrillator inserted. The device was supplied by company X with serial number Y. During the production process, a Blockchain was created to be able to track the device. A hash to identify this unique device is stored in the Blockchain with other relevant information. The hash of the device information is stored in an unchangeable digital ledger. The implanted defibrillator is linked to the patient and the device's Blockchain is updated with information from the hospital and the GP regarding the care of this patient. The device is supported by a number of smart contracts that automatically inform the patient and healthcare providers if the device needs to be adjusted or if irregularities are detected (Nichol 2018).

Blockchain can help solve barriers caused by strict healthcare regulations. This specifically concerns exchanging data (IBM 2018). Blockchain makes it possible to share client data in a uniform manner. Three major challenges concern:

1. Individual autonomy: self-ownership of identity
2. Scalability: chain transactions
3. Interoperability (open interaction between systems)

Individual autonomy concerns the principle that every client is the source and thus the owner of their own identity. Blockchain technology gives clients control over their own identity, access to the data and the authority to determine who can see that data.

Seven Design Principles

Blockchain has the potential to decentralise traditional supply chains and combine them with AI and the IoT, creating new value networks (Tapscott and Tapscott 2018). Data can be used better if they can be used freely and safely within and between the various healthcare domains. The establishment of a shared network between providers, professionals and clients strengthens clinical outcomes of a healthcare process. Fraud can also be prevented.

Blockchain has seven design principles:

1. Network integrity
2. Distributed power
3. Value as incentive
4. Security

5. Privacy
6. Rights are preserved
7. Inclusion

When Blockchain is applied in healthcare, it is a shared platform that decentralizes data using a high degree of security. Blockchain makes it possible to work with a care passport that contains relevant data. The use of medication can also be monitored via track and trace, which shows the quality of care over a certain period of time. By working with portable devices such as smartwatches, clients can provide real-time information for monitoring and realizing outcomes. Through the secure sharing of data, the quality of care plans is improved, thereby simplifying administrative processes and avoiding unnecessary care deployment.

Here, too, the use of smart contracts creates an audit trail with regard to the various aspects of care deployment. In Chapter 4.1, we mentioned Prescrypt. Prescrypt makes it possible for chronically ill people to get prescriptions that are secured on a Blockchain. This gives the client control over his medication and the accessibility of his information. Clients decide which healthcare professionals they want to share their data with and which pharmacy they want to send their medication overview to. This is illustrated in Figure 21.

Philips Healthcare uses Blockchain technology for welfare apps and client ID programs. Blockchain would make a central intermediary unnecessary under specific conditions, or under other preconditions could be limited to the management of partial databases (Czeschik and Stambolija 2018). Another product based on Blockchain is MyClinic.com. MyClinic makes it easy to make appointments, view medical records and schedule follow-up examinations. The objectives are accessibility and control for the client and simple contact between healthcare professional and client (Medicalchain).

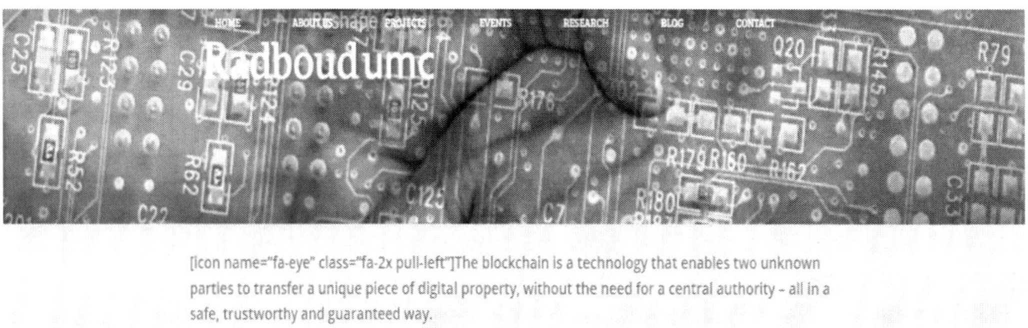
HOME
EVENTS
RESEARCH
BLOG
CONTACT
Radboudumc
[icon name="fa-eye" class="fa-2x pull-left"]The blockchain is a technology that enables two unknown parties to transfer a unique piece of digital property, without the need for a central authority – all in a safe, trustworthy and guaranteed way.

Figure 21. Blockchain in healthcare, Radboud UMC REshape Centre.

Medicaid

Medicaid is a relief program in the United States that provides health insurance for about 74 million individuals and families with low income and wealth. Medicaid is co-financed by the American states and the federal government.

One problem is whether the coverage of care can be continued throughout the year; because the coverage is incomplete, there is no access to the care part of the year. In order to be able to participate, for example, an assessment of the bank's own financial position and a review by the relevant employer are required. This has created a complex bureaucracy in order to arrive at a final verification of the necessary data. This complexity is caused by distributed data files, the right balance between privacy and transparency and the verification requirements. Medicaid is therefore looking at the possibilities of Blockchain to arrive at a different working method.

Medicaid has elaborated this in a study that addresses the five most important changes that can be expected in 2040 (Deloitte 2020):

- Smart medical devices for clients to *empower* their own health and well-being: these are devices that manage conditions for care interventions via sensors and *telehealth*. Think also of programmes to promote lifestyle and medication compliance. And the creation of intelligent healthcare communities that focus on data, technology and behavioural interventions to make the central role of clients possible.
- A national database of health data: the data are interoperable between healthcare providers and healthcare professionals and fully accessible to clients. This creates a more holistic approach to clients that avoids inefficiencies.
- Shift from care providers to organizations focused on quality of life: it is increasingly about prevention and self-management of health.
- Personalized behavioural interventions (preventive healthcare): *precision engagement* connects data, artificial intelligent, algorithms and behavioural expertise to come up with behavioural interventions that are most effective.
- Local care hubs where facilities are brought together: these are centres for prevention, treatment and a more holistic approach to care and quality of life.

Blockchain for the Electronic Health Record

From the perspective of Blockchain, the design of an Electronic Health Record (ECD) requires the seven process steps (Nichol 2018).

1. Receiving a token: a healthcare transaction is received by the Blockchain as a collection of actions recorded in the form of tokens.
2. Determining a base block: the last confirmed block is checked, including an identifier for the block used to create a new block.
3. Ensuring a *peer review*: the token is validated (the collection of care transactions, diagnosis and treatment protocols) and sent to peers to review.
4. The validation of the block: the digital signature of the validators is added to the block; the block is hashed.
5. Token expansion: the initial token is expanded with the validation token to confirm the handling actions.
6. Creating a block: based on the validation token, digital signatures, peer reviews and a collection of care tokens, the block is created by miners.
7. Sending the block: the combined blocks (collection of care actions) are sent to peers.

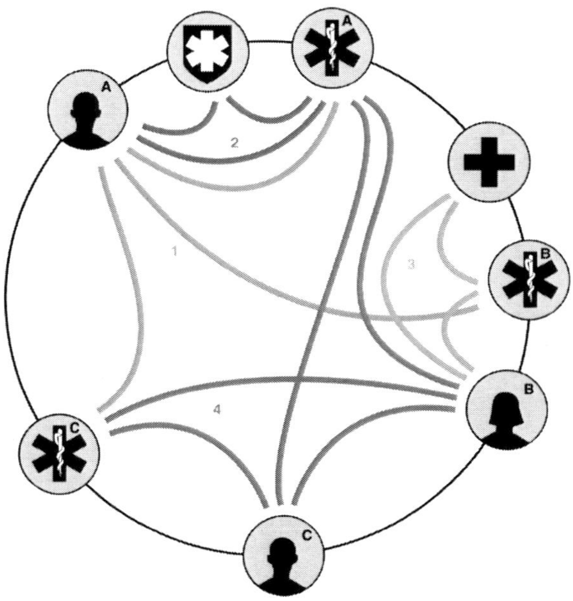

Source: MedRec.

Figure 22. Many mutual contacts.

However, a major problem in healthcare is the lack of interoperability between domains. It turns out to be difficult to unlock and share data. The core of every ECD is that privacy and security are guaranteed. The aim is to provide clients with their own data via an ECD or EHR. The MIT Media Lab has developed the MedRec project for this purpose. Clients have to deal with different healthcare professionals and care providers who also have contacts with each other, as can be seen in Figure 22.

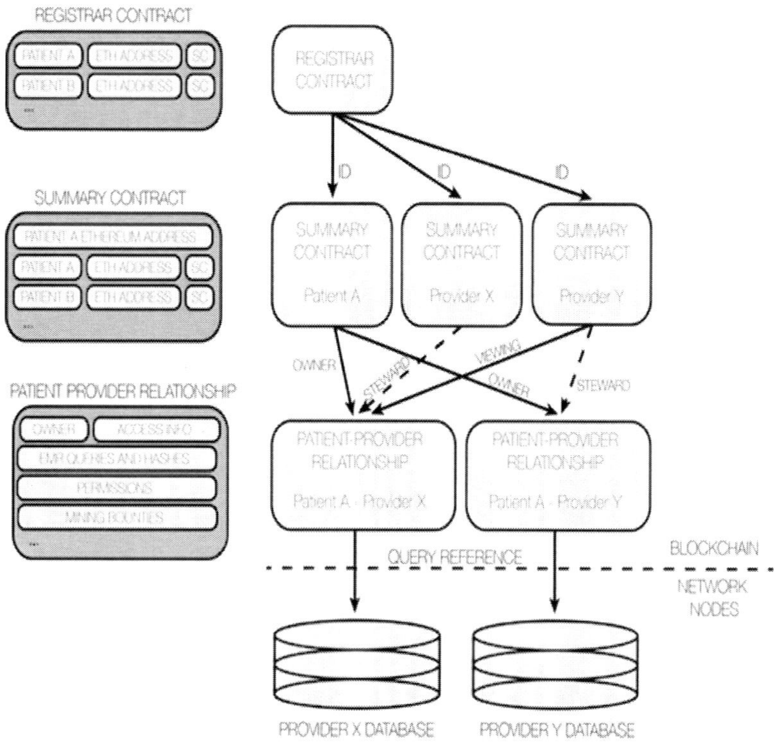

Figure 23. The three contracts of MedRec.

Clients (and their informal caregivers) are therefore connected to different care providers. MedRec offers a combination of a social need and a technological solution. The first implementation of MedRec was developed by using Ethereum Blockchain. The system of smart contracts ensures connection between clients and care providers. MedRec does not store the data, but encodes metadata that make it possible for clients to securely access care data in different domains. The metadata contain information about ownership, releasing data and integrity of the data requested. MedRec 2.0 is being tested. Smart contracts are considered agreements to execute a certain code (source of medical information) under certain conditions. MedRec has three types of smart contracts, see also Figure 23.

- The *registration contract* binds participating parties (clients, care providers, health insurers) to their identity as recorded in Blockchain. Only registered parties can add information.
- The *summary contract* provides insight into the relationships between the different parties. It provides references to the client care provider contracts: current and past connections to different *nodes* in the system. The acceptance or deletion of these relationships is determined by the client. Each participant in the

system can locate a summary of their relationship with other participants. The acceptance or deletion of contacts is checked by the client.

- The client-care provider *relationship contract* connects two nodes in the system where one records medical data for the other.

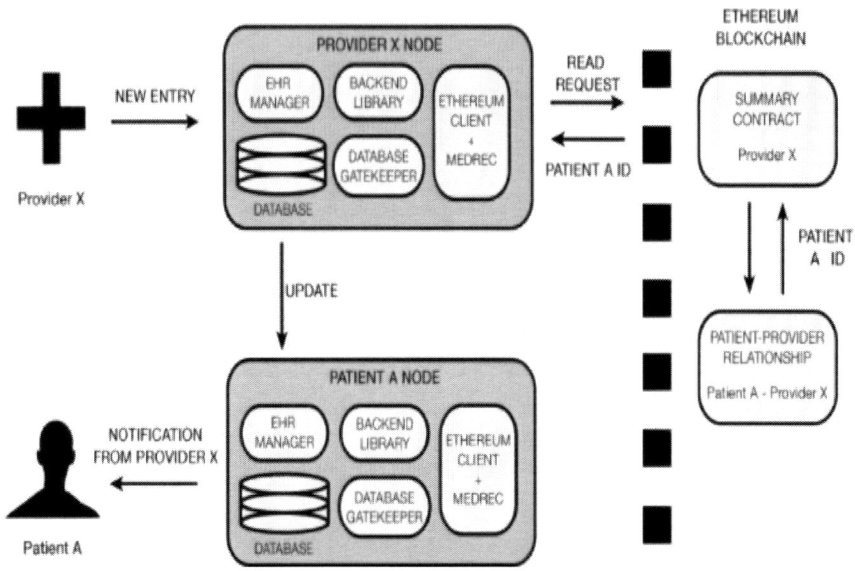

Source: MedRec.

Figure 24. From request for access to the message from the healthcare professional.

MedRec works within a private Blockchain: a private peer-to-peer network of reliable, validated nodes. In order to limit risks related to privacy, the following approach is being worked on. A care provider submits a request for access to the care provider. The Electronic Health Manager ensures an update via the database and MedRec. The Blockchain creates a summary contract and identifies the patient. After completing the entire process, the patient receives a message from the healthcare professional, as can be seen in Figure 24.

Realizing a Good Transfer

Developments in recent years, such as the Landelijk Schakelpunt ('National Exchange Point'), have mainly focused on curative care. Connections with long-term care providers and the social domain remain complicated. For example, general practitioners still indicate that electronic information exchange with home care, district nursing care, nursing homes and social support is almost impossible in a standardised manner, although they would like to do so.

Although data is increasingly recorded digitally, nurses and caregivers are still unable to make sufficient use of the benefits of digital recording. Data are stored in separate systems and are also not unambiguous. As a result, there is no exchange between systems and nurses have to carry out additional registrations. And they still have to manually retype their data when a client is transferred. In addition, the nursing transfer is regularly incomplete. Nursing transfer is therefore a vulnerable part of the care process. This creates risks in the care for the client.

Blockchain enables a new model for the exchange of care information. This reduces the current fragmentation in the various care systems and enables a better view of the results of care interventions. However, the use of connected devices also means an increasing risk with regard to the security of data.

In order to improve the quality of the transfer between nurses and caregivers, an information standard for the nursing transfer has been established by the Informatieberaad Zorg ('Healthcare Information Council'): *eOverdracht* ('eTransfer'). This is a collection of agreements designed to ensure that care information is transferred from one care institution to another with the right quality. With the aim of improving the quality and continuity of the information in the nursing transfer.

Roadmap for Interoperability

Interoperability in healthcare is the ability to allow a large number of healthcare ecosystems to collaborate easily without unnecessary efforts by users and providers within the ecosystem (Nichol 2018: 81). Blockchain is an obvious technology to make this possible.

The future of ICT in healthcare lies in the possibility of interoperability based on unity of language. In this way, information can be shared: for example, in the form of an Electronic Client Dossier (ECD), Electronic Health Record (EHR) or a Personal Health Environment (PHE). Blockchain is an obvious technology to make this possible.

The Dutch healthcare system still has limited interoperability. Blockchain can thus ensure improved interoperability in different ways. A roadmap to arrive at national interoperability (Blockchain Research Institute) contains the following steps:

- set up a secure network structure
- enable verifiable identity and authentication of all participants
- a clear representation of authorisation with regard to access to the ECD

Step 1: Set Up a Secure Network Structure

A well-designed information architecture is characterised by agreements at all levels in the organisation with all parties involved, which is why we discussed the *five-layer model*. If the internal architecture is well designed, interoperability can be achieved between self-employed organisations, such as specialised healthcare institutions, hospitals, GPs and patients. The application possibilities of the Blockchain are already described in the maternity care case about Mijn Zorg Log. A Blockchain transaction goes as follows:

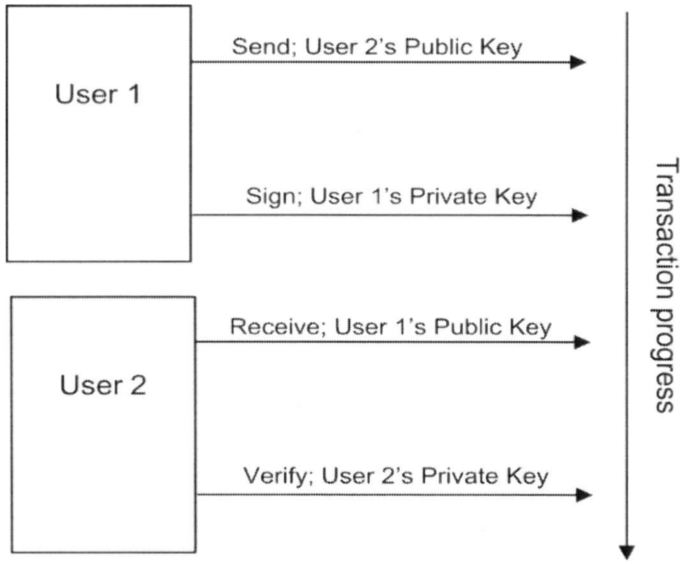

Source: Vazirani et al. npj Digital Medicine 3, 2020.

Figure 25. A Blockchain transaction.

Due to the ability to work with smart contracts, Blockchain is suitable for healthcare. By storing an index of care records, a level of interoperability could be established across the current separate systems via Blockchain. Interactions between client and professional are recorded in smart contracts and temporary access can be guaranteed by tokens created by users and passed on to healthcare providers or health insurers.

Step 2: Enable Verifiable Identity and Authentication

The validation of data and the authentication of participants solve a large part of the problems of data sharing. Administering care data on a Blockchain gives clients control over their data. The use of smart contracts ensures efficient automation of processes: as an example, a client receives a client history questionnaire in advance at the start of a new doctor-patient relationship (MedRec 2020).

Healthcare professionals exchange information electronically during the nursing transfer. The InZicht programme focuses on long-term care through exchange between home care and hospital, nursing home or disability care. The purpose of the programme is to accelerate electronic data exchange safely and unambiguously, so that nurses and caregivers can digitally exchange and reuse the care data relevant to them.

Step 3: A Clear Representation of Authorisation

Interoperability depends on a client's ability to control. Clients have full access to the data via their EHR or ECD. Then there is still the possibility that external parties can access their data. This can be overcome by working with a 'permissioned' Blockchain (see Chapter 1.4). This method limits those who can execute smart contracts.

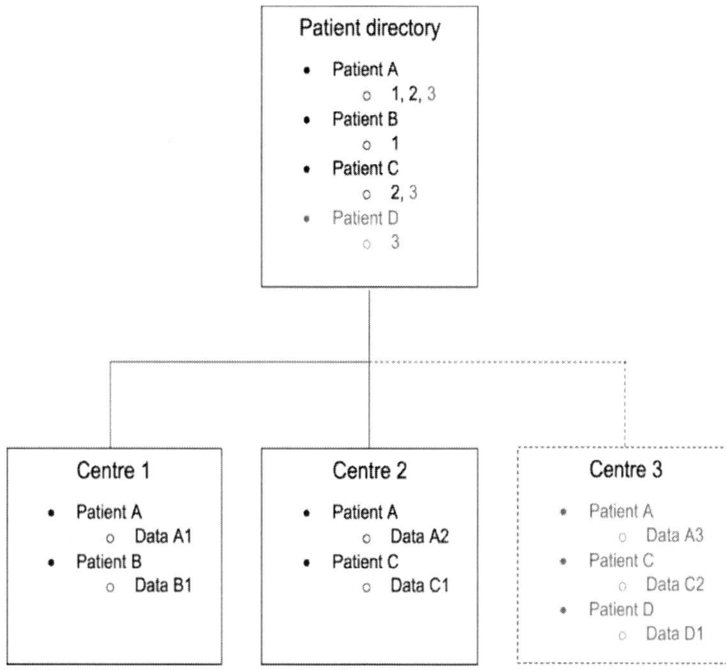

Source: Vazirani et al. npj Digital Medicine 3, 2020.

Figure 26. Connection of independent care providers.

As interoperability needs to be further developed, it is important to consider how different *ledgers* can interact. When individual healthcare providers introduce their own ledger system using Blockchain's API (*application programming interface*), they can be connected to a wider network of Blockchain-based healthcare providers. This is illustrated in Figure 26 (source: https://www.nature.com/articles/s41746-019-0211-0).

Each patient list - numbered 1, 2 and 3 in the figure - represents a Blockchain ledger. The client case register records all pseudonymised client data. The case register connects data to the various centres where a client has medical interactions. Individual centres record their own data containing rules for access to data and more detailed metadata, such as Data A1.

More Effects of Blockchain for the ECD

By using Blockchain for the ECD, the costs are reduced because security is regulated in an efficient manner. The data transfer process takes place at lower costs because data is immediately available. This is particularly important for chronically ill people because their data is available simultaneously for many domains.

It is not practical in terms of speed and storage capacity to store all healthcare records on each computer in a blockchain network. It is an option to use blockchain as a method to access data by systematically compiling a catalogue of all health records. Every time data is added to an ECD by a healthcare professional or client, a reference in a metadata centre is passed on to the blockchain, while the data is stored securely in the *cloud*. A complete index of a person's health record is stored in one location with related metadata. The blockchain with the secure *indices* of files authorises an individual to access the data in the cloud (Vazirani, O'Donoghue and D. Bridle 2019).

The storage and sharing of medical data are essential to achieve better healthcare outcomes. This is reinforced by widespread use of interoperability and thereby reducing administrative costs.

An example of the convergence of technological developments, design principles and interoperability is described in the following case. The GG (Gezondheid en Gedrag ('Health and Behaviour') app) provides feedback on the development of the client and provides the healthcare professional with access to data and insight into how the development process is going.

Case 5: Deventer GROZzerdam Innovates with an App

The Netherlands is undergoing a profound transformation in thinking and doing in the field of health and care. There is a shift from focusing on people's problems and caring for people to people's functioning and participation, so that residents can experience better health and participate more, and the care and welfare system becomes more effective and cheaper. This transformation requires new methodologies, services and technologies.

The municipality of Deventer is at the forefront of this transformation. Deventer is one of the four GROZzerdam locations where the future health ecosystem of the Netherlands is being developed. Deventer GROZzerdam is an innovation community in which residents, professionals, organisations, companies, educational and research institutions, municipality, health insurer and national system parties join forces to realise this transformation.

The emphasis is on an innovative way of working in a number of districts, with one of the results being to reduce health inequalities between people. Residents of the neighbourhoods are working on lifestyle change and participating in new network structures. It also measures lifestyle change and health gains, collecting health data for new interventions.

Improve Your Functioning with the GG App

Deventer GROZzerdam works on the basis of the vision and methodology 'From illness and care to health and behaviour'. Central to this are the values, goals and actions of residents. Professionals connect with those and stimulate development among residents. Functioning is a central concept in this.

The GG app is an instrument developed by Bettery Institute, which is further developed in Deventer on the instructions of the health insurer and the municipality. It is a supportive *e-health tool* that simply activates residents to formulate goals and come up with actions, so that the resident improves his own functioning and that records the development that the resident is experiencing. An instrument that professionals use in the interaction with residents.

With the information he enters in the GG app, the resident receives feedback on his development and the professional receives (if the resident gives permission) information and registration of the resident's process. By focusing on residents, new forms of care and services are created that contribute to a new organisation of care and well-being.

At the 'back side', resident information is classified in the International Classification of Functioning, an international standard developed by the WHO for displaying and registering health. With the help of this classification, exchange with social and medical registration systems is possible.

GG App and Blockchain

Ownership of the resident of his own data is an important starting point of the GG app. Blockchain is essentially a technology that guarantees the ownership and uniqueness of the user. The aim is to organise the underlying system of the GG app on the basis of blockchain. An important point of attention is safeguarding the privacy of the users.

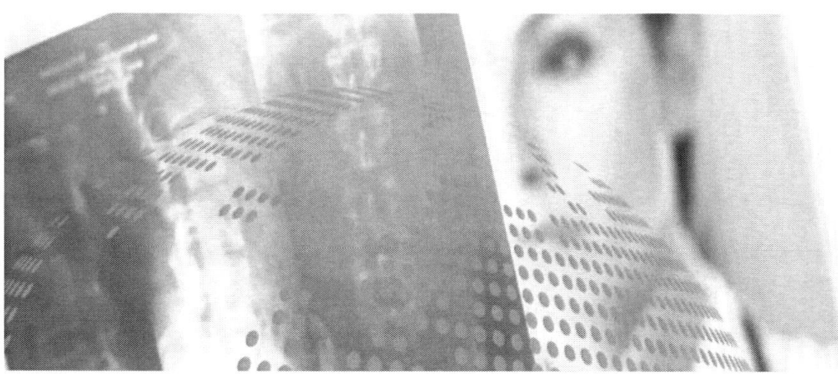

Source: Health Valley.

Figure 27. The first four GROZzerdam regional field labs have started.

Starting in September 2020, the GG app has been further developed in an interactive process with users. Within the '*Wijk voor elkaar*' ('Neighbourhood for each other') initiative, residents and professionals will use the GG app on a small scale – with thirty to seventy users. There is a link to the *Wijk voor elkaar* registration system. The feedback on the use of the GG app provides the information for the development of the next version, after which the use can be further scaled up.

Synchronous to that process, Saxion students developed a basic model for blockchain under the GG app, including further explorations in the area of privacy, data exchange between residents and professionals, etc. The results were presented on the day blockchain & Care on February 4, 2021 in the Saxion Blockchain Week.

POLICY CONCLUSION

In this book, we have demonstrated how blockchain can contribute to addressing the major healthcare issues. These include recording medical data (security, interoperability, accessibility), recording the results of medical research, setting up care chains and ensuring the quality of the medicines.

In current healthcare practice, avoidable errors are still made as a result of the lack of information. In addition, time is wasted on double healthcare activities. Therefore, the electronic exchange of healthcare information between healthcare professionals and healthcare institutions should become the standard (Gateway Review 2020). Electronic data exchange takes place in a very complex environment.

Important developments for the implementation of blockchain include: increasing the agility of organisations and professionals (including due to COVID-19), a sense of urgency to continue digitisation, artificial intelligence focused on early diagnosis and self-diagnosis, standardisation of healthcare activities, and lifestyle interventions. Among other things, COVID-19 needs to accelerate the provision of good information. Blockchain contributes to clear, validated and reliable recording.

So while Blockchain is at an early stage, we believe it will converge with Artificial Intelligence and the Internet of Things (see Chapter 3). This makes a fundamentally different way of organising care processes possible (RVS 2019).

Porter's Agenda

In the thinking of Porter (Porter and Teisberg 2006), it is of great importance that an IT platform facilitates the movement. Despite much effort, there is still limited information exchange and limited availability of reliable outcome measures. Interoperability is of great importance: using the same definitions and setting IT and data standards.

Porter describes this process from a healthcare perspective. Value-driven care is based on the overall care process: consultation, interventions, aftercare and result

(Jeninga and Woldendorp 2019). Measuring and developing the results are central to this. Only by measuring results and having an overview of their costs based on a care chain will the right investments be made. The outcomes of the integrated care process must be recorded safely and unambiguously.

The agenda of Porter (Porter and Teisberg 2006) thus indicates the end goal (Woldendorp and Hoekman 2019): an integrated organisation of care within which relevant outcomes for clients are achieved, where costs and outcomes are known and continuously improved, and in which an integral funding takes place on the basis of the entire care path and the delivered end result, as can be seen in Figure 28.

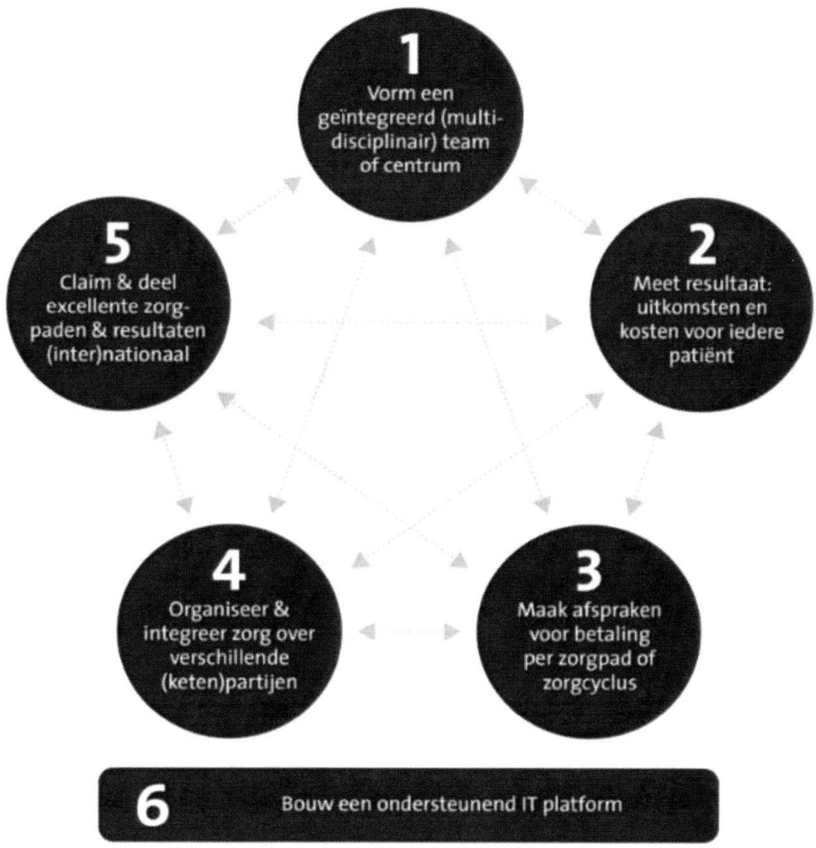
1
Vorm een geïntegreerd (multi-disciplinair) team of centrum
2
Meet resultaat: uitkomsten en kosten voor iedere patiënt
3
Maak afspraken voor betaling per zorgpad of zorgcyclus
4
Organiseer & integreer zorg over verschillende (keten)partijen
5
Claim & deel excellente zorg-paden & resultaten (inter)nationaal
6
Bouw een ondersteunend IT platform

Figure 28. Six steps towards an integrated organisation.

Impact of Blockchain

The introduction of Blockchain is a fundamental change: information is already shared before an interaction between client and healthcare professional takes place. This strengthens communication and the interaction based on it in terms of quality. That leads in turn to a more effective treatment process. Collaboration and coordination between healthcare professionals is greatly improved. For example, in chronic care where clients usually deal with multiple healthcare professionals, cost savings and quality gains can be achieved.

Blockchain can help reduce costs and improve the quality of care. blockchain can also ensure flexibility, interconnection, accountability and protection in accessing those data that are necessary for the provision of good care. Through the application of blockchain, standardisation and transparency can be merged.

The use of Blockchain technology in healthcare makes the difference in data management. The technology will make sharing medical data more effective, efficient, secure and more transparent for all healthcare stakeholders. A network of healthcare institutions can exist without having a patient's personal data.

Blockchain technology makes it possible to work more efficiently and transparently, thereby creating new forms of collaboration. The starting point in healthcare is to arrive at a user-friendly design. blockchain offers a technological solution for working with a shared infrastructure. Advantages of working with blockchain are then:

- The blockchain remains unchangeable and can be traced so that clients can easily send information to healthcare professionals.
- A medical record that is added remains safe.
- Healthcare professionals who want to view data can obtain permission from the client via the blockchain.

The advantage of working with blockchain is that nobody is the exclusive owner, because there is a far-reaching form of decentralisation, but also that the data is recorded once (and cannot be changed), and nobody can do anything to the data. That makes it transparent. Decentralisation is guaranteed by the fact that the network consists of different computers, all of which have a copy of the data. In the event of an adjustment, everyone is informed: no one is the only one who has data available. One of the most important advantages of blockchain is effective and efficient control over healthcare data.

Blockchain technology can fundamentally change the following nine areas of healthcare:

1. medical device data integration
2. asset management
3. client dossiers
4. clinical trials
5. safety monitoring with regard to side effects
6. medication compliance
7. regulatory compliance

8. invoicing and claims
9. contract management

In terms of policy, it is important to note that blockchain offers a lot of potential advantages. Potential, because application possibilities have not yet been used in a combined way on a large scale and have not been proven until then. One reason for this is that not everything is technically possible yet and therefore experiments are needed to make this technology more stable. One way to deal with this is to elaborate possible scenarios in which the formation of decentralised structures is the focus.

By digitally facilitating healthcare professionals in their working environment, there is room for innovation at a professional level. A properly functioning underlying digital infrastructure is therefore a condition for effective and efficient collaboration in a region while maintaining the quality of care. The application of platform technology can create digital and physical networks at local, regional and national levels. This is not only about networks around the patient but also about networks between healthcare professionals both inside and outside the walls of the healthcare organisations.

This means that data increasingly influence the organisation of care processes. The 'value-driven care' model indicates that the purpose of care processes is to create value for stakeholders, primarily the patient. For the healthcare and social domain, this agenda means: close cooperation on expertise around target groups, measuring the results of interventions, making agreements for the comprehensive financing of activities around target groups (including in the WMO, Zvw and Wlz), setting up chains and sharing the measured results. We currently see (too) little exchange of information to undertake joint knowledge development from the transition.

Applications of Blockchain

By organising the information provision close to the client and giving him control over the information, a new healthcare facility is created. It initiates a *patient journey*. The correct information is provided at each step: from the invitation to a consultation to the publication of results. The patient journey is therefore the journey that the client (*care*) or patient (*cure*) makes through the healthcare organisation(s), linked to the activities of the organisation to achieve this.

Blockchain is exceptionally well-suited for facilitating such a patient journey. Traceability, responsiveness and trust issues remain obstacles for more efficient care chains. Blockchain's ability to remove these limitations can unlock value by both reducing inefficiencies and creating new opportunities. The more parties there are working together, the more valuable blockchain is to increase mutual transparency and trust.

Blockchain can also be used for:

- the exchange of data (e.g., between healthcare provider and health insurer)
- access for the patient to his data
- despatch and payment of expense claims
- recording evidence of, for example, medical operations that have taken place (because the patient has confirmed via Blockchain that those operations have taken place)

Blockchain can also be used for traceability of medicines. Not only for traceability of a recipe, but also for counterfeit medicines.

Blockchain can also play a role in *authentication*, for example in the Personal Health Environment (PHE). Ministry of Health, Welfare and Sport has asked the healthcare offices to focus more on innovation in their healthcare procurement policy. For health insurers, the introduction of the PHE system leads to a pooling of information. The health insurers are designing a Digitale Zorg ('Digital Care') knowledge centre. For the exchange of medical data between PHEs and healthcare providers, it is essential that authentication - demonstrating that you are who you claim to be – takes place at the right level. Blockchain technology already makes this possible.

Blockchain also makes it possible to bring together information collected in the social domain and the care domain.

Blockchain is currently being implemented more theoretically than practically. The legal, organisational, social and technical preconditions under which Blockchain can be of value to healthcare require further clarification.

Close Collaboration

Blockchain is about building consensus. Consensus becomes stronger if more parties are involved. This means that Blockchain can make an important contribution to shaping value-driven care.

The more parties there are working together, the more valuable Blockchain is to increase mutual transparency and trust. Blockchain offers new opportunities for collaboration between different actors. We have shown that with Blockchain technology, a more sustainable, safer and reliable digital infrastructure (Veuger 2018b and 2019d) can be built. An example is what network organisation Microbiome Centre has done (see the case after Chapter 2). Precisely because the use of Blockchain can mean that existing processes, data exchange and relationships can (will) change, attention to control is important.

A healthcare network is a coordinated way of collaborating between a group of healthcare providers to improve the health outcomes of a (partial) population. A healthcare network consists of various healthcare providers and caregivers involved in one person with one or more conditions. A condition-specific network concerns a long-term connection of several independent organisations/individuals who provide care and experience with each other around the patient the need to continuously work on improving the quality of care, with the aim of improving the quality of life of persons with a specific condition (ParkinsonNet 2019).

Important reasons for collaboration are (KPMG 2019):

- offering care across domain boundaries
- providing a different form of care
- smart deployment of shared staff
- developing joint innovations
- exchanging information

Such a healthcare landscape requires, among other things, a secure data infrastructure with which clients and healthcare professionals can exchange (medical) data within and between regions, and laws and regulations that support desired changes.

By placing responsibility with professionals, organisational forms can arise around work processes and chains that transcend the boundaries of one's own organisation. Because the information is available, professionals can independently come to: the distribution of (shared) resources, accountability of own resources, mapping effectiveness and efficiency and the elaboration of operational plans.

Safeguarding Privacy

A key issue within healthcare is safeguarding the privacy of clients. It is extremely important that medical data is not disclosed. Only with the permission of the patient may the care information be disclosed to another person.

Our starting point is that with the application of Blockchain technology, patients can choose the care that suits them. But how can a patient do this in a field where complexity is only increasing? This complexity is caused by the fact that a large number of care domains and care providers are involved in many illnesses. By organising the information provision close to the client and giving him control over the information, a new healthcare facility can be created.

Especially in the case of care for people with multiple care needs, where professionals with different professional backgrounds often have to work together across domains, professionals experience insufficient support for the regulations and professional codes. The individual professional codes set their own standards in the field of privacy and professional secrecy, and this can hinder cooperation. It is not always clear when information may or may not be shared and to what extent this is necessary in the best interests of the client. It is then the question which standards or rules are leading.

Blockchain enables a fundamental recalibration of the position of clients: complete control of your own data. In the Dutch context, the movement is aimed at clients and patients managing their own information in a Personal Health Environment (PHE). This system only works if information is standardised, to strengthen communication between professionals, and between clients and professionals. The client determines which information is available to which healthcare professional.

Blockchain for Electronic Health Records

Information and ICT systems are often fragmented per organisation. The ICT systems in which healthcare providers keep data on the treatments of patients are usually purchased and managed by their own organisation. For example, hospitals spend a lot of money on electronic health records per institution. In other sectors too, many healthcare organisations rely on the waves of digitisation and e-health on their own digital files. It is also a logical consequence of the legal obligation for each healthcare provider to maintain their own health record to account for good care and their own actions. In addition, it follows from the legally regulated professional secrecy the obligation for healthcare providers to secure this file in such a way that only authorised persons have access to it.

Although files within healthcare institutions are becoming increasingly accessible to clients and can be shared with relevant healthcare providers within the organisation, it remains difficult to connect the information from these systems across the boundaries of organisations (RVS 2017). Dossiers of patients belong to individual care and assistance providers and therefore too little to the patient himself (RVS 2017). As a result, people do not have sufficient access to and insufficient overview of their own data, which are fragmented across individual files with different healthcare providers.

Supervision

Internal supervision must monitor developments in society and their significance for their own organisation. That certainly applies for technical innovation. In its guide 'De rol van de raad van toezicht bij innovatie - Een brede benadering van technische innovatie' (‘The role of the Supervisory Board in innovation - A broad approach to technical innovation’) (NVTZ 2020), the Nederlandse Vereniging van Toezichthouders in Zorg en Welzijn ('Dutch Association of Supervisors in Care and Welfare'; NVTZ) describes five themes that are relevant in this context, namely: changing views on health, ethical issues, organising in an ever-changing field of forces, the people in the organisation and careful data management.

Change Strategy

In order to arrive at an effective implementation, the Review Team (Gateway Review Report 2020) recommends a clear (adapted) change strategy, in which the relevant parties (multidisciplinary communities) are involved and have the same basic information. Standardisation is the guiding principle for both healthcare professionals and clients. The Ministry of Health, Welfare and Sport is the director in the realisation of electronic messaging. It is essential that linking to other systems is easy to achieve.

The guiding principle in the design of a practical trial is to answer the following six questions:

- Which process should the Blockchain support?
- How big is the application of the Blockchain?
- Who uses the Blockchain, what are the roles (rights and duties) of these different parties, and who is an administrator?
- To what extent is this clear in advance?
- To what extent do you set up permissions in advance?
- Which practical applications are suitable for the various roles and authorisations?

In Chapter 5, we discussed the experiences in maternity care. However, they are too limited to reach clear recommendations. These six questions form a framework for drawing up the change strategy.

Digitalisation through blockchain technology contributes to a transparent, effective and efficient administrative process. In the practical trial, a separate identity service was used due to the lack of a national digital identity for public services. Such a service is indispensable for implementing blockchain in healthcare.

Healthcare is a digital island empire. Blockchain can play an important role in a new relationship between the patient and his data, for example through greater transparency and control over data exchange. By using blockchain, information (anonymised) can be shared irrefutably and in real time with different parties. Blockchain can thus support healthcare processes, make them faster and make them less sensitive to human errors. The technology can help to make healthcare safer, better, more accessible and cheaper.

The Zorginstituut has meanwhile drawn up an action plan to guide the deployment of digital care. This concerns the development and application of quality standards and mapping promising innovations that work across domains.

The NZa has indicated that the possibilities for reimbursing digital care must be expanded. The NZa explicitly states that insurers can play a more proactive role, in particular towards their insured. The NZa believes that insurers can use their communication channels with their insured parties regarding the use of digital applications in the healthcare process and prevention (VWS Progress Report 2020).

The core is that individual citizens are at the heart of the new care model. Blockchain enables a new model for the exchange of care information. This reduces the current fragmentation in the various care systems and enables a better view of the results of care interventions.

REFERENCES

Aa, A. van der and T. Konijn (2001), *Ketens, ketenregisseurs en ketenontwikkeling. Het ontwikkelen van transparante en flexibele samenwerkingsverbanden in netwerken.* Utrecht: Lemma. [*Chains, chain directors and chain development. Developing transparent and flexible partnerships in networks.*]

Adler-Milstein, J. and E. Pfeifer (2017*), Information Blocking: Is It Occurring and What Policy Strategies Can Address It?* https://www.ncbi.nlm.nih.gov/pmc/articles/PMC5339397/.

Aminubaba, M., A. Yusuf, A. Ahmad and L. Maijama (2014), Performance analysis of the encryption algorithms as solution to cloud database security. *International Journal of Computer Applications* 99(14):24-31, August 2014.

Andersson, e.a. eds. (2018), *Managing digital transformation.* Stockholm: School of Economics Institute for Research.

Arbesman, S. (2017), *Overcomplicated. Technology at the limits of comprehension.* New York: Portfolio/Penguin.

Baldwin, R. (2019), *The globotics upheaval. Globalization, robotics and the future of work.* London: Widenfeld & Nicolson.

Bargar, D. (2016), *The economics of Blockchain: a study of its engineering and transaction services marketplace.* Thesis. Clemson University.

Berenschot (2019), *Naar werkende governance op Blockchain in de zorg. Kaders voor verstandige toepassing en ontwikkeling*. Final report. Utrecht. [*Towards working governance on Blockchain in healthcare. Frameworks for Wise Application and Development*]

Blockchain Research Institute, https://www.blockchainresearchinstitute.org/.

Bones, C., J. Hammersley and N. Shaw (2019), *Optimizing digital strategy. How to make informed, tactical decisions that deliver growth.* London: KoganPage.

Bradshaw, D.J. (2018), *Technology disruption and Blockchain: understanding level of awareness and the potential societal impact*. Thesis. National College of Ireland.

Brynjofsson, E. and A. McAfee (2014), *Het tweede machinetijdperk. Hoe de digitale revolutie ons leven zal veranderen.* Tielt: Lannoo.

Capgemini (2017), *Blockchain: a healthcare industry view.*

CBInsights (2020), *The Blockchain report 2020.*

Consensys (2018), *5 Reasons Why Enterprise Ethereum Is so Much More Than a Distributed Ledger Technology.* https://media.consensys.net/ 5-reasons-why-enterprise-ethereum-is-so-much-more-than-a-distributed-ledger-technology-c9a89db82cb5.

Corten, P. A. (2018), *Implementation of Blockchain powered smart contracts in governmental services.* Thesis. Delft: Delft University of Technology.

Davenport, T. H. (2019), *The AI advantage. How to put the artificial intelligence revolution to work.* Cambridge, Mass.: The MIT Press.

Deloitte (2020), *Medicaid in 2040. Five big changes.* https://www2.deloitte.com/us/en/insights/industry/public-sector/the-future-of-medicaid.html.

Diamandis, P. H. and S. Kotler (2020), *The future is faster than you think. How converging technologies are transforming business, industries, and our lives.* New York: Simon & Schuster.

DSCSA (2020), *Drug Supply Chain Security Act (DSCSA).* https://www.fda.gov/drugs/drug-supply-chain-integrity/drug-supply-chain-security-act-dscsa.

Ford, M. (2018), *Architects of intelligence. The truth about AI from the people building it.* Birmingham: Packt.

Francisconi, M. (2017), *An explorative study on Blockchain technology in application to port logistics.* Thesis. Delft: Delft University of Technology.

Fujitsu (2019), *Fujitsu Detects 13 Types of Potential Risks of Enterprise Blockchain System.* https://www.fujitsu.com/cn/en/about/resources/news/press-releases/2019/frdc-0222.html.

Gateway Review (2020), *Elektronische gegevensuitwisseling in de zorg. Spannend om te spreken.* Report (Gateway number 2020-RO-14). [*Electronic data exchange in healthcare. Exciting to speak.*]

Global Data (2020), *Blockchain in healthcare: thematic research.* https://store.globaldata.com/report/gdhcht045--blockchain-in-health care-thematicresearch/?utm_source=email&utm_medium=pr&utm_campaign=200117a_gd_ph_pr_Blockchain_healthcare_thematic&utm_nooveride=1.

Groot, E. de and M. Rosman (2019), *Dare. The mindset for successful innovators in the digital age.* Amsterdam: Amsterdam Publishers.

Gupta, S. (2018), *Driving digital strategy. A guide to reimagining your business.* Boston, Mass.: Harvard Business Review Press.

Health Valley (2020), *Eerste vier regio-fieldlabs "GROZzerdammen" van start.* https://www.healthvalley.nl/actueel/netwerk/vier-regio-fieldlabs-grozzerdammen-van-start. [*First four regional field labs "GROZzerdammen" started.*]

Heuvel, B. van den (2014), *Netwerkzorg. Een nieuw organisatieconcept voor personen met een complexe, langdurige zorg-en ondersteuningsvraag*. Leuven: Acco. [*Network care. A new organizational concept for people with complex, long-term care and support needs*.]

Hoornstra, H. and W. van Lieshout (2019), *Digitale intelligentie. Wat je moet weten, leren en doen in een digitale samenleving*. Amsterdam: Business Contact.

Huizinga, R. (2018), *Blockchange! Hoe overleef je de crypto economie*. TROI Studio. [*Block change! How do you survive the crypto economy*.]

Iansiti, M. and K. R. Lakhani (2020), *Competing in the age of AI. Strategy and leadership when algorithms and networks run the world*. Boston: Harvard Business Review Press.

Idenburg, P. J. and M. Philippens (2018), *Diagnose transformatie. Een toolkit voor grensverleggers in de zorg*. BeBright. [*Diagnosis transformation. A toolkit for frontiersmen in healthcare*.]

Jeninga, A. and H. Woldendorp (2019), *Dit is waardegedreven zorg. Veranderen vanuit een systemisch perspectief.* Amsterdam: SWP. [*This is value-driven care. Change from a systemic perspective*]

Kennisgroep Keteninformatiemanagement (2019), *Blockchain assurance. Blockchain: kans én bedreiging voor auditor.* Norea.

KPMG (2019), *Wie doet het met wie. Het verbonden zorglandschap*. KPMG. [*Who does it with whom. The connected healthcare landscape*.]

Laurence, T. (2019), *Introduction to Blockchain technology. The many faces of Blockchain technology in the 21st century*. Van Haren Publishing.

Ledger Insights (2018), *R3's Corda dominates insurance sector*. https://www.ledger insights.com/r3-corda-blockchain-insurance/.

Ledger Leopard (2019), *How MicroBiome eliminated mountains of paperwork.* https://ledgerleopard.com/how-microbiome-eliminated-mountains-of-paperwork/.

Liezenberg, C., D. Lycklama and S. Nijland (2018), *Alles transactie. Over data, vertrouwen en de ongekende kansen van het transactionele internet*. Tiel: Lannoo. [*Everything transaction. About data, trust and the unprecedented opportunities of the transactional internet.*]

Lim, D. (2020), *Blockchain unlocked. Business transformation with Blockchain technology*. Singapore: Candid Creation Publishing.

Lim, C. L. and A. Janse (2020), *Blockchain basisboek.* Amsterdam: De Boekdrukker.

Linn, L. A. and M. B. Koo (2019), *Blockchain for health data and its potential use in health IT and healthcare related research*. Dragonchain, blog April 30.

Linn, L. A. and M. B. Koo (2016), *Blockchain for health data and its potential use in health IT and health care related research.* https://www.healthit.gov/sites/default/files/11-74-ablockchainforhealthcare.pdfA.

Man, A. P., P. Koene and M. Ars (2019), *How to survive the organizational revolution. A guide to agile contemporary operating models, platforms and ecosystems.* Amsterdam: BISPublishers.

Marcus, G. and E. Davis (2019), *Rebooting AI. Building artificial intelligence we can trust.* New York: Pantheon Books.

McAfee, A. and E. Brynjolfsson (2017), *Machine, platform, crowd. Harnessing our digital future.* New York: W.W. Norton.

Medicalchain, *Inside Medical chain Issue #21.* https://medicalchain.com/en/inside-medicalchain-issue-21/.

MedRec, https://medrec.media.mit.edu/technical/.

Megchelen, J. (2020), *Op zoek naar blockchain: waarheid of waanzin.* https://www.computable.nl/artikel/blogs/security/6860957/5260614/op-zoek-naar-blockchain-waarheid-of-waanzin.html. [*In search of blockchain: truth or madness.*]

Mohammad, A. F. (2019), *Decision analytics using permissioned Blockchain 'commledger'.* Dissertation. Grand Forks: University of North Dakota.

Nictiz (2017), *Blockchain in de zorg.* [*Blockchain in healthcare*]

Odyssey (2020), https://www.odyssey.org/.

ParkinsonNet (2019), *Handreiking aandoeningsspecifieke netwerken.* [*Guide to disease-specific networks.*]

Pearl, J. and D. MacKenzie (2018), *The book of why. The new science of cause and effect.* London: Allen Lane.

Petitjean, F. (2019), *Fujitsu komt met nieuwe handpalmidentificatie.* https://www.computable.nl/artikel/nieuws/security/6765432/250449/fujitsu-komt-met-nieuwe-handpalmidentificatie.html. [*Fujitsu comes with new palm identification.*]

Porter, M. E. and E. O. Teisberg (2006), *Redefining health care. Creating value-based competition on results.* Boston, Massachusetts: Harvard Business School Press.

Raad voor Volksgezondheid en Samenleving (2017), *Heft in eigen hand. Zorg en ondersteuning voor mensen met meervoudige problemen.* The Hague. [*Take matters into your own hands. Care and support for people with multiple problems.*]

Raad voor Volksgezondheid en Samenleving (2019), *Waarde(n)volle zorgtechnologie – Een verkennend advies over de kansen en risico's van kunstmatige intelligentie in de zorg.* The Hague. [*Valuable healthcare technology – An exploratory advice on the opportunities and risks of artificial intelligence in healthcare.*]

Rabobank, *Blockchain toepassen: tips van een ondernemer met ervaring.* https://www.rabobank.nl/bedrijven/groei/innoveren/blockchain-technologie/. [*Applying blockchain: tips from an entrepreneur with experience.*]

Radboud UMC, REshape Centre. *Blockchain in healthcare.* http://radboud reshapecenter.com/portfolio/blockchain-in-healthcare/.

Rathenau Instituut (2018), *Waardevol digitaliseren. Hoe lokale bestuurders vanuit publiek perspectief mee kunnen doen aan het 'technologiespel'.* The Hague.

[*Valuable digitization. How local administrators can participate in the 'technology game' from a public perspective.*]

Russell, S. (2019), *Human compatible. Artificial intelligence and the problem of control.* New York: Viking.

Sacolick, I. (2017), *Driving digital. The leader's guide to business transformation through technology.* New York: Amacom.

Sahota, N. and M. Ashley (2019), *Own the A.I. revolution. Unlock your artificial intelligence strategy to disrupt your competition.* New York: McGrawHill.

Serrurier Schepper, M. and T. Hiddink (2019), *Artificial intelligence in actie. AI-oplossingen bedenken en implementeren.* Culemborg: Van Duuren Management. [*Devise and implement AI solutions*]

Shena, G. (2017), *Scalability analysis of Blockchains through Blockchain simulation.* Dissertation. Las Vegas: University of Nevada.

Sidu, I. (2016), *The digital revolution. How connected digital innovations are transforming your industry, company and career.* Old Tappan: Pearson Education.

Tapscott, D. and A. Tapscott (2018), *Blockchain revolution. How the technology behind bitcoin and other cryptocurrencies is changing the world.* New York: Portfolio/Penguin.

Taylor, J. (2020), *Cloud storage comparison: Top 4 fastest cloud storage.* www.imobie.com/cloud-manager/fastest-cloud-storage.htm.

Tilooby, A. (2018), *The impact of Blockchain technology on financial transactions.* Dissertation. Atlanta: Georgia State University.

Topicus (2019), *Future of IT. Trendrapport Q2 2019. IT-beslissers over Blockchain: de Nederlandse markt in cijfers.* [*Future of IT. Trend report Q2 2019. IT decision makers about Blockchain: the Dutch market in numbers.*]

Topol, E. (2019), *Deep medicine. How artificial intelligence can make healthcare human again.* New York: Basic Books.

Vasarhelyi (2017), *Three essays on audit technology: audit 4.0, Blockchain, and audit app.* Dissertation Neward Rutgers: State University of New Jersey.

Vazirani et al. (2020), *Blockchain vehicles for efficient Medical Record management.* Digital Medicine 3, 2020. https://www.nature.com/articles/s41746-019-0211-0.

Veuger, J. (2020a), Sole Editor *Blockchain Technology and Applications II.* Peer reviewed. Nova Science Publishers Inc. New York USA. ISBN 978-1-53617-931-6. https://novapublishers.com/shop/ Blockchain -technology-and-applications-ii/.

Veuger, J. (2020b), *Blockchain Convergentie.* Lectorale rede op 17 januari 2020 (84 p.). Deventer: Saxion University of Applied Sciences. https://www.saxion.nl/binaries/ content/assets/onderzoek/ meer-onderzoek/Blockchain/Blockchain-convergentie-jan-veuger-2020.pdf. [*Blockchain Convergence*]

Veuger, J. (2019), Sole Editor *Blockchain Technology and Applications.* Peer reviewed (262 p.) Nova Science Publishers Inc. New York USA. May 2019. ISBN 978-1-

53615-288-3. https://nova publishers.com/shop/Blockchain-technology-and-applications/ Book reviews: https://novapublishers.com/shop/Blockchain-technology-and-applications/.

Veuger, J. and G. Garritsen (2020), *Healthcare Governance Design in Blockchain. International Journal of Applied Sciences,* Vol. 3, no.2, June 2020. https://j.ideasspread.org/index.php/ijas/article/view/601/550.

Veuger, J. and G. H. Lap (2020), *Blockchain in Healthcare. Journal of Archives of Business Research.* Vol. 8, no. 6, 202-227. https://journals.scholarpublishing.org/index.php/ABR/article/view/8490.

Vishnoi, M. (2020), *MedFabric4Me: Blockchain Based Patient Centric Electronic Health Records System.* Thesis Arizona State University USA. Approved by prof. dr. Dragan Boscovic and Kasim Selcuk Candan and Maria Grando.

VNG (2017), *Gemeentelijke Blockchainpilots 2017.* The Hague. [*Municipal Blockchain Pilots 2017.*]

VNG (2019), *Blockchain. Een praktische handleiding voor overheden.* The Hague. [*Blockchain. A practical guide for governments.*]

VWS (2020), *Voortgangsrapportage Innovatie en Zorgvernieuwing.* [*Progress Report Innovation and Healthcare Renewal*]

VWS (2020), *Nadere toelichting actielijnen innovatie en zorgvernieuwing.* [*Further explanation of action lines for innovation and care renewal.*]

Wachter, R. (2017), *The digital doctor. Hope, hype and harm at the dawn of medicine's computer age.* New York: McGrawHill.

Wadhwa, S. (2019), *Decentralized digital identity management using Blockchain and its implication on Public Sector.* Dissertation. Dublin: Dublin Business School.

Wallin, A. J. (2018), *Rethinking digital transformation of healthcare. The role of technology and institutions in service innovation.* Aalto University: dissertation.

Woldendorp, H. and J. Hoekman (2019), *De weerbarstige praktijk. Een evolutietheorie van het sociaal domein.* Amsterdam: SWP.

World Health Organization (2017), *A study on the Public Health and Socioeconomic impact of substandard and falsified medical product.* https://www.who.int/medicines/regulation/ssffc/publications/SE_Study_EN.pdf.

Zorginstituut Nederland (2018), *Praktijkproef Blockchain kraamzorg met Mijn Zorg Log.* The Hague. https://docplayer.nl/93363076-Praktijkproef-Blockchain-kraamzorg-met-mijn-zorg-log-rapportage.html. [*Practical trial Blockchain maternity care with My Care Log.*]

Zorginstituut Nederland and Pels Rijcken (2019), *Blockchain in de zorg in relatie tot de AVG.* The Hague. [*Blockchain in healthcare in relation to the GDPR.*]

In: Blockchain and Health
Editor: Jan Veuger

ISBN: 978-1-68507-232-2

Chapter 3

TRANSFORMATION OF ELDERLY CARE AND IMPACT OF DIGITALIZATION

Harry Woldendorp*

Knowledge Partner Research Group Blockchain,
Saxion University of Applied Sciences, The Netherlands

ABSTRACT

The interaction takes place in a context that is rapidly transforming. New forms of care provision are emerging through technology and digitalization. This may involve predictive care, but also clients who organize themselves via, for example, a platform in order to gain more influence on the care process. This is about the connection between technological innovation and social innovation. Technological innovation has various components: Home, Garden and Kitchen Technology, but also the application possibilities of artificial intelligence. Social innovation is reflected in, for example, healthcare cooperatives. Social innovation is expressed in various ways to achieve more autonomy. An important part is that clients have access to their own health information. In terms of policy, it is about interpreting demand-driven management: the organization of care on the basis of an equal position between client and care professional, whereby the client has the relevant health information available. Interacting with each other in a certain way creates a form of life however, it can also be interpreted differently. For both, it is about finding meaning in which the unequal roles lead to equal people. Important elements are: understanding of each other's position, reflection on the own position, provision of information that matches the client's wishes and approach of the care professional, information provision that meets the needs of informal caregivers, funding model that facilitates equivalence and space for professionals to handle variety (innovation of regulatory space).

* Corresponding Author's E-mail: harrywoldendorp@platformvmz.nl.

Keywords: digitalization, transformation, elderly care, impact

INTRODUCTION

Individual Control

More and more innovations and new healthcare concepts are finding their way to the (healthcare) market more easily (Bakas 2017). Innovations in the area of E-health, home automation and robotics are gaining attention (Idenburg and Van Schaik 2010; Idenburg and Van Schaik 2013). An example of the possibilities of healthcare technology and digitalization can be found in Scandinavia (Nies 2019). The Danish healthcare system has been thoroughly digitised. In Sweden, technology and e-health are seen as auxiliaries to allow independent living at home for as long as possible. Finland makes frequent use of monitoring instruments and telecare. Norway has a strategy for healthcare information technology.

A recent report also indicates that large scale use of digitalization and healthcare technology may lead to more individual control, a higher quality of life and a more efficient use of scarce healthcare professionals (Commissie Toekomst Zorg Thuiswonende Ouderen 2020).

The most important lesson for technology for the elderly is to 'keep it simple' in all aspects, such as design, functions, use, explanation, support and understandability; make costs clear and organized. The most important preconditions for the use of healthcare technology and digitalisation are as follows (LUMC 2020):

- Technology, growing older and living longer at home go together perfectly if approached from the side of demand.
- The elderly are open to technology if it is properly introduced and supported. Accessibility of technology is crucial
- Good matching is crucial and if technology is the answer to a need, there will be an effect.
- Support for or during the introduction of (digital) technology is crucial.
- The involvement of users during the development and/or implementation of technology
- Personalisation is essential for the use of digitalization and healthcare technology. Implementation will be based on the need (for long-term use) and on observing the personal context of a person's residence. This is even more relevant for new technology that is often unfamiliar to the target demographic. The presence of informal caregivers is required for this.

For the client, self-organization therefore is about being able to shape the content of care. Self-organization involves making a system work with as few rules as possible (conversely: as much space as possible) (Groot 2010). The start-up is used in the research to connect sensemaking and uncertainty in a new way (Beek and Huizenga 2017). In this way, space is created to refocus the interaction between client and professional. This strengthens the client's position in order to organize his or her own life. The same applies for the professional in order to shape the interaction with the client from this perspective.

Interaction Client and Professional

The quality of care is largely determined by the quality of the relationship between the client and the care professional (RVS 2017). Clients must be given a more central place in monitoring and promoting the quality of care. This is possible by designing the care process in such a way that clients can give positive and negative feedback (RVS 2019b). The RVS states that 'putting the care relationship between client and care professional at the centre makes solidarity less anonymous and leads to less calculating behaviour and improper use of care' (2017, 54). The healthcare professional and client are central in the Action Plan: (De)regulation of Care (VWS 2018) for making healthcare more effective.

The direct interaction between client and professional is becoming more important. This is facilitated by the influence of digitalization (information provision) and technology (support in the home situation). In elderly care, the interaction between client and professional is usually interpreted from a demand-driven perspective (Van der Kraan 2006).

Impact of Competence

The key question is how, in those shifting roles, the position of the client can be strengthened and the professionalism of a healthcare professional has the most value in the use of technologies (hardware) and digitalization (software) creates opportunities for the autonomy and self-reliance of the elderly. The impact of technology and digitalization is often still unclear for healthcare professionals (SCP 2019b: 78).

The healthcare practice will change, so healthcare professionals need a different working method. However, the elderly and the healthcare professionals may lack the required skills for e-health and robotization. Today, healthcare users are often not aware of the choice or the possibilities, while the healthcare professionals experience ambiguity about the use of applications, causing its use to fall behind the supply and preventing a scale-up (PBL 2019). Looking at the impact of digitalization and technology it is about systems, empowering, design rules and values (Schwab 2018).

In addition, for the client, care deployment contributes to the quality of life. An important element in this is a sense of competence: something lets someone feel and perform better (Caris 2013). A sense of competence, control or direction leads to sensemaking (Machielse 2016). The design of the interaction is therefore important. Experts manage models of reality instead of reality itself (Beer 1978). However, the point is to arrive at the reality in which the interaction takes place (Van Gigch 1991).

The changes that are coming involve complex interactions between technological, economic, political and social forces (Baldwin 2019). The increasing complexity that characterizes healthcare (Kernick 2004; Lindberg, Nash and Lindberg 2008) results in part from the effects of digitalization and technology (Topol 2019).

Agility

Organizations and professionals are confronted with innovations happening faster than they can process with current organizational forms (Beckford 2016). They face uncertainties about the impact of digitalization and new technologies on the work they do (Kane, Phillips, Copulsky and Andrus 2019). Schwab: 'we are at the beginning of a revolution that is fundamentally changing the way we live, work, and relate to another. In its scale, scope and complexity, what I consider to be the fourth industrial revolution is unlike anything humankind has experienced before (2016: 1)'.

The healthcare world is constantly changing and requires agility (Pinkroccade 2013; Poiesz and Caris 2010; Kerklaan 2016, SCP 2016b). Healthcare can be described as a digitized business, but not a fully digital business. A digitized business implies that the delivery to a client is in a digital format. To be digital is: the end-to-end processing is done digitally and the commerce to acquire the service is digital (Sacolick 2017: 7).

Organizations deal with complexity by applying forms of self-organization or self-management (Beer 1978; Beer 1979; Beer 1981; Beer 1985; Malik 2009; Malik 2011b; Malik 2016). The effect thereof in turn impacts the interaction between healthcare professional and client. Within the interaction between healthcare professional and client, it is key that the preconditions for autonomy, control over structure and organization of demand-driven management be met.

Through insight into system principles and making maximum use of information, a new balance in the interaction between a client and a professional is achieved. Working on the basis of self-organizing principles (with the caveat of sufficient and adequate support via an ICT infrastructure) is seen as an effective design within elderly care (Brafman and Beckstrom 2006).

Disruption is an innovation that makes things simpler and more affordable (Christensen 2009). Technology is a way to combine materials, information, labour and energy in an output that has a higher value. The massive arrays of sensors (InternetofThings) makes it possible to aggregate data and process macro and micro responses (Sacolick 2017:156).

The introduction of medical innovations appears to be a social phenomenon characterized by interactions between different stakeholders (clients, healthcare professionals, financiers, regulators and citizens) and by a heterogeneity of value perspectives. There is also an interaction between the promises and the practices of an innovation (Abrishami 2018).

More and more developments in the field of home automation and sensor technology (fall detection) are happening in the home setting (TNO 2019). Healthcare technology is increasingly being used in the home setting (Burns 2005). However, there are also obstacles to applying home automation (Ehrenhard, Kijl and Nieuwenhuis 2014). E-health and home automation contribute to self-reliance and comfort at home, an efficient use of healthcare professionals and the early detection of possible calamities (PBL 2019).

Clients place increasingly higher and new demands on the service (Van Montfort 2016). The tension between the need for control (legislator, health insurer, management) and the need for autonomy (professional and client) is increasing further. Working with digital technology can reduce that tension. The accounting must be done in consultation with clients and professionals.

Adaptive System

The assumption is (Begun 2003) that healthcare is a complex adaptive system, where changes are constantly taking place. These changes are caused by increasing variety. Due to the increase in variety, the relationship between client and professional will change fundamentally (Malik 2016). As a result, the system term of variety becomes central.

Adaptability can be described as follows (Ackoff 1999): a system is adaptive if a change in the environment or internal state leads to a reduction in efficiency in achieving one or more goals that determine the system's own function and to responding to that by changing its own internal state or the relationship with the environment such that efficiency increases in relation to the goals.

Dutch society is experiencing increasing complexity that places ever greater demands on the ability of citizens to cope (WRR 2017). More and more people are struggling to deal with this. In this context, the WRR (2017) speaks of a self-reliance paradox: the great emphasis on own strength, control and responsibility actually reduces people's self-reliance. In the case of major life events (illness, loss of partner), this complexity enters into one's own world without taking into account the mental burden that people can handle (WRR 2017, 14).

According to research by Morgens (2019), future care for the elderly will be characterized by: regionalization: network care from cure and care; real estate: as long as possible at home; care is purchased by the client: the elderly (or their caregiver) choose the type of care, the care professional, the time, the date and the location where care must be provided. According to the research, the use of technology leads to 20% or more time savings for healthcare professionals. The issue here is that over half of the informal caregivers think that professionals do not pay them enough attention (SCP 2019).

Variety

Woldendorp (2018) describes the following trends in elderly care in the Netherlands (Woldendorp 2018):

- Strengthening the personal directorship of the client (autonomy is central; support by technology)
- Customization: personalized care (professional perspective, thinking and action are focused on the needs, wishes and requirements of the client)
- Network structures: organizing support and elderly care and optimal coordination between informal care (informal caregivers and volunteers) and formal care
- Innovative power: creating innovations together with the elderly and using (available) digital technology capabilities.

This has a number of consequences for the position of client and professional:

- The position of clients is strengthened: that is about concepts such as autonomy, self- direction, management of (the quality of) my life, personalized care.
- The position of professionals is both strengthened and weakened: on the one hand, it is about forms of self-organization and domain shifts; on the other hand, it is also about the pressure to provide personalized care (and therefore to be more flexible) and about digital developments. The position is strengthened by working with self-organization. However, due to the increasing requirements of clients, the autonomy of the professional (as a result of self-organization) is restricted.
- The position of care organizations is changing: it is increasingly about network care. The focus is not on the organizations, but on the way in which care is provided (Kernick 2004).

The strengthening of the directing role of clients translates into greater variety in the interaction with the professional. This is not only about the role of the client, but also about the possibilities that the care offers. Precision medicine is about applying interventions that exactly match the specific illness of the individual patient. It is expected that additional and more specific drugs or treatments will be developed that are focused on the individual context of a client (Blijham and Hillen 2019).

Healthcare is becoming more individual, more personalistic, more specific and more contextual. The required support in healthcare and wellbeing differs per person: the intensity of the required help for two elderly people with a similar diagnosis can vary wildly.

The needs assessments performed in the elderly care should be seen as nothing more than a general estimate, to be developed by the healthcare professionals. This requires a development of healthcare policy by healthcare professionals close to the elderly (PBL 2019).

For healthcare professionals, this means that a more specific, individual assessment must be done in relation to the client. This reduces the importance of standards and protocols in the care process (Van Montfort and Wylick 2019b; 2019c).

There is a great diversity in the relationship between context and practices of clients, healthcare professionals and organizations. The deployment of care relates to the coordination between care time (care professional) and personal time (client). The starting point is dealing with diversity of needs and having insight into what is going on for a client at a given moment (Verbeek 2011). For healthcare professionals, three elements are decisive for this coordination: direct coordination with the (time) demand of individual clients; flexibility; and collaboration with other healthcare professionals.

Elderly care therefore does not develop solely from a professional perspective but from a shared perspective of clients and professionals. An interactive change strategy is therefore needed: from experience to learning to improvement to implementation to repetition (Kramer 2001).

COVID-19

At the beginning of 2020, many new experiences with digital care were gained due to the corona problem: rapid growth in the use of image calls and new forms of digital care. However, the Raad voor Volksgezondheid en Samenleving (Council for Public Health and Society; August 2020) indicates that it questions the durability of these developments.

The applications mainly concern a scaling up of existing digital forms of care. Innovative forms of digital care emerged mainly locally and in places with which experience had already been gained. However, where the knowledge and experience with digital care was lacking, care also decreased. The value of the digital care that is offered is still difficult to assess at the moment. The characteristic of a transformation is that the end effects are not yet clear. It is therefore important to apply design principles that allow flexibility.

In many places, the regular form of care is restarted. It is therefore not possible to determine whether developments in the field of digital care will continue. The RVS proposes that more focus be placed on investing in digital infrastructure and scaling up existing applications to stimulate a learning practice in which digital care can be developed in a targeted manner.

According to the RVS, the following four elements are essential for public policy in the short term:

- identifying the main substantive priorities to which digital care should contribute, instead of quantitative ambitions for specific forms of digital care
- creating sustainable forms of funding for digital care for existing providers
- providing space for innovative digital forms of care
- continue to actively learn and evaluate to find out whether the intended goals are also achieved

Based on experiences from the period March – June 2020, accelerated digitization of care is noticeable at all levels. Image call functionality plays a key role in supporting working at home by healthcare professionals and to enable communication and information exchange between (IC) doctors, hospitals, general practitioners, VVT institutions, patients and family.

For example, the facilitation of secure video connections (patients and their family members at home) has been implemented because corona patients receive few or no visits. In the situation from June, regular care for a large number of patients has been relaunched. Hospitals rapidly started monitoring patients remotely.

Digital care can involve various forms of care and support: remote communication (e.g., consultation via video calls or information exchange via online communication platforms), but also active or passive monitoring (e.g., via sensors or apps), triage and diagnostics remotely or digital forms of treatment or support (digital daytime support or online therapy). It can be used as a means within existing healthcare processes, or as a means to achieve innovation in healthcare processes (RVS 2020).

A year's experience has now been gained with the impact of COVID-19 on the healthcare system. The main lesson of the coronavirus crisis lies in the experiences gained now that many healthcare providers and clients have actually worked with applications for digital care.

It has been found that the future-proof digitization of care is not yet actually demonstrable. Many examples emerged, locally and in that context where experience with digitization had already been gained. However, this book assumes that we will see a different structuring of care. The preconditions that are necessary for this are elaborated.

The essence is that technological and social innovation are linked from the start. A key issue is that both healthcare professionals and clients have direct access to data. Clients will be able to take more decisions themselves.

Effects of Digitalization: The Importance of Information

Advantage of Digitalization

This section discusses the impact of digitalization. On the basis of the available literature, it becomes clear that data health works if it is part of an (integrated) care practice. That means a lot for the way professionals work. Strategic success is determined by developing a digital strategy that works in practice (Bones, Hammersley, Shaw 2019). Clients, professionals increasingly have access to information they may not have had before. Digital systems blur access and decision rights (Kane, Phillips, Copulsky and Andrus 2019:230).

Technological and social innovation are connected with each other. These developments give the patient more and more access to their own health information. The effects of digitalization on elderly care will also increase at an accelerated pace (Nadella 2017). The influence of digital technology is increasing in all sectors: shops, travel, banks and insurers, mobility etc. (Kaplan 2015).

Healthcare innovation is defined as: the adoption of those best-demonstrated practices that have been proven to be successful and implementation of those practices aimed at improving treatment, diagnosis, education, outreach, prevention and research, and with the long term goals of improving quality, safety, outcomes, efficiency and costs' (Iyawa, Herselman and Botha 2016: 247).

The impact of technology on healthcare professionals leads to automation (direct access to data) and innovation (new professional dividing lines; new working methods; new organizational forms; phasing out professional domains; building new professional domains) (Susskind and Susskind 2017). Emergent technologies are Artificial Intelligence, robotics and Virtual Reality (TNO 2019). The use of AI offers opportunities to bring a lot of information (medical, social, psychological) about a client together and to convert it into more personalized advice. Healthcare is one of the focal points of A.I. (Sahota and Ashley 2019).

The advantage of digitization in general is:

- Infinitely scalable
- Connection (at almost zero marginal cost) to other digital activities
- Digital activity can embed processing instructions (Iansiti and Lakhani 2020).

A key question in this context is what problems can be solved with AI and what possibilities there are (Davenport 2019). The dynamics in healthcare revolve around the interaction between client and healthcare professional. The true challenge of the effects of digitalization and technology is the different rates at which clients and professionals adapt to change (Kane, Phillips, Copulsky and Andrus 2019: 29).

Freedom of Choice

This relationship and freedom of choice must be central. The client's freedom of choice should be initiated by autonomous developments around that client. Current regulations offer little or no room for these autonomous developments. Clients will make far more decisions themselves and (partly) take care of implementation or arrange it themselves. And of course the – increasingly easily accessible – medical treatment information from the professional will continue to play a major role in this (Van Montfort 2019b).

The user becomes part of organizations that are focused on new living and care models (Mohammadi 2017). By experiencing and using the needs and uniqueness of users, opportunities arise to redesign the social, spatial and technological context: empathic design (Mohammadi 2017, 8). In this context, empathy is about creating an environment that is capable of imagining itself in the context of a person in need of care. It is about 'experiencing' his or her needs, wishes, actions, motivation and feelings and acting on that basis (Mohammadi 2017, 24).

Huijsman (2013) recognizes the following trends, among others. Empowering clients by promoting, restoring and maintaining self-management of citizens and directing the direction or end of their own lives in close interaction with immediate relatives (strengthening informal care). In the living situation, an emphasis on longer self-reliance at home with personalized medicine through technology and robotization of care. This concerns the deployment of ehealth, self-diagnosis, telecare, home care technology, home automation and do-it-yourself care; molecular medicine, nanotechnology, genetics and DNA profiling; biotechnology, medical nutrition; ICT, EPD, health information technology; health gaming; prevention and aftercare.

Care in the Right Place

The impact of technology on healthcare professionals leads to automation, such as direct access to data, and innovation, such as new professional dividing lines, new working methods and new organizational forms (Cozijnsen 2001). The fastest-growing quantity on earth is the amount of information that is generated. Gupta: 'we create 2.5 quintillion bytes of data every day. Put differently, 90 percent of the data in the world today has been created in the last two years' (2018: 214). Information is everywhere. More and more people prefer to address questions to their online networks. Smart networks offer a knowledge advantage. The speed of collaboration, customer service and innovation determines the continuity of an organization (form) (Lanting 2013).

Policy in the area of information sometimes requires unexpected effort of clients and healthcare professionals. The recent replacement of the Dutch Personal Data Protection Act (Wbp) with the General Data Protection Regulation (GDPR) leads to difficulties for the cooperation between the general practitioner, district nurse and informal caregivers, because there are more restrictions on sharing files. This may thwart an efficient and effective healthcare for elderly living on their own (PBL 2019).

It is essential that information is in the right place at the right time (Care in the right place): ehealth promotes self-management, decision making together, networking together and network care; information at the right time in the right place is an integral part of good healthcare; give people their own data in their personal health environment (PGO); provide a quality framework for the electronic exchange of data; encourage the evaluation of the effectiveness and efficiency of new innovations; strengthen the digital skills of people and professionals.

It is precisely in the home situation that care must take place. That is one of the elements of the necessary transformation of care. This requires a different definition of healthcare provision: it concerns clients, healthcare providers and communities (KPMG 2016).

Digital Tools

Working with a digital tool promotes the broad sharing of information. Agreements are better enforced, and healthcare professionals have a better idea of which family members and other professionals are involved in healthcare. Informal caregivers in particular find it a safe idea that communication can be done quickly and directly. When such systems are used, this ensures more frequent contact between healthcare professionals, informal caregivers and the client.

Conditions for using such a tool are (Broese van Groenou 2015):

- Proactive client or informal caregiver;
- Complex healthcare situation that requires a lot of consultation or includes an agenda function;
- Care situation that can be urgent from time to time;
- Multiple users for whom it is important to be aware of developments in the healthcare situation;
- One user who lives nearby for follow-up steps;
- Knowledge of digital communication for all users;
- Client or informal caregiver see the added value of digital communication and attach to contact between client-informal caregiver-care professional.

International research shows that caregivers need knowledge to be able to navigate within the overall health system. The most important factor that reduces the burden on informal care is to have a sense of control in the decision-making process regarding their position as informal caregiver. Information provision plays a major role in this (Njoku 2015).

Active consumers are therefore a force for change. Client feedback is therefore also an important source for ideas and research. It is important that client-oriented technology be easy to use. For health apps, it is important to consider in advance how data can lead to information (influencing behaviour). The model for this is PKB: patients know best. Integration can be achieved by offering the client the option of self-management.

The elderly must play an active role in determining the type and extent of care they receive. For professionals, they must be able to deal with complex care and welfare needs.

Current society is characterized, among other things, by the fact that actors attach increasing importance to individual control and self-determination as a counterforce (Hooghiemstra 2018: 18). Many stakeholders want to exercise more direction over the collection and management of healthcare data. Technology makes that possible, for example in the form of a personal health environment ('persoonlijke gezondheidsomgeving'; PGO). Six developments also play a role (Hooghiemstra 2018: 31):

- increasing need for and opportunities for personal health environments;
- increasing mobile health-related services for people via smartphones;
- changing role of healthcare providers: joint decision-making and specialization;
- big data, merging with other new technologies such as artificial intelligence, Internet of Things and blockchain;
- increasing private providers outside the traditional semi-public organizations and healthcare professionals; and
- increasing influence of the government.

Convergence of Developments

The convergence of Blockchain, AI and the IoT will form an impactful combination of security, interconnectivity and autonomy and lead to fundamental changes in the way processes run (Diamandis and Kotler 2020; Veuger 2020). Many healthcare organizations do not use efficient and effective methods to deal with healthcare data. Blockchain has the following possible consequences for healthcare: storage of medical data (safety, interoperability, accessibility), medical research, clinical trials, the supply chain and the quality of the medicines.

Hooghiemstra (2018: 201) indicates that these developments lead to greater power capacity over health data from companies and government. This must then be balanced by the countervailing power of clients.

Although there is much talk about the directing role of clients, the healthcare provider appears to be decisive for the deployment of the care. The directing role therefore remains with the healthcare professional (Bosma 2013). A future-proof organization focuses much more on anchoring the role of the client. Bosma: 'Directorship, and therefore decision- making authority, lies with the citizen or subsequently with the executive core of an organization' (Bosma 2013: 49).

Quality of care is a multidimensional concept with distinct aspects such as effectiveness, safety, patient orientation, timeliness and efficiency. These aspects also apply to eHealth (Nictiz 2017). Definition of consumer eHealth: 'information and communication technology offered to the consumer directly on the market without the intervention of healthcare providers, which aims to support or improve the health of users'. Professional eHealth concerns information and communication technology that has been developed by, for or with care providers and is applied within the treatment relationship or in a formal care context (Nictiz 2017: 5).

However, digital developments do not lead to a single logical business model. The client ultimately determines which model is the most successful. New(-er) core values in healthcare are contributing to the quality of life and enabling self-directorship. This includes strengthening self-organization among professionals, setting up network structures, application of new technological options and achieving a new distribution of knowledge and skills.

Position of Client

Self-Management

This section describes the basic principles in policy that lie behind the pursuit of autonomy. The need for self-management is increasing.

One of the opportunities of medical technology lies in providing tools that strengthen client engagement and self-management. Home automation is aimed at strengthening the autonomy of the user through technology. It appears that individuals adopt new technology faster than organizations. More than half of the knowledge workers have better technology at home than at the workplace (Lanting 2013). Online social networks have significantly higher transaction costs for exchanging data and knowledge than organizations.

This technology is focused on the citizen/client and thus not only on healthcare providers and healthcare professionals. The movement is from the outside in. Entrepreneurship is about connecting from outside to inside (De Bree 2017). As soon as someone becomes responsible for a task, this leads to an experience that can turn out positive or negative.

The literature studied describes in different ways the extent to which more technology deployment will play a role in supporting self-management and monitoring and thus moving part of the care towards the client. Proper care probably requires more and/or a more efficient deployment of care professionals. Strengthening monitoring via technology is likely to influence the capacity to be used. More use of technology is expected to have the effect that clients (or caregivers) will take on a larger part of the care provided through self- care and will take more control of their own care. There are also developments in which care becomes part of other domains: for example, sectors such as plumbers pay attention to interactions with vulnerable elderly people.

Normative Practice

The normative basis of many policy principles within healthcare is the autonomy of the citizen. This basis is difficult to translate into a policy context in which there is a lot of pressure on the available resources (Woldendorp and Hoekman 2019). In order to achieve effective policy, the policy preparation for change must be designed from a multi- perspective approach (Houppermans 2011). It is not about applying a dominant perspective, but about looking at potential solutions from an open system (Otto and De Leeuw 1994).

Citizens' personal directorship takes place within the conditions set by the government and the market (Feenstra and Wansink 2009; Maljers and Wansink 2009). Expert group: these conditions have a restrictive character in shaping the interaction between client and healthcare professional. From the vision of market thinking, citizens are rationally acting customers focused on their individual interest. However, this does not do justice to current developments in healthcare (Tjeenk Willink 2018).

Tjeenk Willink (2018: 76) states that 'policymakers start with assumptions that are apparently normative, but are in fact budget-determined: the competent citizen who directs his own life and health, preferably as long as possible – also alone – continues to live at home, takes rational decisions, is able to use modern techniques'.

More and more initiatives between the government and the market arise from citizens: housing initiatives by parents of children with disabilities, neighbourhood and care cooperatives et cetera. Tjeenk Willink (2018) indicates that a common characteristic of this is that they must conquer their space in both the government and the market.

Taking Initiative

These developments require a new way of working. At the core of this way lies that the various parties have to cooperate much more: policy makers, citizens, clients, healthcare professionals, researchers and social organisations (RVS 2020: 47). For clients, this means that they have more control over their lives, among other things. There are four policy assumptions for the elderly care (Nivel 2014):

- Elderly people want to live self-reliant as long as possible
- They want to and can pay more for support and care
- Informal care and volunteers can largely replace professional care
- Use of technology helps in letting the elderly live self-reliant

However, far from all the elderly fit these assumptions. That is why it is important to account for diversity in organising elderly care. The elderly care requires customization and a larger diversity in care provision (SCP 2019b). This requires an open, interactive attitude, in which all relevant actors are involved from the start. By not applying problems and goals as fixed concepts, but rather as guides, interaction is promoted. (Mintzberg, Ahlstrand and Lampel 1998).

Van Montfort (2019) argues that 'Citizens are increasingly well-educated, they are getting older, their income position has improved considerably compared to the previous generation, they are more assertive and generally know how to formulate their own preferences better. In addition, we see that the "new technology" compared to the "old, complex" technology is equally high in quality, but is much smaller, easier to operate, more user-friendly and relatively cheaper. That means that we as consumers are increasingly becoming our "own producer." These developments will have major consequences for direct care provision and for the relationship between healthcare client and healthcare provider.'

To organise healthcare yourself, you need the following: awareness of the care need, knowledge of what is required and possible, knowledge of who can help, and, finally, knowledge of how to organise that care. Research by the SCP shows that a little less than half of people over 65 sufficiently possess these healthcare skills (SCP 2019b: 44).

The group that takes the initiative has to deal with hurdles regarding cooperation, rules and legislation, finances and internal organisation. There is often a lack of recognition as a full party by cooperation partners (RVS 2020: 49).

Position of Professional

Skills

The increasing influence of clients has an impact on how healthcare professionals deliver care. This leads to a completely different approach to the interaction between client and professional. Professionals play the central role in (starting to) work with the client as director. In addition to the appropriate competences and skills, they need more professional space for this and a corresponding organizational structure (network structure) (Blommaert 2014).

The more competent the professionals, the better the care. The question is now twofold: Where should a professional be competent? And how is it ensured that the highest level of competence is achieved (also in changing circumstances)? (Bennett and Miles 2010; Smid 2001). The impact of technological advances will affect the size, skills, and training needs of the professional workforce (Chapman, Miller and Spetz 2019.

Chairman of the Executive Board of a VVT (Care, Nursing and Homecare) institution (interview May 2, 2019): there is a high degree of client focus within this nursing home. What goes wrong are mainly organizational issues that are caused by management and the supporting departments. Essential to organizational change is responsibility for the wishes of clients. The healthcare professionals have sufficient collective cleverness. In the nursing home sector, it is about a contribution to a full life. Professional healthcare is only part of that.

For clients, technological possibilities will increase. However, this requires clients to keep abreast of technological developments, digital skills and their own interpretation of data (Morgens 2019). Emerging technological advances hold potential in navigating the social, cognitive, and physical changes associated with aging (Chapman, Miller and Metz 2019).

Digital and technological skills are also needed for care professionals (www.digivaardigindezorg.nl; www.anderswerkenindezorg.nl). Vulnerable groups such as the elderly are often less able to find and use ehealth applications. This can lead to greater inequality in healthcare (Bolman 2019).

However, almost 10% of healthcare professionals are low-literate (Stichting Lezen en Schrijven 2018). Clients' knowledge capacity is limited by being able to read and understand health information. In the Netherlands, 3 in 10 Dutch people have problems with health information (Rademakers 2016). My own work practice shows a high degree of diversity with regard to working in a digital environment.

Organization of Care

No matter how good the professional quality is, if activities do not match, the result is insufficient (Caris 2013, 11). Responsibilities must therefore be integrated, and the effort must be aimed at integral goals. Influencing takes place on the basis of expertise (heterarchy). Heterachies are formed by networks in which all participants have the same 'horizontal' position of power and authority. This creates equal relationships (Caris 2013), calling for greater freedom and more responsibility for professionals. That is the reverse of a hierarchical model. The third method of influencing takes place via (internal) networks. Distribution of influence is based on reference power: a combination of prestige, competencies and behavioural characteristics. Within networks, it is less about expertise but more so about strengthening one's own competencies (Caris 2013).

The healthcare professional must be free of organizational dependencies: it is about the interaction. The organization of healthcare and support is a precondition; demand-driven management goes further. Clients have the skills and decision-making capacity. The client's position must be strengthened from this framework.

Network Structures

In healthcare, work is increasingly being done in network structures (Boonstra 2007). Network structures are about making connections that lead to consensus with regard to solutions (Malik 2017: 210). The definition of a network is: a network is a form of cooperation aimed at better solutions for clients.

Healthcare chains arise from, among other things, the sensemaking and actions of the various actors involved. This increases the complexity. The question then is whether you can reduce the complexity of chains by increasing the directing role of the client.

Currently, networks are mainly established around vulnerable elderly people. Depending on the situation of this client, a circle of care professionals and informal caregivers arises around the vulnerable elderly person. A properly functioning underlying digital infrastructure is a condition for effective and efficient collaboration in networks while maintaining the quality of care. In the future, digital and physical networks will be created at local, regional and (inter-) national levels (Ramo 2016). This is not only about networks around the patient but also about networks between healthcare professionals both inside and outside the walls of the hospital. As a result, bulkheads will disappear, and specialisms will merge into one another.

Providing care in networks requires a different way of healthcare provision and organisation by healthcare professionals. This role comprises not only informing and providing care, but also facilitating discussions (RVS 2020). This changes the character of the interaction.

Healthcare and elderly care are moving towards the development of healthcare networks of healthcare professionals, both physically and digitally (Dautzenberg, Curfs and De Bakker 2013). A care network takes the needs of the client as a starting point; different players in the network can add value at different times (Van der Krogt 1995). In this way, a network of various professional expertise and informal contacts is created around a client, contributing to the care process and the quality of life.

The role of the district nurse is more focused on directing the network: from other professionals but also from the client's network. The nurse is able to use a change strategy that is aimed at bringing clients and professionals together to achieve awareness of the added value of a new method. Elderly care therefore does not develop solely from a professional perspective but from a shared perspective of clients and professionals.

The interpretation of the interaction between client and professional requires a self-organizing system. Complexity is not so much caused by the number of variables but by how these variables are interrelated. In an increasingly complex world, it becomes increasingly difficult for a controlling system to make the right choices (doing the right things well) (Schaveling, Bryan and Goodman 2012).

Client-Professional Interaction

Frame of Reference

This section discusses the mutual positions of client and professional. Clients, professionals and management work within the same system, but from a different position and a different frame of reference (Rosmalen 2016). The same things are interpreted in different ways (Daft and Weick 1984). Every interpretation leads to different feelings and different behaviour. That is why attention is devoted in the theoretical elaboration to the concepts of language game and form of life (Wittgenstein 1992).

Hauwert's research shows that, based on theoretical assumptions, actions are determined by what someone thinks and how someone speaks. It can be said that the actions of aids are generally not consciously focused on tracing, recognizing, stimulating and developing personal directorship for people with multiple disabilities (Hauwert 2018: 161).

Common Meaning

Sensemaking is conveyed by language. That is why clear concepts and having a sense of the meaning of words in a certain context are so important. In addition, many buzz words are used in healthcare that displace meaning. In the care domain, the following buzz words are mainly used: 'resilience, empowerment, autonomy, self-direction, independence, freedom of choice, participation, strength-oriented and recovery-oriented work, shared decision-making, dialogue-driven planning, customized support' (Baart 2018: 57). Baart: However, there is seldom dialogue or shared decision-making, and it is not possible, either. The difference in knowledge, the professional's overview, familiarity with alternatives and familiarity with effects are far too great: the professional (always) knows better (Baart 2018: 58). There is therefore hardly any space for another language game. The conceptual device used has the form of an ideology.

Within the elderly care, a business model is sought that makes future-proofing possible (Boonekamp and Woldendorp 2006; Van Schagen and Woldendorp 2003). An example is the introduction of self-management (with the establishment of Buurtzorg as an example).

Buurtzorg is, nationally and internationally, a well-known and successful example of how self-management can be organized. The success focuses on shaping professional autonomy, where interaction with the client plays an important part. The client's autonomy is a point of attention. Within the outlined developments in care for the elderly, self-management is both introduced and phased out. More and more healthcare activities in (complex) elderly care require network structures where different disciplines work in a multidisciplinary and possibly interdisciplinary way. Working with platforms is increasingly starting to take off.

The point of departure is that there is a tension between policy standardization, namely that healthcare is very complicated and the practice, namely that part of the healthcare in the home setting, is usually not complex. There has been a shift here. The starting point is that the vulnerable elderly citizen can continue to live in his or her own living environment for as long as possible (Bovenkamp 2010). With age, the vulnerability (of a part) of the population increases, and the complexity of the demand for care increases.

The question is to what extent you can achieve common meaning in the relationship between client and professional. Important instruments for this are the dialogue and the structure of the interaction (De Bruijn 2014). It is precisely at the interface between baseline, first, second and third line is that it is desirable to arrive at an effective implementation of care domains. In other words, how do you bring the directing role of clients (Van Montfort: prosumer) together with the expertise of professionals.

Quality, Effectiveness and Efficiency

Demand-driven management has five central elements (Van der Kraan 2006: 261):

- Sovereignty of the care recipient;
- Control of the care recipient over the care offer;
- Skills of the care recipient to exercise control;
- Responsiveness of the supply side with regard to the demand perspective;
- Mutuality between field parties in the pursuit of demand-managed care.

The new generation of the elderly will increasingly take the lead in innovation. Both the client and the environment will change in interaction. Another factor is that generations use different values (Becker 1992; Bontekoning 2014; Boshma 2010). Innovation comes in the form of: products (medication or medical technology), services (treatment methods), models (financing and collaboration) and social changes (culture). Elderly care is characterized by the fact that views, applications of (information) technology and positions of professional expertise change and innovate simultaneously (Breedveld 2013).

On the side of both the client and the professionals and in the interaction, shifts will take place in the future (future environment). For the client, three criteria apply for assessing the care:

- Quality of healthcare: Does the professional offer good care?
- Effectiveness of healthcare provision: Does the professional offer the right care?
- Efficiency of healthcare provision: Do I get value for money? (Porter and Teisberg 2006)

Quality, effectiveness and efficiency take place in interaction. The client has a central role in that: it is about how the client experiences the various interventions and what possibilities they have for professionals. Clients are active givers of meaning: they construct their reality themselves and assign meaning to their environment (Hauwert 2018: 50). Guba and Lincoln (1989) assume that it is not only about individual interpretation and giving meaning, but also about the interpretation and meaning sought in dialogue.

Grounded theory was developed in a school of nursing (Glaser and Strauss 1965). The aim of grounded theory is to generate a theory (Glaser and Strauss 1967). By understanding underlying processes professionals can intervene to help resolve client's concerns (Glaser 1978). Grounded theory was influenced by symbolic interactionism: a client and a professional act towards things on the basis of the meanings that these things have for them (Charmaz 2008). There are many versions of grounded theory (Calam 2006).

Conceptual Model

What is needed is 'inclusive model making', which can provide insight into interaction (Van Twist 2018: 125). People mould models, but models also make people. This is because models have the pretension of mastering professional practices (2018: 133). Inclusive modelling is about building models in interaction with those involved and stakeholders. Vermaak (2017): modelling is construction work. Models have a function to create a provisional order that enables insight, deepened in interaction.

Reality is not unambiguous and is open to different interpretations (Charmaz 2010). This applies to interactions between clients and healthcare professionals, but also between different clients and between different healthcare professionals. Self-organization: a system may be said to be self-organizing if it can alter its internal structure to increase its level of adaption (Beer 1979; 1981; 1985). Variety: is the number of possible states or conditions of a system and is an indication of the complexity of a system. Interaction: focuses on mutual influence between client and professional to strengthen the client's directing role. Client: a client is someone who is able to formulate a question based on self-management to which an (professional) answer is possible. Professional: a professional is characterized by being able to take responsibility, through self-regulation and based on professionalism, for his or her own actions aimed at solutions for clients. Information: information is a difference that makes a difference in the interaction between client and healthcare professional.

There are no certainties in advance in the interaction between client and professional. The same expression can be used in different contexts: its meaning is determined by its use in different contexts. If the environment changes, the self-organizing system must change as well in order to remain adaptive. There are no certainties in advance in the interaction between client and professional. However, (implicit) rules are applied: for example, the care provider who puts the focus on his or her own expertise.

Cybernetic management means self-organization: organizing a complex system in such a way that it will be able to adapt (Malik 2016: 27). The key problem of cybernetics is therefore the question as to how systems of any kind can cope with the complexity of their environment which results form permanent changes and the speed of these changes (Malik 2016: 108).

Personalized care and positive healthcare reinforce each other. Preventive and lifestyle support are reinforcing in reducing the vulnerability of the elderly. Healthcare technology and remote monitoring are aimed at increasing quality and improving the effectiveness of care deployment (Vilans 2014). Technology works when its supports the professional practice (Vilans 2016b). For the professional, it is about creating a working environment that guarantees quality of care (and offers opportunities for improvement), for optimal digital support (reduction of administrative burden and possibility of feedback on one's own professional actions) and for a method of organization where self-organization is paramount.

Demand-driven management is defined as the organization of healthcare based on an equal position between client and healthcare professional, whereby the client has access to the relevant health information (based on Van der Kraan). Quality of life is about physical well-being, emotional well-being, social well-being, giving meaning, material security, autonomy and relationship between care provider and client (ZonMw 2015). Network is a form of cooperation aimed at better solutions for clients. A platform integrates competencies and functions so that services can be delivered based on technologies, infrastructure, agreements, competencies and protocols (following Kreijveld, Deuten and Van Est 2014).

Personalized care and positive healthcare reinforce each other. Preventive and lifestyle support are reinforcing in reducing the vulnerability of the elderly. Healthcare technology and remote monitoring are aimed at increasing quality and improving the effectiveness of care deployment (Vilans 2014). Technology works when its supports the professional practice (Vilans 2016b). For the professional, it is about creating a working environment that guarantees quality of care (and offers opportunities for improvement), for optimal digital support (reduction of administrative burden and possibility of feedback on one's own professional actions) and for a method of organization where self-organization is paramount.

The concept of self-organization forms the core of the interaction between client and professional. The methodology of grounded theory was chosen because it was not clear in advance how the interaction between client and professional would shift. To give substance to that shift as a result of digitalization and technology, a qualitative approach is chosen. The regulation and connection of changes within complex systems happens through information and communication (Malik 2017: 195).

Directing Role of the Client

Context of Position Client

Importance of Perception

The description of the elderly determines our perception of someone: an elderly person creative, wise, has a lot of life experience, is a mentor or an elderly person is demented, confused, dependent etc. A painter with rheumatism in his or her hands can be appreciated for his or her understanding of art, the way the world is perceived, the sense of colour etc. For elderly people who (unknowingly) look at themselves from negative stereotypes, it appears that they adopt a more dependent attitude, professionals take over things unnecessarily, and institutions organize their care system on the basis of (too) great a care dependency.

We like to take some work off the hands of the elderly ('No, just stay put, I'll do it for a while'), out of good intentions or simply because it is faster to do something yourself than to wait for an elderly person to do it themselves. Researchers such as Ellen Langer (2010) show that this attitude also has a huge impact on the behaviour and well-being of the elderly themselves. Their self-reliance diminishes, and people rely more on care. And that costs money and reduces quality of life.

Our ideas about what elderly people can and cannot do limits people in their options, says Langer (2010). Small things can make a huge difference. In inpatient settings, for example, it appears that if elderly people can make a number of decisions independently and have to take care of plants themselves, their physical and psychological health will improve. It is not the physical condition that hinders, but the way we think about our limitation that causes us to become dependent. She starts from the psychology of possibilities (Langer 2010). Perception plays an important role in what we (think we can) do. For diseases, we often use categorization, the impact of which we easily underestimate. The descriptions of someone who has cancer or depression makes those involved feel that their illness is the same as their person. With a cold or headache, we describe ourselves as we feel at a certain moment and not who we are.

We can describe the current situation with someone's limitations well, and these descriptions are often the basis for care (life) plans and indications. This perspective can easily be a hindrance. Langer (2010) advocates starting from what someone's capabilities could be. The assumption is that we do not know in advance what we can do. Encourage people to try different things without immediately judging whether they can or cannot do something. If it does not work, then you know it was not successful that time in that way. Perhaps the same goal can be achieved in a different way. Langer's plea is that we learn to experience. An activating environment is also important. This combination of environment and responsibility leads to a new perspective on their own capabilities, and with that, on their physical and mental health. It is therefore essential that the elderly themselves play a role in policy development and the organization of care processes. Langer (2010): Everything is the same until it is not. Kets de Vries (2008): An actual journey of discovery does not consist of seeing new landscapes but of looking at things differently.

Empowerment

Empowerment is described by Machiel as 'a process in which vulnerable people no longer feel alienated or powerless, but are once again able to make conscious choices about their own lives. The point of departure is that vulnerability and dependence can go hand in hand with control and directorship' (Machielse 2016, 39). The new generation of elderly people want much more control over their lives and their relationship with the professional. The elderly are citizens who (can) make their own contribution to society: the best example is the care of grandchildren. Instead of assuming someone's limitations, it makes more sense to start with what someone can do. Solely the fact that someone is getting older and is perhaps less mobile does not affect the desire to structure your own life and to make independent choices. This also applies to people who are dependent on care. It therefore requires a switch in thinking, both from policy makers and from professionals in care and welfare, as well as from the elderly themselves.

Empowerment requires a form of reflection aimed at learning to analyse one's own actions from the relational relationships with other people within a specific context (Linders 2019). Empowerment is aimed at increasing the capacity of people to shape their own lives, their own context and the desired changes therein. Linders indicates that empowerment is not a method, but an approach on which the professional can base his or her actions (Linders 2019).

The client is characterized by: person, own context, specific; diversity, heterogeneity, variety; elderly, chronicity, multi-issue; income position (relatively) improved; better educated; more empowered, clearer preferences (Van Montfort 2016). However, there is also a large group of vulnerable elderly people who are completely dependent on care. The positioning of elderly people who operate independently is facilitated by technology, with a shift from old to new (Van Montfort 2016). The client is not only a consumer but also co-creates: prosumers. Rotmans: a proactive consumer who also produces (Rotmans 2017: 35).

Old	New
High-quality	High-quality
Complicated	Simple
Client-unfriendly	Client-friendly
Alienating	Connecting
Expensive	Inexpensive
Large-scale	Small-scale
Curative	Preventive
Consumer	Producer

In this context, the client's own directorship (Van Montfort 2016) means:

- healthcare choices: client
- organization of care: client
- healthcare purchase: client.

Personal Directorship

What does the outlined perspective mean? For clients, experiences are becoming increasingly important in their valuation of care providers: interpersonal aspects, no waiting times, clear information etc. Experiences are especially appreciated if there is an authentic (identity-related) service provision. Clients' assessments are largely determined by their own experiences.

Hauwert: 'The increased reliance on personal directorship, the weakening of social relationships, the shrinking of the welfare state, and an inadequate vision of healthcare and service organizations due to increasing market forces mean that social integration of vulnerable citizens requires innovation and varied forms of support' (Hauwert 2018: 14). There is a dominant discourse of autonomy and personal directorship and on the other hand the problematic practice of healthcare (Hauwert 2018).

Patients are opting with increasing awareness for certain healthcare providers. The recent FWG trend report (2017) shows the most important trends for the coming years: more concrete realization of innovative power, offering coherent care with added value for the client; space for the individual, personalized care; integrated approach. Cohesion is the key: the whole person with their own context; the client's own world is the starting point. Not everyone can keep up: there are also clients with limited self-sufficiency. The key is therefore to create coherence around individual questions where one's own lifestyle is central. Resilient older adults draw support from social contacts, invest in younger generations, taking actions to manage or improve socioeconomic conditions, valuing own's skills, persevering and resigning oneself to adversity (Kok 2019). Directorship does not apply for everyone: there are clients who cannot fulfil that role (Hauwert 2018).

When implementing self-management and self-directorship, it must be taken into account that there are also vulnerable groups in society that are unable to direct their own care. People with low health skills (29 percent) need support in this (RIVM 2014). In the RIVM study, a distinction is made between care for one's own health (for healthy citizens aimed at staying healthy, and for patients to retain directorship over their own care (self- management) and care for others (role of informal caregivers and volunteers).

This is indicated with the term 'vulnerable elderly': that involves both physical characteristics and physical and cognitive (dys)function (Machielse 2016). Almost all people over the age of 75 have contact with one or more healthcare professionals. About a quarter of them receives support from the WMO (Social Support Act) and a quarter receives district nursing (Dutch Healthcare Insurance Act) (SCP 2019b).

Balance

Platform technology makes other forms of life possible (Dijck 2016). Although there is always an unbalanced relationship between a care recipient and a care professional, it is important to make that relationship as balanced as possible. As self-organization of the client increases due to platform technology, the role of the healthcare professional is focused on setting up and structuring the interaction. Platform technology makes it possible to position the client as a 'healthcare institution'. A new form of life is hereby created. The client determines the choice of care provider and planning and monitors the budget. The role of the client and healthcare professional will change fundamentally. To facilitate this, it is essential to link the cash flow to the demand side (client) and no longer to the supply side (Van Montfort 2011).

The relationship between the client and the professional is always central. In the interaction with the care professional, the client becomes more like a care institution that sets the framework for the activities of the care professional. The entrepreneurship of the professional is aimed at handling variety.

In order to be able to continue living at home longer, the cohesion between the social network, personalized care and care technology is essential (SCP 2016). Government policy is expected to increase the reliance on informal care, while at the same time the possibilities for informal care support and respite care will decrease. The economic value of informal care (in the sense of savings for the government) is estimated at 4 to 8 billion a year (De Coole 2009).

Person-Focused Care

Due to the increase in multiform care needs, the required network must be set up individually. Due to the multitude of requirements and preconditions set by the various health care systems, it is becoming increasingly difficult to keep a grip on one's own life. Support is needed that is focused on one's own individual situation and that, despite the multitude of rules, makes it possible to manage the care process. It is about realizing a person-oriented approach (Council for Health and Society 2017).

For clients, it is important to use a broad perspective. Then it concerns aspects of what the clinical picture is, whether there are psychological problems, what the social system looks like, and how the living environment is structured. It is clear that client situations have complexity that is not reduced to one simple issue. The model of person-focused care consists of the following three core elements: the care relationship, the context in which care is provided and the results. Daily care is provided in the interaction between client and healthcare professional. The point is that care professionals pay attention to each individual elderly person (Emmelot 2019).

The context in which care is provided is designed in such a way that personal care is the starting point. The results of personal care are the core element; what matters is the effect on clients. The care for self-reliant elderly has three types of bottlenecks (SCP 2019b):

- Personal strength and possibilities of elderly and their networks are overrated
- Receiving care and support is complex: there are different types of care, provided by different domains, each with their own access criteria
- Healthcare provision is insufficient: personnel shortage and lack of specific expertise

The client experiences his or her own competence when the healthcare professionals see them as individuals and act accordingly. Then the values do not have to be the same. The complexity of elderly care can be felt by both clients and healthcare professionals. To ensure that innovations work for the elderly in a positive way, it is important to take the living environment of the elderly (their preferences, wishes, experiences and their meaning) as a starting point for changes (Luijkx 2014, 19). Activities that involve both socialising and cognitive activities help to give meaning to people's lives (SCP 2018).

Proper care to self-reliant elderly regards offering personalized, proactive and multidisciplinary care and support. Vulnerability is a dynamic concept that varies in complexity of healthcare and support needs and in diversity of domains in which there is vulnerability. If personal control is the starting point, there should be no obstructions for elderly to indicate what they need. This requires an open, listening attitude of the parties involved (Wind en Te Velde 2019).

In order to better answer the care demand of the client and to facilitate self-care, the current boundaries between null, first, second and third line are becoming blurred: there are more and more care networks. Multidisciplinary collaboration means that every healthcare professional makes his or her own specific contribution. Good collaboration between care professionals and informal caregivers becomes crucial. This will place different demands on the competencies of healthcare professionals.

Self-Management

Complex problems do not require a simplifying approach but a broad diagnosis (Buurman 2018, 8). It is essential to involve clients with a complex demand for care in improving care and using technology (Buurman 2018; Zwakhalen 2018). This means:

- Client experiences must be actively used to achieve improvements in healthcare.
- Justice must be done to the complexity of the demand for care.
- Healthcare professionals and healthcare organizations are jointly responsible for the outcomes of healthcare.

- Healthcare professionals are facilitated by the training of competencies (Buurman 2018, 9).

Self-management determines the quality of life and is increasingly emphasized by the chronically ill and (vulnerable) elderly. Self-management is about 'the capacity and skills of a person to experience a certain degree of balance and well-being even in old age despite age-related losses, with the aim of maintaining or achieving the best possible quality of life' (Vilans 2007). The core of the interaction is that the client and the care professional find a way of working that best suits the client and his situation. In care (chronic and long-term care), the focus is on self-reliance, participation and being part of society. Value-driven care takes shape in care in the treatment plan in which it is determined together with the patient what his ambitions are for living, working and leisure time. Care, often expressed as increased self-reliance, is measured qualitatively afterwards by means of observations and questionnaires that are completed together with the patient.

The results of cooperation within healthcare for clients are mostly aimed at quality of life in combination with objectives such as 'self-reliance' and 'control'. The results of cooperation within healthcare for professionals are creating short lines between healthcare professionals and improved coordination of the execution of care provision for vulnerable elderly (Van Linschoten en te Velde 2016).Healthcare for vulnerable elderly is particularly personalized care. However, in most cases it is unclear how the alignment to the preferences, control and participation of the elderly/informal care provider is given shape (Van Linschoten en te Velde 2016: 51).

Society is changing: current communication options offer more openness and demand speed; it is expected that there will always be an immediate response; clients and their families are more assertive. This puts value-driven care at the centre. Support for people with disabilities must be value-driven as well as effective and efficient. Efficiency is the realization of a process with a minimum of wasted resources. Effectiveness concerns the use of the right resources to achieve the result that meets the client's requirements (Hoebeke 1994).

Integrated Care

The research of Saskia van Dijk (2017) focuses on how stimulating self-reliance within the nursing context influences value-driven care. Nurses indicate that self-reliance mainly leads to an improvement in the quality of life. In addition, if it is well integrated into the nursing process, it can lead to a reduction in costs, for example through fewer consultation moments. Within elderly care, value can be expressed as health outcomes and experiences divided by costs (or: Value = Health results (outcomes)/€).

Mirella Minkman (2012; 2017) states that integration must be central: people must be viewed by the professional from an integrated perspective, and the care surrounding them must be organized and managed in this way. The goal of integrated care is to achieve better (experienced) quality through customized care (Schrijvers 2017). Integrated solutions require a lot from internal and external cooperation.

Personalized and integrated care seems to be a way to improve quality and to keep costs under control. Bloem (2012) has elaborated on personalized care: the care contributes to health gains in the person's own perception. This is possible if the care is transparent: What is the effectiveness, quality and cost of care? What should happen around them? It is about facilitating the person's own decisions: What do I want, and how do I achieve that? Integrated healthcare involves bringing prevention, care and well-being together to facilitate (the maintenance of) the client's function (Baan 2015). This involves an effective set-up of self-management support, multidisciplinary collaboration, evidence-based care provision and clinical information systems.

However, integrated care is difficult to realize for a client who has to deal with independent domains and separate financing. That is why it is necessary that collaboration be shaped from the different domains. As the case becomes clearer, customized arrangements will develop into generic arrangements within the three domains involved.

Participation

In addition to having capabilities and possibilities, participation is also about the self-image of citizens and clients (Van de Wijdeven 2012). In today's society, active citizenship is less organizationally embedded than in previous decades. The breakdown of factions has played an important role in this. Social involvement is often based on solving concrete problems in one's own physical or social environment. Van de Wijdeven emphasizes that insight is needed into the 'dynamics of doing' (2012: 315).

According to Jager-Vreugdenhil (2012), it is desirable to map out the participation contexts in which people are active and what their motives are. This means that self-organization and government interventions are disconnected. The network society is responsible for a shift from government to society. The collaboration of people on specific issues will be central. It is then about supporting citizens with those solutions. The same applies to healthcare; see the aforementioned development of healthcare cooperatives.

Van Montfort (2019): '"Citizen initiatives" come in all shapes and forms. We thus have the care cooperatives, member associations of home care organizations, senior associations, pensioners' associations. These are all initiatives that deal with issues such as "care, quality of life and living etc." for their members or in their neighbourhood or municipality. They have all kinds of legal forms as well as different "fields of activity." It is estimated that there are many hundreds of thousands of "members." The association "Nederland zorgt voor elkaar" (NLZVE) encompasses nearly 600 "care cooperatives." In

2019, there will be nearly 1000 of these types of cooperatives. These are all private initiatives.' (Smelik and Bardoel, 2018).

Informal Care

In the coming years, an appeal will increasingly be made to individual responsibility and also to the municipal responsibility for care and welfare. Informal care is the care that, from a personal relationship and often unpaid, is offered to people with a (chronic) illness or disability. These are partners who look after each other, children who look after their parents, parents who look after their children and friends or neighbours who help each other.

Collaboration with family and informal care around healthcare and support are becoming increasingly important in elderly care. When setting up network structures between professional care and informal care, there are four roles that an informal caregiver can play: as a colleague, expert, client and neighbour. Which role is most prominent may differ, for example, due to the phase of the disease or the living situation of a patient. The emphasis on collaboration is different for each role. A lot of attention is paid to digital systems to support the collaboration. Platform technology reinforces the role of the informal caregiver.

The interdependence between informal care, deployment of volunteers and professional care has a dynamic nature. There are shifts from different perspectives: from the control options of a certain target group, from the policy vision, from the place where care can be provided (nursing home care in the home situation), the way in which care is organized and the possibilities for digital technology. The number of informal carers in the Netherlands is approximately 4 million people (one third provide both intensive and long-term care) (InvoorMantelzorg). The pressure on informal caregivers is expected to increase. Sharing information is important for the position of informal caregivers (SCP 2019).

Quality Framework

The focus on strengthening social networks is more important for living at home longer than for adapting homes. Citizens are increasingly thinking about how they live and want to arrange care in their own neighbourhood or village and take action. There are initiatives that focus on mutual assistance and socializing; others purchase care or arrange the *Wet maatschappelijke ondersteuning* ('Social Support Act'; Wmo) applications themselves. In short, an infrastructure is needed that can support the diversity of initiatives (a logical consequence of personalized care).

In the outline agreement for district nursing 2019 - 2022, the foregoing is detailed as follows:

- The directorship of citizens is central. Healthcare providers handle the delivery of effective care and the support of good quality and therefore put the quality and efficiency of the district nursing care first. Healthcare providers are responsible for the quality of their own professional practice and for making a good indication.
- It is about the functioning of people, physically, psychologically and socially. It is about promoting proper functioning (prevention) and, in the event of illness, limiting the consequences thereof and, if possible, reversing such consequences (through support, guidance and treatment). This requires timely identification, health skills of clients, broad triage and adequate referral at the right time, more time for clients, consultative cooperation and good follow-up and specialized care in which the care needs of people and the possibilities to regain directorship over their own functioning are central (ownership).
- Financing follows the client.
- Collaboration within the medical domain and between the medical and social domain; reducing unwanted practice variation; utilizing technology; electronic exchange of client data/PBL; exchange of data; development of outcome indicators.
- The district nurse, together with the general practitioner and the Wmo expert, forms the connection between the various domains together.

Quality models have been developed for both care at home and care in an inpatient setting. For home care, this has been worked out on the basis of personalized care in a partnership between client, family and care professionals. For the intramural sector, it is mainly about guaranteeing the quality of life. The position of the client is strengthened in both models.

Elderly care increasingly organizes itself as person-oriented care:

The quality framework for nursing home care has ten principles: client as a person, emphasis on learning, supervision and accountability aimed at quality improvement, strengthening trust in professionals (Kessels 2012), learning together, reducing bureaucracy, safety for clients, extra attention to staff composition, quality principle (WLZ), more and better quality.

In this quality framework, we see a shift to the client's perspective. The intention of the new quality framework is to be part of daily care practice: interaction between clients, professionals and their organization. The perspective of the client and primary care is leading.

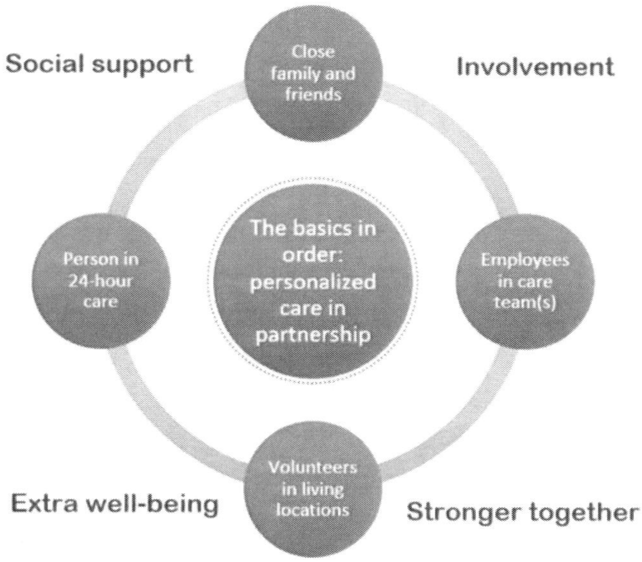

Figure 1. Personalized care (Kennisplein Chronic Care).

The quality framework for nursing home care (Zorginstituut 2017) is based on the following integrated model:

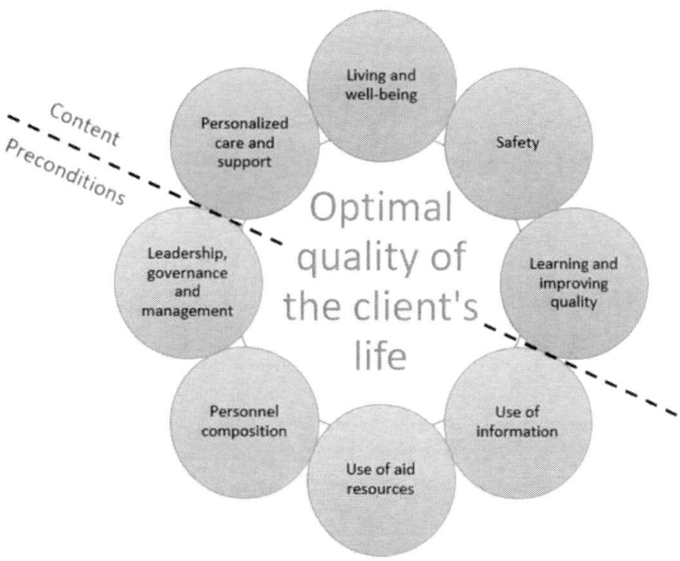

Model 1.

There is a high degree of diversity among the elderly: on the one hand, people who remain vital until later in life (80%); on the other hand, people who need more care and support. It is desirable to start from the individual circumstances. Nivel (2014) distinguishes four profiles:

- Proactive elderly (46%): these elderlies highly value deciding over their own life and they have the network and resources to do so. The previously mentioned policy assumptions best fit this group.
- Care-desiring elderly (28%): have the feeling that they could decide over their lives, but do not regard self-reliance as highly
- Hesitant elderly (10%): they have the feeling that life washes over them. They often have a poor quality of life and lower education. They attach little importance to self-reliance, act dependently and easily accept help
- Helpless elderly (16%); this group also feels like life happens to them. They often live alone, have little money, have a low education and a poor quality of life. They want to live self-reliant as long as possible but cannot without professional support.

The Elderly

The possibilities for longer independent living are only increasing: technological developments, new treatment and care interventions, social neighbourhood initiatives and forms of ehealth (Van Campen 2017). This leads to the following distribution based on Actiz data:

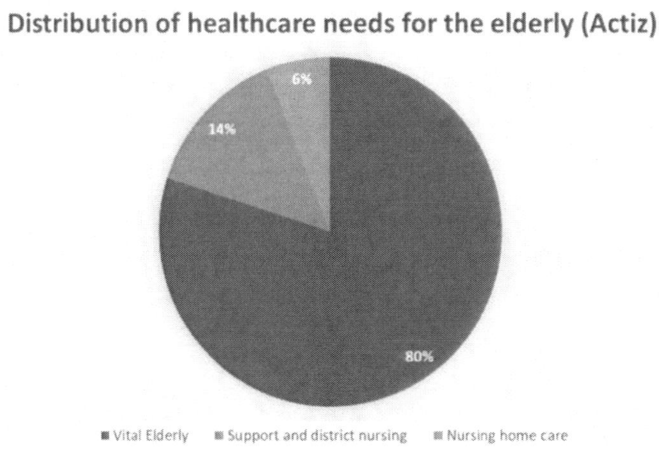

Figure 2. Distribution of healthcare needs for the elderly (Actiz).

Based on this distribution of care recipients, this leads to the following development of clients and professionals: in 2016, 270,000 clients received home care, and 110,000 clients, more intensive (nursing home) care. In 2025, it will be 350,000 clients in home care and 141,000 clients in nursing home care. Based on these figures, the growth in professional deployment is as follows: 15,000 new home care professionals are needed each year (3,000 as a result of growth; 12,000 as a result of replacement). For nursing home care, there is an annual additional deployment of 13,000 professionals (3,000 as a result of the growth of more intensive care, and 10,000 to replace outflowing professionals) (Actiz data).

At this moment 40% of people with health impairments (4.5. million adults) do receive some form of care and support (SCP 2019). Most elderly live at home (94%) (NZa 2018). The financial impact is that 80% of the expenses of healthcare is for 20% of the elderly (NZa 2018). The group of migrants in care for the elderly will increase: in 2011, there were 78,000 people aged 65+ with a non-Western background; in 2050, it will be around 520,000 elderly people. In 2000, there were about 8 thousand people over 65 from Morocco and Turkey in the Netherlands; now more than 47 thousand elderly Moroccan and Turkish migrants live in the Netherlands (CBS 2018). According to the population forecast of the Central Bureau of Statistics, this number will increase to around 144 thousand in 2040 (CBS 2017b). Moreover, this increase will quickly become visible, because Moroccan and Turkish over-65s live in a highly concentrated way in the larger cities (no less than 41% live in Amsterdam, Rotterdam, The Hague and Utrecht), and within these cities, in certain neighbourhoods. Furthermore, Moroccan and Turkish over-65s are also reaching an increasingly old age, with an increasing need for care as a result. The share of over-75s in this elderly migrant population has increased from around 10% in 2000 to 39 and 37% in 2018 and 2040 respectively (Fokkema 2019).

Value-Driven Care

The responsibility for care is provided in consultation with clients and professionals. In this case, value-driven means that support must provide an answer to the question of the citizen and is not only inspired by the professional opinion of the help provider. Porter (2006) states that in order to make healthcare more effective, you must connect competition with value for the patient. Value is determined by taking as a starting point the specific medical condition of a patient over the entire chain of care (Modig and Ählström 2017): from monitoring and prevention to treatment up to and including aftercare (recovery or chronicity). The measurement and development of the results are central to this.

Value-driven care is therefore about measuring the value described as delivered care outcomes divided by costs incurred. Patient value concerns the outcomes that are relevant to the patient divided by the costs required to achieve these outcomes.

Porter describes a medical condition as: ‘a set of patient health circumstances that benefit from dedicated, coordinated, care. The term medical condition encompasses diseases, illnesses, injuries, and natural circumstances such as pregnancy (Porter 2016, 44). A study (interview with 22 people involved) by Koeijer and Hazelet (2017) shows that four preconditions are crucial for a broader and successful implementation of value-driven care: a patient who is able to help decide about his or her care, available and reliable data and financing based on outcomes (value). The research shows that value-driven care is primarily seen as improving the quality of life of the patient and delivering appropriate care at the right time and in the right way. In addition, regular reference is made to the concept of positive health (Huber 2014), namely health as the capacity to adapt and to play the directing role in the light of the physical, emotional and social challenges in life.

Interaction with Professional: Autonomy of Client

Participation Ladder

There is great belief in individual control of one's own life. However, the care arrangements sometimes fail to meet that requirement (Putter 2017). Moreover, support options and the ability to deal with them are unevenly distributed. Putters: the contrast is growing between those with an accumulation of resources and those with an accumulation of defects. This includes the capacity for both thinking and doing (2017: 32). For a long time, it was mainly about the difference between the haves and the have-nots and the compensation through care, labour and income to be able to participate in society. Today, it is much more about the cans and can-nots, so about whether a client is really helped with the care provision or care allowance and whether a client can find his or her way in the complexity of rules (Putters 2017: 31).

The following definition is used for directing care: someone (or multiple people) has directorship when they decide how the care is organized (Verver, Merten and Wagner 2016: 7). The interpretation of participation is shown on the basis of the participation ladder. The participation ladder (Binkhorst 2009) distinguishes five forms of participation:

1. Information: the client also knows. The (care) process is started, and the client is kept informed. The professionals have a positive attitude towards patient participation, but there is no real involvement.
2. Consultation: the client thinks and talks along with the professional. The professional determines what happens, but actively seeks the opinion of the client. The client is a serious discussion partner, but the professional is not directly committed to the results from the discussions.
3. Advice: the client advises and the care provider decides. Clients' opinions are actively sought, and they are explicitly asked for an opinion. The proposals and ideas of clients count and the professional in principle commits to the results, but may deviate from this in the final decision-making (with substantiation).
4. Partnership: the client participates in the decision. An equal cooperation is created in which clients have their own role, and there is joint decision-making with care providers. For example, clients and professionals jointly determine

what they want to talk about. In principle, the professional commits to the results of this consultation.

5. Direction with the client: the client determines and the care provider supports. The client (or better the community) determines the goals and priorities of an activity or organization. The directorship over healthcare is primarily the responsibility of clients. The professional is in fact given an advisory role and tests the preconditions set in advance.

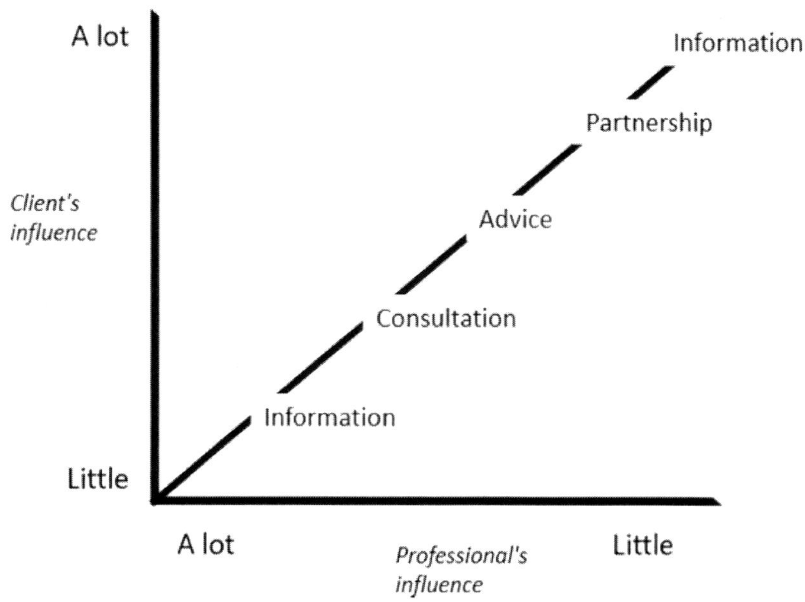

Figure 3. Participation ladder (Binkhorst 2009).

The participation ladder provides a theoretical framework. Practice is characterized by mixed forms. Supply and demand have a reciprocal relationship. It is always about finding the optimum connection. The key is the proper coordination between the question asked and the possible supply (Poiesz and Caris 2010). Coordination supported by IT is essential. It is about creating new roles that contribute to the total chain of work processes (Minkman 2010). Essential elements are: shared goals, shared knowledge and mutual respect.

Importance of Autonomy

Human behaviour is socially determined. Therefore, action usually takes place without any form of reflection. In a form of life, forms of self-evident, non-reflective behaviour are learned. Many professionals assume their own autonomy, but do not recognize the autonomy of the client. Slaets (2017) makes a distinction between normative frameworks (set of norms, rules and procedures in care) and narrative frameworks (telling, presence). From the normative framework, there is negative well-being: we are talking about illness, symptoms and limitations. The narrative framework is about the meaning of existence: positive well-being.

Slaets: 'Giving meaning to life with joy and suffering is the core of good care'. He states that the new (current) quality framework for elderly care is out of balance with an excess of guidelines and obligations. I elaborate on that quality framework later in the book.

Personalized care leads to self-reliance and self-management. Self-reliance is more about general daily activities: washing yourself, taking care of your house, maintaining contact with others. Self-management is not only about being able to cope well illness and its consequences but also about living well with a disease (Kennisplein Chronic Care). The *Zorgverzekeringswet* ('Healthcare Insurance Act'; Zvw) stipulates that healthcare insurers arrange nursing and care. The Wmo provides that municipalities will provide support and guidance to and from the home. The Wlz is aimed at the most vulnerable elderly and disabled people in institutions. This concerns care in kind, a full package at home and a personal budget. This division of tasks between three control systems does not fit with personalized care (SCP 2019). Much of the elderly receive different forms of care simultaneously.

Personal Directorship

The system around a client wants professionals who are knowledgeable, but also professionals who can apply this general knowledge in everyday life. This includes support with self-reliance and support with self-management. An important part of self-reliance and self-management is personal directorship, or self- directorship. Personal directorship is about making your own decisions about your life and care and support. The central question is: What do I want? Personal directorship means: the ability to arrange your own life and necessary support and the practical ability to be self-sufficient in physical, social and psychological terms. Personal directorship involves the following four aspects:

- Starting from the positive: What can I do as a client? Where does my strength lie?
- Strengthening the client through insight into his or her own drives and situation: In which areas is it going well? In which areas is it not going so well? What do I want to do or would like to be able to do again?
- Leave control over support and assistance up to the client as much as possible: What do I want with my life? What do I want to work on? What help do I need? And what do I want that help to look like?
- Strengthening and enabling informal and social networks.
- The narrative approach is increasingly becoming a normal approach within elderly care: it is about the use of life stories, talking with the client and family

about wishes and needs to get a good picture of the person, the background and the world of the care recipient.

The sense of personal directorship is the extent to which a person experiences managing events himself or herself. This is important for being able to handle setbacks. Research shows that elderly people with a low sense of personal directorship are more likely to transition from no care to professional care. Van Campen (2017): 'nearly half of those over 65 who experience little directorship no longer live independently fourteen years later. That is nearly one and a half times as many as among people who experience more directorship.' When implementing self-management and self-directorship, it must be taken into account that there are also vulnerable groups in society that are unable to direct their own care. In the outlined perspective, other forms of advocacy are therefore also needed.

People with low health skills (29 percent) need support in this (RIVM 2014). In the RIVM study, a distinction is made between care for one's own health (for healthy citizens aimed at staying healthy, and for patients to retain directorship over their own care (self- management) and care for others (role of informal caregivers and volunteers).

Authenticity

The implementation of care processes, based on the capabilities of people as a whole instead of their limitations, requires a high degree of authenticity. Standing on one's own strength (individuality) and being involved with each other (sociability) must be connected in a balanced way. Zwart and Middel (2005): 'In social life, there must be more practise with new forms of connectedness'. Care is asymmetrical: those who provide care and those who depend and rely on the care of others. Power is hidden in giving care (Baart 2018: 21). In the presence-based approach, a professional comes in without a fixed agenda (Baart 2011: 735). The professional chooses an accessible approach. It is about offering yourself and showing interest. The key is open and free attention and recognition and confirming what the care recipient shares. The professional tries to reconstruct, out of stories, behaviour and actions, what is central to the world for the personal involved (Baart 2011: 743).

Presence-Based Model

Connections are realized out of respect for and insight into each other's autonomy. The personal contribution is also decisive here. As Kets de Vries (2008) puts it: 'Talking about bulls is not the same as standing in the arena'. The core of presence-based theory is that, as a care provider, you start with the other person and not only with your own good intentions (Senge 2015). The question that you always have to ask from the presence-based theory is whether your own good intentions are actually good (enough) in the case of that specific patient and his or her family. That requires not only good listening and looking but also the preparedness to actually adapt the care.

Baart describes professional care as an aid bureaucracy: the cultures of professional aid and care provision are usually the same. That is why we encourage entrepreneurship from the PlatformVmZ. As an entrepreneur, you focus on the wishes of the client. You look at your profession differently: the client must be served and not so much the regulations. A risk is also that highly vulnerable clients are left out of the picture. Baart: 'the market does not demand some things at all, yet they must be done, given and made available, or there are questions asked for which there are no 'fixing' answers and that require something very different than a market-oriented response'.

The professional also has an eye for the network and plays an active role in it. There is an unrushed pace and loyalty to the client. Baart: 'the relationship is symmetrical when it comes to controlling the goals of life to be pursued, but professional when it comes to the roles' (2011: 783). Care provision is a form of service provision, where the idea of production (form of life) is often disastrous according to Baart:

- The client is no longer a consumer, but a co-producer.
- The 'product' is not fixed in advance but must be discovered.
- The end product is not always perceptible: the service takes place in the communicative process.
- It is about finding the human dimension; a predetermined plan is counterproductive.
- There is learning during the service provision; space is needed (Baart 2011: 824).

Complexity of Care

Current care provision is characterized by four obstacles (Baart 2011):

- Impeded accessibility: clients find it difficult to find care.
- Decoupling care tasks: care tasks and values diverge.
- Increased significance of bureaucracy: involvement, work qualities, core activities and stories are constricted.
- Misplaced business structure of care provision: dilution of the distinction between providing and producing a care service.

The practice of healthcare is extremely complex and requires complex thinking. Professional work is becoming more complex and more ambivalent (Kanne 2016: 21). Good care can never be determined according to a standard model because everyone is different and no two contexts are the same. This means that there can also be conflicts in what is good conduct in a certain situation (Kanne 2016: 323).

The narrative identity plays a pivotal role between the ethical identity and the actions of a person: listening to and telling stories is therefore of great importance for the development of a professional identity (Kanne 2016: 328). A question is whether quality is a characteristic of care or precisely the meaning that the care provider and/or care recipient attach to that care at a certain moment (Baart 2018: 28).

During the provision of care, someone's identity comes into the picture: relational action is about the identity of the care provider and the care recipient. Good care is then care that achieves what the other agrees with. The assessment of whether care is good depends on the situation, the relationship between care provider and care recipient and the moment (Baart 2016: 15).

The core of presentation theory is providing relational care. Baart's development takes place on the basis of:

- Providing relational care: it is about understanding the relationship and the care recipient understanding the capabilities of the care provider.
- Cultivate quality awareness: by means of a well-maintained and critical awareness of quality among care providers (narrative quality test).
- Work practically and wisely.

Baart indicates having worked out a system of thinking around this (2016: 271). The relational interpretation of care has five types of relational interpretations:

- Care that is designed *from* the relationship: care relationship
- Care that is designed *as* a relationship: care relationship
- Care given *in* relationships: biographical relationship
- Care provided *by* relationships: institutional relationship
- Care provided *with an eye* to relationships: finality relationship.

According to Baart (2016: 213), relationship-oriented working is undervalued due to the commercialization and methodification of care. Working in a relationship-oriented manner leads to results that can only be achieved in this way: coordination and prevention of mismatches, obtaining recognition etc. It also ensures that professional perpetuation is reduced and prevents people from becoming more dependent and making the need for help endless: the care trap (2013: 104).

Quality of Policy

If there must be an understanding of a certain situation then it is desirable for that understanding to be both for what is said and what is done. It is therefore about being able to talk (listening) and being able to observe (form of life) (Schatzki 1996). It follows that the position of clients can be strengthened by embedding the voice of insured persons and patients in the healthcare procurement process (RVZ 2014a). The Ministry of Public Health, Welfare and Sport is currently working on an amendment to the Health Insurance Act (pending): 'Opinions and wishes of the insured must become more central to the policy of the health insurance company. It is important that the insured have input in the healthcare procurement policy' (bill 34971). Patient associations and associations for the elderly advise more direct forms of influence and feedback (reactive 20 May 2019).

Participation of the elderly in policy development can be achieved in many ways. By conducting research, but also by letting elderly collaborate and participate in policy initiatives as equal (discussion) partners. Then they also see the dilemmas that policy makers face, and they can brainstorm - well informed - about creative solutions. Good collaboration in the care network seems to have a positive connection with the quality of care. Having joint control over the care and the feeling of having a grip on life is positively related to the perceived quality of life. For a better quality of care, it is important that both informal and formal care providers invest in good cooperation with each other (Cooperrider 2003; Masselink 2008).

Research from the VU (Zwart-Olde 2013) shows that 35% of the elderly can direct their care with the help of others. These are relatively often elderly people who find it important to play a directing role. 45% of the elderly indicate that a formal care provider directs the care network. This can greatly benefit the quality of the policy and the chosen solutions. Policymakers are usually people in the prime of their lives, for whom different things are important than for the elderly. This was also apparent from a study into the housing needs of elderly people with dementia: Would they rather live in a house in a residential area or in a care institution?

People between 70 and 75 were interviewed, as well as people between 40 and 50. It turned out that the elderly, based on their experiences with dementia, had very different ideas about what good living facilities are than the people between 40 and 50. The latter group preferred residential facilities in the neighbourhood. Cosy, with other neighbours. The elderly preferred a small scale but then in or at a care institution. In a house in the neighbourhood, a demented resident cannot go out the front door, because then he or she is on the street, and that is dangerous. Moreover, it is much more difficult to join in activities. In short: it unnecessarily limits someone who is demented in their options. This is a perspective that was not included in the policy.

The core of Langer's (2010) ideas is that we see variety. If we have a certain perspective about the dependence of the elderly, it usually determines what we see and how we will behave. However, if we realize that everyone is different and that we are different from ourselves at different times and with different people, our perspective is considerably broadened.

The design of regular aid emerges from the implementation of policy principles. The tricky thing about that is converting a client's demand into an action plan. Because there is often a translation, the authenticity of the demand is somewhat lost. It is thus about being able to hear the other person. Baart (2011): the structure of involvement is that of question and an answer to it and not another question.

Logic

From this perspective, there is a tension between the logic of professional organizations and the logic of citizens. The previously described standards of professionals who work within the municipalities, but also within the collaboration parties, do not or insufficiently match the standards of citizens (Van Gunsteren 2008).

This is further complicated because healthcare operates on three sets of logic: healthcare logic (appropriate care in a certain (changing) context); logic of rules (application of rules and frameworks); and distribution logic (distribution of resources). This often complicates access to healthcare for clients (RVS 2019d).

Due to the increase in multidisciplinary cooperation, the client has to deal with more and more care providers. This also requires that the client keep an overview in the care process; this also applies for the caregiver. IT plays an increasingly important role in directing the care process (comparable to developments in the travel industry (booking.com) and retail (Albert Heijn/bol.com). Management and healthcare professionals differ in their vision of the duties of informal caregivers. In general, there is little contact with (non-resident) informal caregivers (Van Wieringen 2014).

Professional care organizations are dealing with strengthening cooperation with informal caregivers to improve the quality of care and with increasing the share of informal caregivers (and volunteers). Informal caregivers see opportunities for improvement in the area of a better interplay between informal and formal care. This also requires healthcare professionals to take on a different role. Not only for clients, but also for informal caregivers, support must contribute to one's own choices (Walstra 2011).

Interventions

Formal caregivers more often perform nursing and caregiving tasks; informal caregivers more often help with relocating out of the home or arranging help. The formal and informal caregivers often help together with the household tasks. According to the majority of older people, it is the professionals who now manage a healthcare network (Zwart-Olde 2013).

The question is how to handle this effectively. Interventions should be based on a good balance between the perspectives of citizens and those of professionals. Five interventions are important (Huygen 2013): sufficient action space for the professional but also for the citizen; for the professional, being able to connect to the citizen, and the citizen, to society; a sense of belonging: a sense of belonging or having room to belong; boundaries and trust.

For the professional, boundaries refers to where interventions are possible. Topol has developed a 'doctorless patient model' in which diagnostics and monitoring are primarily the responsibility of the patient (Topol 2015). For the citizen, it is a question of support where autonomy ends. Trust relates to the interpretation of each other's roles, in respect for each other and respect for mutual expertise and input.

Technology is used on the one hand as a supplement to professional assistance; on the other hand, technology can be used to improve self-care. However, working with digital solutions requires that the working methods of care professionals and the approach to informal care can be challenged. In the care process, the patient often has an information deficit relative to the care provider. In the case of chronic diseases in particular, it appears that the patient has an information advantage over care providers in the aftercare phase.

Positive Health

The concept of quality of life is central within elderly care. An important model is the development of positive health by Machteld Huber (2014): 'health as the capacity to adapt and to fill your own directing role, in the light of the social, physical and emotional challenges of life'. In many cases, a client-oriented approach has a positive effect on the quality of care. In the case of personal care, the client is looked at as a whole, not just the disability, and responsibilities are more divided between the care provider and the client (Rademakers 2016).

It is important to see the preservation of functionality and self-reliance of individuals in conjunction with the social network in the living environment. Informal caregivers and relatives play an important role in maintaining vitality, recovery or preventing deterioration. Their role is not taken over by care providers and only becomes smaller when care is provided further away from home. For a request for care, the general practitioner holds the director role throughout the entire chain.

Research shows that transparency with regard to outcome (both client-related and professional-related) can lead to quality improvement. Quality improvement focused on client-related topics seems to benefit from a centralized approach; professional quality improvement benefits more from local initiatives (Winters 2014). A certain degree of framing for clients therefore seems necessary. Quality has a number of dimensions: safety, effectiveness, efficiency, client orientation and timeliness.

What does this mean for caregivers and nurses? For personal healthcare assistants, this means: they often work in an outpatient setting; care technology has a fixed place in the work (remote care; home automation). The coaching role towards volunteers and informal caregivers is strengthened. The (basic) nurse also works mainly in the outpatient setting. Here too, the broadening of the application possibilities of care technology applies (Kort 2008).

Vision of Care

The nurse specialist also works in first-and-a-half-line care. The treatment responsibility is increased. The balance between care provision and efficiency is not only about organizational models, but also about the way of thinking. The quality framework offers a mix of old thinking and new thinking. The question is whether we can no longer take steps towards a future-oriented approach with care technology and digitalization (Kanter 2001). It is again about the relationship between client wishes and professional behaviour.

As it has become clear by now: the client's question and thus the client's influence on the performance of (service) tasks are central: Which services are offered (housing, care, treatment and welfare)? How are they delivered (time, treatment, quality level)? How do capacity and costs play a role (waiting time, flexibility)? And in which context are the services delivered (lifestyle-oriented living, kitchen <-> restaurant)?

A central element for success is that care technology is part of the vision of care (Technologie in de verpleeghuiszorg 2019). We are currently seeing the coming together of various technological improvements: application possibilities for mobile phones, tablets and PCs. A large number of digital services are available on the internet. Sensoring makes it easier to track people, among other things. Social networks increasingly use digital solutions (Topol 2012).

Information: Preconditions for Achieving Autonomy

Vulnerability

Vulnerable elderly people do not always receive the right care. There is a lack of coordination and cooperation between professionals. There is insufficient insight into each other's competence. A great deal of consultation is needed on the financing of health care: within the demand for district nursing but also between the health care domain and the social domain. There is no regulation with regard to integrated cross-domain care for clients at home (Zorginstituur 2018). A new method of organizing care requires innovative funding modalities.

Vulnerability: vulnerability among the elderly is a process of accumulating physical, psychological and/or social deficits in functioning that increases the chance of negative health outcomes (functional limitations, admission, death) (Social and Cultural Planning Office 2011). From the latter, the relation between client and professional, the funding model within which the interaction between client and professional takes place is essential. A start has already been made in Gezondheid 2.0 (RVZ 2010). To arrive at the open model outlined above, a form of funding is required that does justice to basic care and makes a translation possible to the (individual) individuality of clients. That is filled in by this final chapter.

What does the new quality framework mean for the IT structure of complex elderly care? The key question is relatively simple: How well is it going? Value addition is about: how staff are deployed, what they are asked to do, how they are organized, and how they actually spend their time. Within personalized care, as much money as possible goes to direct care activities. The question is always: how does this decision contribute to an increase in value for a client (in a bed or at home).

Assessment Framework

An assessment framework has been issued for elderly care. This assessment framework has the following themes:

- Client-centred: need for care established in consultation with client; client has insight into care process; strengthening self-reliance and directorship;
- Integrated care: the client experiences that professionals have mutual contact and that the care is coordinated;
- Informal care: caregivers can count on professionals taking their capabilities into account;
- Safety: risks in the area of the home/living situation, medication safety, domestic violence reporting code, medical aids and medical technology are signalled in time by the care provider.

The wishes and desires of the client are the starting point for providing care. Characteristics of the relationship between professional and client are: professional knows the client (history, what is important etc.), relationship is balanced and respectful, listening ear for the client and his or her loved ones, and the client fulfils the directing role.

At the end of 2016, this framework was established for networks of professionals who provide care to vulnerable clients who live at home. The most important starting points are:

- Client perspective: contribution of care to his or her adaptability and personal directorship
- Networks: working in conjunction between professional care providers, informal caregivers and volunteers
- Vulnerable clients: testing specifically against citizens with the greatest risks
- Standards: from the client's perspective
- Role of IGZ: quality of care

In network medicine, patient care is central; together with informal caregivers and care professionals, he or she directs his or her own health (Metz 2016). The healthcare professionals and the caregivers guide the patient through clinical recovery and social recovery. In addition, a properly functioning digital structure is a condition for effective and efficient collaboration in networks. The patient can give informal caregivers access to their own healthcare file.

The client manages his or her own medical and health data in an electronic client file. The focus is therefore on self-management for physical well-being, psychological well-being, participation in society, self-determination and self-direction and daily functioning. Wachter (2017): 'One can envision a day when patient-centred communities and clinician-centred ones blend together, with patients gaining information and support from peers while periodically being counselled by credential experts' (2017: 200).

Stamtafel

Digitization creates new forms of information. The division of roles between client and professional shifts because the client has more control (information). This has a twofold effect: the variety for the client decreases (since the client gets more control), while for the professional it increases (since the professional deals with individual questions). The impact of COVID-19 is accelerating developments already underway. The question is how this can be done effectively. A first elaboration can be seen in the field of video calling: between professionals, between professionals and clients (and their family) and between clients and their family. New forms of contact arise (e.g., De Stamtafel: www.stamtafel.nl). The Stamtafel (regular table) is an online social (care) platform to connect people with family, friends, member associations, villages, community centres, nursing homes and volunteer organizations. They support in personal and everyday contact. The Stamtafel is easily accessible to use and at the same time offers a safe and high-privacy environment.

The digital, social Stamtafel has been set up for this vulnerable group. Via the App, people can share information and assistance requests with family, friends and caregivers. It helps initiate social contacts and increases involvement with the neighbourhood. The advantage is that they maintain control over what is shared. It is also sometimes easier to ask for help digitally. In this way, the digital Stamtafel aims to combat loneliness, support independence, increase the scope of interaction and ensure the feeling of self-direction with regard to care, contact and safety.

Interdependence

Due to the increasing connectivity and accessibility of information, there is an ever-growing group of informed and empowered patients (and caregivers) (Njoku 2015). For example, the Patiëntenfederatie Nederland has developed an instrument for elderly to indicate what they value themselves at Mijnkwaliteitvanleven.nl. Joint decision-making takes place at various stages of the care process. Together with the care professional, the patient directs a personal health record with the care professional.

Although there are an increasing number of digital solutions, these are only effective if they fit the needs and skills of a caregiver. Home automation concepts make it possible to remotely monitor daily activities of a client and to easily intervene in them. It is important here that the available functionality is at the service of the informal caregiver and that proper guidance on the technological possibilities and a good backup system are ensured (Adler 2014).

This results in increasing interdependence: it is therefore important to invest in your own (digital and social) networks (Zorg voor 2020). Increasingly, the client will decide for himself or herself how and when he or she makes contact with care providers. In addition, the distinction between patient and consumer is narrowing: there is also an increasing ability for healthy people to collect information about their own health. It is always a question of the extent to which support is actually provided in a customized way to the needs and wishes of an individual informal caregiver. On the one hand, support must take place throughout the entire network of informal and formal care support, and, on the other, it is about enabling an individually focused approach.

Informed Clients

This concerns access to information but also the way in which the information is delivered. The information ensures that there is clarity regarding the informal caregiver's own role, the role of the professional, the organization of care, the evaluation and improvement of care and the way in which adjustments can be made. The collaboration between informal caregivers and care professionals is about having insight into everyone's position, expectations, emotions and capabilities. The involvement, input and (co-) management from the network are central to this. Healthcare uses an available digital infrastructure. On the one hand, self-reliance also means that professionals are engaged in a timely manner. On the other hand, the route to a more self-reliant society also means that professionals can help with taking that step. Current professional support is used differently (Peeters and Cloïn 2012).

Due to the increasing connectivity and accessibility of information, there is an ever-growing group of informed and empowered patients (and caregivers) (Njoku 2015). Joint decision-making takes place at various stages of the care process. Together with the care professional, the patient directs a personal health record with the care professional. In network medicine, patient care is central; together with informal caregivers and care professionals, he or she directs his or her own health. Consistent and clear communication are key. It seems simple, but it is complicated. How do you handle the (permanent) changes in legislation and regulations and the changes in the environment? How do you handle (changing) views of professionals?

Adapting the Environment

Elderly care is characterized by the fact that views, applications of (information) technology and positions of professional expertise change and innovate simultaneously. The new generation of the elderly will increasingly take the lead in this innovation. In the home setting, there are more and more developments in the field of home automation and sensor technology. The effects of robotization in healthcare will still be limited (Ford 2015). Organizing is supported by the new core values in health care: contributing to the quality of life and enabling self-direction.

Technology can be used to adapt the environment to the needs of citizens. Living independently for longer is based on the human dimension and creating a balance through embedding in the social, technological and spatial context (Mohammadi 2017). As a result, care provision in the home situation becomes part of an ecosystem. Research by KPMG (2017a) shows that robots are particularly capable of supporting the elderly in household tasks, helping them to undertake their own activities, contributing to social interaction and playing an important role in collecting, analysing and distributing medical data.

In the area of internal mobility, KPMG (2017a) expects that the following functions can be performed by robots: assistance with going to the toilet, helping with administering medicines and performing light household tasks. A description of robots shows that a contribution can be made to the cost-effectiveness of care: a machine that can perform multiple tasks, increasingly smarter and cheaper (De Vlugt 2016).

Although healthcare technology is often based on standards, it is desirable to take into account clients' skills and needs, degree of willingness and independence and physical environment, as well as the presence of social networks in relation to the individual health situation. In addition, effort is also a matter of good timing and sustainable support.

Research by Peek (2017) shows that the role of grandchildren with, for example, 'take a picture for me' is helpful. A majority of the (future) elderly (71%) say they would like to use ICT if this means that they can continue to live at home longer (Van den Broek et al. 2016, 123).

Impact Technology

Due to technological developments, consumers, clients and citizens have less and less need for organizations (Lanting 2011). It is about organizing: setting up smart networks, chains and communities (Lanting 2014). There is a difference between different healthcare domains: in the hospital world, the influence of technology (robotization) is increasing rapidly; in elderly care, this is (even) more limited (Geisler 2003).

The impact of these technologies on elderly care in the coming years is still unclear. It is clear, however, that technology has more and more influence on the organization and structure of healthcare processes (Kurzweil 2005). Examples are the increasing use of smartphones and iPads; inventory management via sensors (including incontinence monitoring), increasing risks (data breach); shifting to Home, Garden and Kitchen technology (Van Montfort 2016), whereby clients purchase tools themselves; and self-measurements (health check), raising issues around privacy protection.

Mobile healthcare applications, in particular, will experience significant growth (Roland Berger 2016). Due to the increasing influence of clients, the healthcare ecosystem will change fundamentally. An increasingly interactive approach between client and healthcare professional will change the healthcare system. For healthcare professionals, it is essential to have insight into the goals that can be achieved with digitalization and healthcare technology and to identify the means to achieve those goals (Roland Berger 2016).

New 'technologies', such as smartphones and smartwatches with health monitoring, ensure that clients take on tasks themselves. Due to new scientific developments, healthcare is becoming more individual, specific and context-bound (personalized medicine). The significance of protocols, guidelines and trial research is therefore going to decrease considerably. Variation in practice will have a more positive meaning in the coming years (Van Montfort 2019b). In addition, within value-driven healthcare, specific interventions involve a reduction in practice variation to increase quality (Jeninga and Woldendorp 2019).

The clients of professionals are increasingly present on online social networks. Professionals use issues in their work to achieve a sense of group. This does not require a hierarchical system, but a platform in which I encounter colleagues who are interesting to me (Molenaar 2017).

Create Coherence

Patients are opting with increasing awareness for certain healthcare providers. The recent FWG trend report (2017) shows the most important trends for the coming years:

- More concrete interpretation of innovative power: providing coherent care with added value for the client;
- Space for the individual: personalized care; integral approach;
- Cohesion is key: the whole person with their own context; the client's own world is the starting point;
- Not everyone can keep up: there are also clients with limited self-sufficiency.

The key is therefore to create coherence around individual questions where one's own lifestyle is central. Directorship does not apply for everyone: there are clients who cannot fulfil that role. The shift to personalized care will become increasingly stronger. The starting point is and remains that the vulnerable elderly citizen can continue to live in his or her own living environment for as long as possible. With age, the vulnerability (of a part) of the population increases, and the complexity of the demand for care increases. It is precisely at the interface between baseline, first, second and third line is that it is desirable to arrive at an effective implementation of care domains.

The RVS (2017) advocates a personal life plan. Preconditions are:

- Client determines who gets access;
- The Client determines which information may be exchanged;
- Plan is available digitally.

Depending on the care situation, the client can appoint a proxy to take on this role. Healthcare professionals are authorized: the client determines which information is accessible to them. A collaborative attitude may be required of healthcare professionals.

Strengthening Client Position

Wicked Problem

To shape the interaction, a different position of the client is required in order to achieve equality. From the client's perspective, it is about the combination of quality of life and quality of care and the way in which that is designed. The reform of long-term care has the following goals at system level (Kromhout, Kornalijnslijper and De Klerk 2018). Better quality of support and care, greater involvement in society (more care for each other) and financial sustainability of long-term care and support. Although there is much talk about the directing role of clients, the healthcare provider appears to be decisive for the deployment of the care.

Dierendonck (2015, 7): if researchers want to produce results that contribute to the quality of life of the elderly, it is essential to involve those elderly in such a way that their own understanding of and experience with aging and the services available to them are optimally shared with researchers and professionals; they often have a completely different picture of the care needs of the elderly.

Affordability of healthcare is an example of an unstructured (wicked) problem: there is a fundamental lack of consensus about values, norms, objectives, statements and facts (Vermaak 2009). As a result, this type of problem is not solved, but instead made manageable (Jeurissen, Maarse en Tanke 2018: 420). What follows below is the specification of a proposal in which the perspective of the client is central.

Funding Model

The Nederlandse Zorg Autoriteit ('Dutch Healthcare Authority'; NZa) (NZa, 2019) notes that the current funding model for district nursing based on different hourly rates for different forms of care no longer meets the requirements of care practice: 'the funding stimulates the use of hours of care, without a need for client to be central' (2019, 5). The volume of ZWV expenditures for nursing and care is (expected) € 3,690,000,000.

The current funding model has services with maximum rates per hour:

Personal care:

- On-call care
- Nursing
- On-call nursing
- Specialized nursing
- Advice, instruction and information

In addition, there are services with a free rate and a contract requirement:

- Chain care for dementia
- Customized compensation
- Regional availability function for unplannable care
- Mutual services.

Within the policy rule experiment on funding nursing and care, it is possible to agree on an integrated hourly rate. This is often applied by health insurers: 95% of the contracted care providers work with an integrated rate. Budget ceilings are used for this. In addition, it is possible to make agreements within the policy rule based on a fixed amount per client per month. This project funding system is being tested in pilot form at a number of places (approximately € 158 million in total). Only within the context of non-contracted care is the 'regular' performance described above still used.

Hourly rates mean that healthcare providers' management of healthcare professionals is mainly based on the production of a sufficient number of hours. Conversely, a care provider that manages on improving the self-reliance of a client is 'punished' by a drop in turnover and low productivity. The same mechanism also works with the use of labour-saving technology (2019, 13). The final perspective for a new funding model must be based on the care that a client needs. Cost effectiveness involves combining expected effects with expected costs (Kievit 2017). Room for variation in care at the individual level is not unlimited (Kievit 2017).

Cost Control

In healthcare, it is also about policy options for cost control (Stadhouders 2019):

- Regulate and limit the price of care.
- Limit healthcare volume.

- Limit the total of prices and volumes through budgeting.
- Influence market processes that ultimately determine prices, volumes and healthcare expenditures.

A widely used model is to focus financing on the outcomes of care. These are defined by five related dimensions (Eijkenaar 2015):

- Good quality of care: content of care/technical quality and patient satisfaction;
- Cost-conscious behaviour: prevention of over-treatment and unnecessary expensive care;
- Good coordination and efficient substitution: To what extent is there good multidisciplinary collaboration and well-coordinated care?
- Cost-effective innovation: To what extent are innovations that lead to lower costs with the same health stimulated?
- Effective prevention: keeping the demarcated population healthy as much as possible.

Adequate outcome funding concerns: an as simple as possible, demand-driven funding system that is explicitly aimed at stimulating care providers to achieve good outcomes of care in terms of quality, costs, coordination and prevention and that also stimulates cost- effective innovation and contains no incentives for undesirable behaviour (Eijkenaar 2015: ii). There are two components to this (basic and performance funding):

- Integrated, multidisciplinary per insured person (population funding);
- Explicit financial incentives for good quality through performance reward (pay-for- performance).

The system design is based on a combination of standardization and customization: care is based on continuous 'healing' relationships; customization takes place based on the needs and values of clients (Hagel 2012); the client is the source of control; knowledge is shared; decision making is evidence based; safety is a feature of the system; transparency is necessary; needs are dealt with proactively; wastage is constantly being reduced; collaboration between doctors is a priority.

Population Financing

When adjusting the funding system, the starting point is that clients are the solution - not the problem. An active client is a force for positive change: their feedback can provide valuable ideas for improving care (KPMG 2016a).

Technology can contribute to improving productivity (and quality) as follows (KPMG 2016b):

- Reduction of practice variation through decision support systems and standardized work processes;
- Provide clients with instruments that facilitate self-management (client portal, care networks) (PatientsLikeMe);
- Reduction of costs through more proactive care (sensor technology);
- Preventing fragmentation through better coordination of care (Patients Know Best: management);
- Easier access to specialist expertise and advice (telehealth);
- Improvement of resource management through the use of digital planning processes;
- Permanent learning curves.

Population financing is a model for achieving this because this type of funding includes a strong incentive to control costs. A problem is that there is no clear definition (Pomp 2013). That is why it is difficult to draw up specific preconditions (Versleijen 2012). Two common effects: with capitation, the care provider receives a fixed amount per insured person per month or per year. 'All' often means hospital care or first-line care. With shared savings, one or more healthcare providers agree with one or more healthcare insurers that they may keep part of the savings against a benchmark. With shared savings, healthcare providers run no financial risk for budget overruns; with capitation, they do. With partial population funding, there is a strong incentive to reduce costs within the own organization; with integrated funding, there is an incentive to refer to the cheapest provider. An indirect but potentially important effect of integrated population funding is that it encourages competition between healthcare providers. This is due to the increased price sensitivity of referrers who gain an interest in finding the cheapest provider. This search behaviour leads to competition and possible innovation (Pomp 2012). Preconditions for implementation are (Versleijen 2012):

- Clear definition of population funding;
- Letting go of the structure of null, first, second and third line: integrated care;
- Attitude and behaviour of healthcare professionals (partly responsible for cost development);
- Clear vision and permanent role for the government.

Population funding is a management tool:

- Fixed (or negotiable) amount for demarcated population (target group or area);
- Amount is based on severity and/or characteristics for that population;
- Amount is used to achieve a predefined package of results for that population;
- (main) provider has freedom in spending the budget and acting within it;
- (main) provider is accountable for the agreed results to be achieved.

Challenges:

- Demarcation of population and definition of responsibility of contracting party;
- Budget determination for the population;
- Managing on results (definition, measurement, contracting);
- Innovation.

Context of Individual Client

This framework offers possibilities for taking the context of an individual client as a starting point. At present, the most commonly used basic funding methods are: funding per healthcare activity (fee-for-service), funding per healthcare bundle per client (bundled payment), funding per healthcare bundle per insured person (capitation payment) and a fixed amount per period (salary or budget) (NDSD, 2016). Integrated funding implies that the funding does not take place per activity, but per condition, client or insured person.

The NZa (2019) concludes that a mixed funding system could possibly be the ultimate destination:

- Integrate population funding corrected for risk characteristics with risk sharing for one or more predefined populations.
- Multidisciplinary funding per client for a number of delineated care episodes (e.g., certain elective procedures and complex emergency care).
- Stimulating performance reward for good quality.

Care consumers must play the following role in the development of the system: involvement in their own care trajectory (drawing up and following care plans) and measuring quality outcomes. In addition, it is about participation in personal care and the development of care standards. It is also important to make a distinction between allocation and use. Allocation is the process by which resources are allocated for a specific purpose (in the described system model system 3): macro level. Van Montfort (2019b): at the national level, it is about determining how much money is spent on solidarity and generally accessible care. Today, the allocation is laid down in outline agreements.

Use is about deploying the resources obtained to achieve certain goals (system 1): micro level. The use therefore takes place at the individual micro level of the client/patient and the healthcare professional. A care plan is drawn up in that relationship.

Resources follow the line of: you get a lot of what you pay for (Van Montfort 1995). If you get extra money for waiting lists, waiting lists are created. It is about using the resources around the real needs of clients. By giving much more space at the micro level for choices, space is created for renewal and innovation and for quality development and efficiency (Van Montfort 2019b).

New Funding Model

For the long term, the NZa assumes full funding for healthcare networks around the client. This is partly based on value-driven care: 'care that contributes to improving the quality of care, improving the health of a population and reducing the costs of care per capita' (2019, 10). Care providers and health insurers must be given space to shape the organization of care around the client and in the neighbourhood.

A description of population management is a proactive, integrated approach from care to well-being through participation, involvement and targeted interventions around a population over the entire continuum from healthy through palliative phase. The appropriate population funding is a 'disease-transcending, multidisciplinary funding of defined forms of care for defined populations'. This integrated coherent care offer must of course be in line with the needs of the population (Meeuwesen 2018).

The NZa indicates that research (Eijkenaar 2015) shows that interdisciplinary funding per healthcare bundle, combined with rewarding good outcomes, is the best way to achieve good healthcare. A healthcare bundle applies to a defined group of comparable clients within the care chain or the network. The healthcare bundle is then described independently of existing partitions and is also funded independently of budgetary frameworks. This promotes:

- Health
- Good incentives for an optimal care volume
- Prevention
- Optimal coordination between healthcare professionals

The NZa has taken a number of steps in preparation. The following is planned from the 'wetenschappelijke programma wijkverpleging' ('scientific programme on district nursing'; WPW) (2019/2020):

- Identifying predictive individual characteristics and client groups
- Gaining insight into characteristics and risk factors of care recipients

- Research into relevant and influenceable outcomes of district nursing care; this information forms an important part of properly functioning funding based on an amount per care period per client
- Developing and applying a measuring instrument through pilots with healthcare providers

Activities of the NZa itself concern:

- Evaluating the operation of the policy rule experiment on funding nursing and care: consequences for a new funding model
- Collecting information to achieve a level playing field
- Researching the organization and funding of system functins (unplanned district nursing in the evening, night and weekend)

A new funding model for home care may be funding based on case-mix classification (Bulck 2017). For this, clients are divided into subgroups according to care needs based on various characteristics. The division into subgroups can then be based on clinical characteristics, such as a condition that someone has, but also on personal characteristics and environmental factors. By financing home care in this way, we can strive to provide customized care.

Within the framework of this book, a combination of population funding and a self-regulating system of individual funding is sought. In the first case, it is about allocating resources; in the second case, it is about the use of these resources (Van Montfort 1986; Van Montfort 1995). To arrive at a sustainable and affordable system, an integrated approach to care, housing, income and well-being for the elderly is needed to arrive at creative network combinations around individual clients (Huijsman 2013, 63). Involving clients in considerations regarding the healthcare provision leads to less care consumption (Klink 2012: 17). The possibility of self-regulation is made possible by decoupling the macro budget and the actual deployment of resources (micro budget). On the basis of the macro budget, it is possible to determine what is available for a specific region or target group.

Interactions form the core of platform technology. Applying this technology in care for the elderly breaks through the current obstacles in which the professional domain is dominant. Platform technology also strengthens the ability for clients to collect information and seek contacts with other clients. From that perspective, an appropriate financing basis is also considered. This is based on a system of person-bound funding in which in the start-up phase is realized at the level of groups of clients (target groups).

Indicators are developed within that target group or region that are appropriate. These indicators are presented to professionals and clients. They commit themselves to arriving at care within the available resources. Both client and healthcare professional participate in innovation processes. Resources that may be released remain at the disposal of the region or the target group. In this perspective, innovation focuses specifically on the use of resources.

The choice was made to base this model on the development of a theoretical framework that can be applied nationally (Bisognano 2012). When looking at healthcare interventions, the question is which criteria can be applied to make an assessment of effectiveness and effectiveness (Trusko 2007). What is striking is that there is increasing interest in the system perspective of Triple Aim.

Pricing

The current funding is strongly focused on rates: it is mainly about the relationship between price and costs. The costs determine what space there is for care deployment within a region or target group. The cost price is determined by fixed and variable costs. The variable costs for deploying platform technology become lower (marginal) with greater use of the platform. The cost price is jointly determined within the region or target group: it is about value for money.

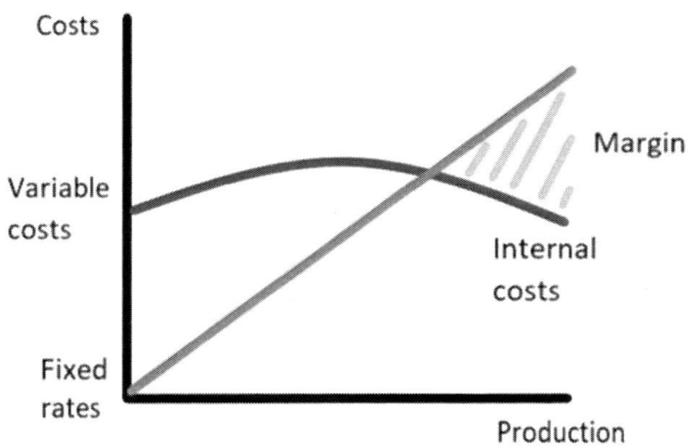

Figure 4. Internal cost price (Van Montfort).

Current thinking often leads to 'cost-driven pricing'. From the costs, it is necessary to come to a certain price. To avoid this in healthcare, it is desirable to switch to 'price-driven costing' (Malik 2017, 124). After determining the rate (price), a margin is deducted from this for the continuity of the activities. The remaining amount determines the entire structure of the care process. The available budget is determined at the macro level; at the micro level, space is created for the use of resources based on individual choices. The combination of price-driven costing and management based on an internal cost price makes integrated care possible. Van Montfort (2019b) indicates that allocation based on budgeting is the most effective form of funding.

By decoupling allocation and use, the space is created for forms of client-bound funding, while at the macro level a form of system control remains possible.

Professionalize Entrepreneurship

Focus

The previous chapter described the preconditions for a care practice in which the identity of the client is the starting point for the design of the interaction. In this chapter, the perspective of the professional is worked out. This chapter is based on literature (focused on entrepreneurial action), dissertations, policy documents and work practice.

A professional is characterized by being able to take responsibility for his or her own actions aimed at solutions for clients. Professional acting has entrepreneurial aspects but has a different focus than entrepreneurship. The start-up methodology is used as a metaphor for professionals dealing with the uncertainty that results from increasing variety. Because of this variety and the possibilities of care technology, the professional will increasingly be confronted with questions and issues that require reflection. It is about the way in which professional behaviour can handle variety.

Entrepreneurship and professionalism have a different focus. Care for the elderly requires the agility that characterizes entrepreneurship. It is about being able to cope with increasing variety by individualizing care and integrating the impact of care technology and digitalization into the professional domain. From the literature on entrepreneurship, the start-up method (Woldendorp and Woldendorp 2019) offers a perspective for realizing the above. This method shows how variety, changes and uncertainty can be handled.

One of the characteristics of professionalism is working with standards that have been established. Due to the increasing variety, however, it is also desirable to have a self-regulating capacity to be able to independently realize the interaction with a client. This is reinforced by the fact that not only is the variety among clients is increasing but more and more new forms of care provision are also emerging.

Reflection

It is important that in the interaction, there is always reflection on the actions of the professional. The client is not only a consumer but someone asking for the solution to an issue that affects their own identity. The development towards a Personal Health Environment means for the position of the professional. By enhancing the client's autonomy, their own professional position also comes into the picture. Personalization of care and the model for joint decision making make the context of each client increasingly important. Entrepreneurial action and innovation are central to the interpretation of the professional role in the interaction with the client. Central is regulatory space (autonomy), flexibility (adaptive capacity) and innovation. Just being good in one's own field is no longer sufficient.

Central to this chapter are the concepts of professional, personal entrepreneurship and start-up approach. The above-described increase in variety in the care process requires, according to the elaborated system principles, two approaches: damping the variety through standardization of care and strengthening the variety by increasing professionals' room to manoeuvre. We see a struggle to deal with this in care organizations: on the one hand, forms of self-management and self-organization are chosen; on the other hand, those forms are being phased out. The choice is to have the interaction between the person requesting care and the care provider take place by strengthening the position of the client and strengthening the position of care professionals. Organizations are then hardly needed. Working with platform technology facilitates clients and healthcare professionals in that.

What is needed is for professionals to increase their learning capacity. This requires an innovative working environment and a learning model that is focused on results. The increasing complexity of care requires that the logic of the professional and the logic of the client become aligned. The starting point for this is acting on the basis of trust and accountability. Personal functioning is central. In the interaction with the client, insight is always needed into the specific context in which that client is located. A better digital and technological working environment can support the professional in the organization of care. The added value of artificial intelligence (AI) is still seen as limited for this form of care. Digitalization and healthcare technology work effectively if it is a normal part of healthcare practice.

Shared Decision Making

For the information that is collected and shared by the professional, the values of the client must be embedded from the start. This includes values such as autonomy and direction.

Work processes are therefore also adjusted from that perspective in consultation with the client. Tools for this approach are the Shared Decision Making (SDM) model and the PGO (Personal Health Environment). Here too, platform technology is supportive. Information can be offered in an accessible, tailored and understandable way in the platform. The SDM model must be based on the client's context. In this perspective, the client is in fact the guide for the professional to make information accessible to that context. This requires new skills from the professional, whereby sensemaking is an essential part. The introduction of the PGO also changes the way the professional works. After all, the client's directorship over their own data is strengthened. Determining the indicators to be used is not an objective process. Here too, sensemaking comes into play.

Regulatory space can be filled in from entrepreneurial action. Here action, responsibility and accountability are central. The competencies and skills that are expected from a healthcare professional fit well with personal entrepreneurship. A model that allows reflection on this personal entrepreneurship is the start-up method. This is about being able to deal with uncertainty and being able to show resilience and courage.

Context of Position Professional

Regulatory Space

Evelien Tonkens (2004) states that professionals must meet clear professional requirements. However, management often translates these requirements into performance criteria that do not do justice to the discretionary context of professional reality. Although a professional in principle performs standard acts, she or he can never regard and treat them as standard. The issue is simple: if professionals follow the management logic, they short-change the client. Management and the client pull hard on the professional but in opposite directions. This leads to a terrible split (Tonkens 2004).

Existing healthcare organizations will increase the regulatory space for professionals. Operations and information management will be more structured to support professionals. Due to the increasing severity of care, there is even more attention for the distribution of expertise: role of (district) nurse and role of personal healthcare assistant.

New Business Models

Due to digital systems, fewer patients will be seen by doctors and general practitioners, shifting instead to nurses who receive digital support with diagnostic and treatment tools. The impact of technology on healthcare professionals leads to client portals (direct access to data) and innovation (new professional dividing lines; new working methods; new organizational forms). Expected developments include: assistance with mobility, tracing people with dementia and increasing communication options. (Topol 2015).

Healthcare institutions find themselves in a changing world. Cornelis (1990) states that hierarchy (rule-guided management) is not suitable for finding solutions in a world that is changing. The rule does not change, so it is invalid, and the new solution, which fits into the new situation, requires adjustment. However, adjustments can only come from people who know the situation.

Within the Nursing, Nursing Homes and Home Care ('Verpleeg-, Verzorgingshuizen en Thuiszorg'; VVT) sector, there are conflicting movements: on the one hand, the trajectory of self-managing teams is continued, and, on the other hand, the trajectory of working with self-managing teams is stopped (Laurens; Cordaan).

Organizations or groups of can quickly increase in size to introduce new applications (Ismail and Van Geest 2015). This results in the creation of new business models in healthcare (Kemperman, Geelhoed and Op't Hoog 2014; De Man, De Man and Stoppelenburg 2015). The realization of new forms of governance also immediately plays a role (Strikwerda and Ten Wolde 2017). Changes in the healthcare market are going faster and deeper, under the influence of advancing digitalization, more complex customer behaviour, new entrants in the competition field and changing business models (Sidhu 2016). Anyone who wants to have a right to exist in the future must therefore think fundamentally differently (Hoogveld 2017).

Learning Model

Organizations and professionals function as systems. The task of this system is to achieve organizational goals (Aukes and Woldendorp 1994). This is achieved because people deliver performance that produces results for customers. A learning model has been developed for this that looks like this (Reijerse and Woldendorp 2000):

Organizations and professionals produce results for customers (or clients). In order to be able to do that, performance must be delivered that produces a customer-oriented result. Performance presupposes competencies (Mulder 2002). In changing circumstances (increasing complexity), competencies require learning (Arets, Heijnen and Jenning 2015). Learning can in turn best be done by gaining experiences that result from the process and the outcome of achieving results (Ruijters 2006; Ruijters and Veldkamp 2012).

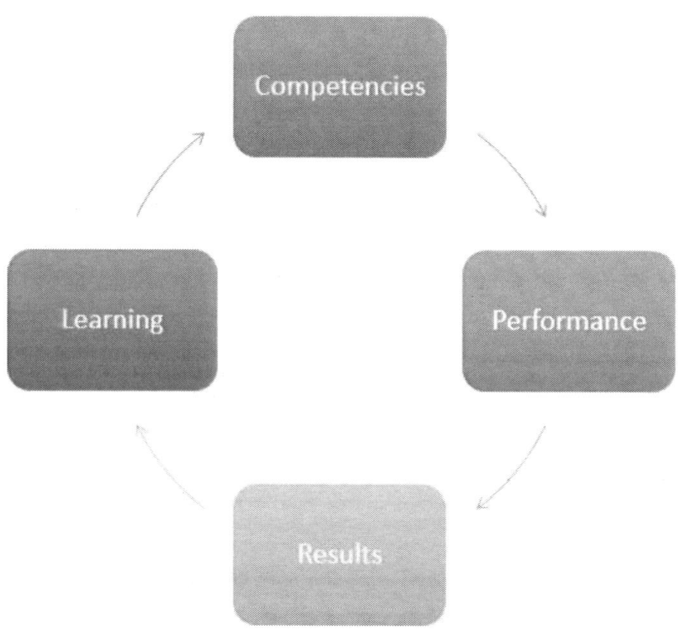

Figure 5. Learning model (Reijerse and Woldendorp 2000).

'Doing better' is only possible if nurses, nursing specialists and carers work in a professional and innovative working environment. That environment is increasingly supported by healthcare technology and digitalization. A working environment must be aimed at ensuring that newly developed knowledge and innovations can be applied in healthcare practice (Vermeulen 2019).

Management of performance and results depends on four preconditions:

- There must be an objective that can be evaluated.
- Effect of interventions must be known.
- Sufficient information (intelligence) regarding the (current and future) environment must be available.
- The capacity to process the information must be sufficient.

Working and learning reinforce each other through the available technology (Marr 2010). It is precisely professionals who must be able to enter into a dialogue with management, colleagues and clients about their own contribution (Ertel and Solomon 2014). Professional forms of self-regulation are assumed in which the willingness to take responsibility for one's own actions is central (Hoekstra 2005).

Game Rules

Healthcare professionals have to deal with different game rules (RVS 2019a, 19):

- As a service provider in a (semi) public sector, they are expected to be cost effective and lawful.
- As a professional service provider, they have to deal with professional standards and guidelines.
- As a private party in a regulated market, they must adhere to the rules of the market.
- As a social organization, they know different stakeholders (local residents, chain partners, etc.).

Care is increasingly characterized by complexity. More and more people have to deal with multiple needs that are highly dependent on the specific context in a given time.

The complexity requires a reconsideration of the current care offer. An integrated and multidisciplinary approach is needed. The core of this is that the preferences and needs of clients will play an increasingly important role (Ruwaard 2012). In addition, safe care can be seen as a value between other values: the context in which care is provided and the position of the care professional in this context create further complexity. This requires room to make assessments and learn from mistakes that are also made in practice. The interaction between client and healthcare professional is always about assessments at the individual level (CEG 2019).

Where regulatory space is created, it is not self-evident that healthcare professionals will also use it. They are not trained to think broadly, but to become a specialist and to avoid risks; it is precisely working within frameworks that provides guidance and certainty (Bussemaker 2019). In order to make healthcare future-proof, it is about clarifying which goals must be achieved and, in particular, which normative principles lie below those? (Bussemaker 2019).

The Dutch healthcare system operates on three sets of logic (RVS 2019): the logic of healthcare, the logic of rules, and the logic of distribution. In practice, these logics clash. A more effective organisation of that practice requires focusing on the value of human dignity. This can be achieved by letting healthcare professionals enter into a meaningful relationship with the client or citizen. Two preconditions for this process are an improved cooperation between healthcare professionals and a different approach to limitations. What is important is understanding the client. It is important for healthcare professionals to jointly develop new ways to treat the client (Bussemaker 2020).

Trust

The concept of trust thus comes to the fore: 'trust is an issue if an actor to achieve something depends on another actor, whereby he cannot fully control or predict the actions of that other' (Stoopendaal and Bouwman 2018, 7). The relational aspect of the interaction between the client and the healthcare professional will be central. Trust has different dimensions (Meurs 2014): performance (providing evidence for a result); competence (required qualifications and expertise); and intention (believing in each other's good intentions). Meurs: 'resilient relationships only come about if we focus on performance, competences and intentions' (2014, 10).

Resilience is the ability to adapt to changing circumstances while maintaining core values. Resilient relationships arise when investing in mutual relationships, putting content at the centre, modesty, experimenting and learning and appropriate accountability (Meurs 2014). For healthcare professionals, this means that they are forced to opt for a personal approach. In addition to this choice, care is increasingly being given in formal and informal partnerships such as networks and platforms. Technological developments have a major and unpredictable influence on how healthcare is organized and delivered (RVS 2019a, 36).

Accountability

Accountability, aimed at improving care, should therefore be the core of professional action (RVS 2019a). The interaction between healthcare professional and supervisor, buyer and government must be reciprocal. Complexity requires embedding accountability in an iterative process: taking action together, reflecting and adjusting plans. This creates preconditions for care professionals for a learning care practice: joint decision making by the client and care provision meaning for both professionals and clients.

It also helps healthcare professionals to respond to the specific context of healthcare demand. Being accountable requires self-reflection from the healthcare professional, a dialogue with the client, a dialogue with other professionals and organizations and a dialogue with external stakeholders (RVS 2019a). Elements in this are furthermore horizontal supervision of professional conduct and mutual intervision (Kraaijeveld 2018).

Elberse (2012): health research is driven by the ideas and interests of researchers and professionals. This is partly due to the supply-driven nature of the healthcare system. A system innovation is required to change this system to a needs-oriented system (De Haan 2017). However, patient participation only takes place on a limited scale.

By placing responsibility with professionals, organizational forms can arise around work processes (chains) that transcend the boundaries of one's own organization (Homan 2005).

Interaction with Client: Autonomy of Professional

Work Practice

Professionals also have to deal with a different position of clients. This leads to, among other things, an increase in more assertive behaviour, a strengthening of the client's autonomy and a need for as much customized care as possible. The perspective of professionals forms the basis for the structure of the organization. Management provides a working environment in which common standards and values are used. The point of departure is a strong common interest.

That is why, in addition to a business-oriented (instrumental) approach to change processes, an approach aimed at the development of professionals is also desirable (Ardon 2011). In terms of management and implementation, the foregoing requires the minimum- intervention principle. The core is that as many decision-making powers as possible are placed as low as possible in the organization.

By defining the client in terms of his or her own personal context, a different form of life is created and, with that, openness to a different interaction. The language, spoken and written, shows how reality is interpreted, how reality is handled, what is assumed to exist in the world and how action can be taken in reality. Understanding is seeing connections and therefore coherence. In the interaction between the client and the professional, understanding each other's language expressions is essential. The conceptual apparatus of start-ups in particular makes a new interpretation of the interaction between professional and client possible.

The care context of the client and the interests of different stakeholders (informal care, general practitioner etc.) can best be seen at the level of basic units (professionals, teams, departments). It is precisely at this level that a better balance can be realized between the deployment of resources (people), the planning to be used and the costs (Almekinders 2006). The learning capacity of care professionals is put to the test by the variety of care arrangements, the emergence of new types of professionals and the emergence of all kinds of intermediaries (Putter 2017).

Innovation

Professionals do not automatically become familiar with technology. Working with technology and digitalization must therefore be part of work practice (also in the education) (Zorgpact 2018). The application of innovative technologies requires a mutual adaptation of technology and society (ECP 2019). Innovations in healthcare only work if they become embedded in society. This means that they are part of the care and technology system, of laws and regulations, codes of conduct and protocols, values and routines of users (Rathenau Institute 2019).

Digitalization is primarily a technological phenomenon. Within care for the elderly, it is mainly about increasing productivity. What is also needed, however, is a value-driven approach (Wallin 2018).

Technological solutions help healthcare professionals and clients work in a different way (Vilans 2019). Creating the right framework conditions appears to be essential for a successful implementation of healthcare technology. The number of applications for eHealth is around 325,000 (Idenburg and Emonts 2019).

Hinssen (2017) expects that five technologies will have an enormous impact:

- Artificial intelligence: ability to perform independent analysis;
- Internet of Things: devices are connected with each other and with data in a smart way;
- Networked intelligence (blockchains): reliable networks that allow secure decisions to be taken in a network;
- Augmented and virtual reality: changes in the structure of reality;
- Quantum computing: an enormous (and fundamental) increase in computing power.

Convergence

Vilans (2018) describes 12 trends which will have impact on the elderly care: online connections, consumermarket, big data, artificial intelligence, risk solutions, robotics, cyborgs, drones, reality technology, blockchain, 3-D printing and biotechnology. Artificial intelligence (AI) is about smart technology: technology that is aimed at direct care to the patient/client and that can (partly) replace the care provided by a human care provider (RVS 2019). For example an experienced physician is no longer required to predict the onset of diabetes in a patient (Siebel 2019: 39).

The combination of AI and blockchain changes the way data are created, how they are distributed and how execution upon data is realized (Laurence 2019: 98). The use of Blockchain technology in healthcare makes a difference in data management. The technology will make sharing medical data more effective, efficient, secure and transparent for all healthcare stakeholders. A network for healthcare institutions can thus exist without having a patient's personal data. Patients are identified in this network via Blockchain technology. As a result, the Blockchain can also form a platform for exchanging patient data.

Healthcare records stored on a Blockchain can help healthcare stakeholders bring all parts of the health data together in a clear way. Another area of healthcare where Blockchain and healthcare can be used is traceability of medicines (Veuger 2020; Veuger en Woldendorp 2021)).

AI relates to six systems (Serrurier Schepper and Hiddink 2019):

- Image: recognizing image
- Text: understanding and producing text
- Speech: understanding and producing spoken language
- Prediction: predicting and making suggestions
- Virtual assistant: chatbots and virtual assistants
- Robotics: mechanical aids

Artificial Intelligence

Big data (ability to store, process and analyse data) lays the foundation for the broad adoption and application of AI: medical image diagnostics, automated drug discovery, disease prediction, genoime-specific medical protocols, preventive medicine. (Siebel 2019: 92).Almost all current applications still fall under 'narrow AI' (Nictiz 2019). This means that they are intelligent computer systems that perform one specific task, particularly in the field of medical imaging.

Contemporary AI is in the adolescent phase (Sahota and Ashley 2019: 104). What is lacking is a 'broad' intelligence aimed at problems that are new and variations that were not present before. Real life is open-ended: no single data point reflects the ever-changing world. In an open, finite world, there are never enough data points.

AI therefore currently has three gaps between ambition and reality:

- Believability gap: we think computers look like humans in terms of intelligence.
- Progress illusion gap: we think AI solutions to simple problems also work for complex problems.

- Robustness gap: we believe that when AI sometimes works, it is thought to always work (Marcus and Davis 2019).

Narrow AI is the situation where an AI system exhibits a certain level of intelligence in a certain field, but it remains a computer system that performs highly specialized tasks for people within that narrow field. For example, it is about predicting lung cancer, predicting the outcomes of a patient in intensive care, recognizing dermatological abnormalities. The added value of AI lies in areas such as more personalized treatments and preventive health care. AI in healthcare offers new possibilities to make advice personal.

These recommendations are based on personal data from apps, consultation and medical data. AI is that part of computer science that focuses on systems that perform functions that we normally associate with the human brain, such as learning, dealing with ambiguity, solving problems, recognizing emotions and being creative (Nictiz 2019).

Examples of AI techniques that lead to improvement in healthcare (TD Connect 2018):

- Big data: treatment based on your own file and a large number of comparable cases
- Sensors: continuous breathing test at home signals early stage of cancer
- Robots in the body: nanobots in the bloodstream that remove clots
- Virtual Assistant: AI assists physician with diagnosis and treatment
- Recognizing an epidemic: recognizing an epidemic based on satellite images
- Help with dementia: remembering when to take medication

The expectation of FME (2018) is that the deployment of AI, home automation and ehealth can reduce the staff shortage in healthcare. The e-intensive care unit (e-ICU) of Philips is mentioned as an example: with a form of telemonitoring, multiple beds can be monitored from a central post. Cost savings are not in fewer staff but in fewer interventions through better monitoring. AI is used for wearable technologies, sensors offering real-time readings on for example heartrate and blood pressure. AI can also be used in developing learning plans tailored to individual professionals (Sahota and Ashley 2019).

Ford: 'my own view is that artificial intelligence gradually proves capable of automating nearly any routine, predictable task, regardless of whether it is blue or white collar in nature' (2018, 5). This will create new jobs, but many jobs will also disappear (Ford 2015). A study by PwC (2019) shows that applying artificial intelligence on a large scale can lead to more efficient and accessible healthcare. Examples of savings are:

- Obesity: more effective self-monitoring to prevent obesity
- Dementia: higher diagnosis percentage in primary care
- Breast cancer: early detection, reduction of direct involvement of doctors in any repetitive tasks

The development of big data and artificial intelligence in healthcare is still in the initial phase. Most technological advances 'arrive and change our world in a steady incremental rate'. (Browne, 2019: 302). Davenport (2019:81):'Many cognitive technologies are close to being good enough to change business models, but aren't quite there yet'. Realizing the calculated benefits does not seem to be achievable easily in practice. Humans are especially good in things like judgment, empathy, intuition and comprehension of complex interactions. (Baldwin 2019: 236). These are central for giving care. Technological developments contribute to three movements: empowered clients: more control over their own health and care; bionic human: restoration of the human body; autonomic systems: computers take over parts of care phases (Idenburg and Emonts 2019).

Healthcare Landscape

Whatever influence these technological solutions have, they must fit into the right care. Proper care is defined as (KPMG 2018): sensible (appropriate), in line with guidelines; accessible to anyone who needs it within the standards for maximum acceptable guidelines; to be determined of the same or better quality on the basis of outcomes of care and support on both a clinical level and on patient experience; for the lowest possible integral costs (over the entire chain).

Based on this, a successful healthcare landscape is characterized by (KPMG 2019): organization of the right care in the right place; technical infrastructure for data exchange and interconnectivity; regulations concerning data exchange; governance in the region; new delivery models where the focus is not on the infrastructure, but on the client and the client's needs.

Information: Preconditions for Achieving Autonomy

Responsibility

From the (more) dominate position of clients, there is a shift from organizations to organizing. This includes strengthening the personal directorship of clients and strengthening self-organization among professionals, setting up network structures, application of new technological options and achieving a new distribution of knowledge and skills.

Network care as a natural evolution of chain care offers more opportunities to cope with the increasing complexity. While chain care focuses on optimizing care within the existing first-, second- and third-line bulkheads, network care offers the opportunity to organize care based on the integral care demand of a patient/client, working around and over the bulkheads. Collaboration between cure and care is necessary. This integrated approach improves the quality and perception of care at lower costs (Valentijn 2015).

Within the care for the elderly, the district nurse plays a pivotal role, in the sense that they fulfil a central function in the neighbourhood through contacts and collaboration with general practitioners, other and informal caregivers. From this perspective, the client serves as the centre of care, and district nurses as the leading professional, both in the care of their clients and within the neighbourhood (De Groot, Maurits and Francke 2018). This also makes their role in the interaction decisive.

The role of general practitioners and medical specialists is much more focused on responsibility for the care process. The district nurse is an essential link in shaping the interaction. They are connected to general practitioners and possibly to medical specialists. The network of healthcare professionals adapts as the health and demand of the client changes. Depending on the type of care and the needs of the patient, the role of the medical specialist can vary from an active leading role to a more supportive role or sharing specific knowledge. Depending on the situation of the vulnerable elderly person, a circle of care professionals and informal caregivers will develop around the client (FMS 2017).

When designing a digital health management, it is important that values such as autonomy are included in a design. Research by Denktank IZO (2019) shows that citizens have difficulty understanding the input of professionals in the area of information provision. It must work for different groups of people (variety). The design must offer (privacy) protection (Niezen and Verhoef 2018). Since May 2018, the General Data Protection Regulation (GDPR) has been in effect, stipulating that explicit permission must be requested for storing and processing all data of persons.

Ehealth

Healthcare will move towards the outcomes of data streams. It is noted that the Dutch healthcare sector is moderately positive about the current IT innovation level. The level of ambition is high (Neomax 2017). Ehealth can support care processes to improve quality, continuity and a person-oriented approach (Swedish society for nurses 2012).It is important that healthcare professionals play a role in the design of eHealth applications: 'nurses have a professional obligation to interact with and care for patients in a way that adheres to core nursing values, which is also the case when eHealth is used' (Swedish Society of Nurses 2012, 11).

Ehealth refers to healthcare that is delivered via technology with or without the intervention of healthcare professionals. Citizens' self-reliance requires a different vision of ehealth than is currently present in practice: that practice is characterized by a multitude of tools and applications. However, ehealth is a way of thinking, an attitude to improve care with the help of information and communication technology (Van Gemert-Pijnen 2015). It is about integrating technology into the work process. The technology must be better anchored in health interventions. This involves having a good view of the actual functioning of technology and having knowledge of influencing behaviour (acceptance and adoption of ehealth).

The Council for Public Health and Care defines ehealth as: 'the use of new information and communication technologies, and in particular internet technologies, to support or improve health and healthcare' (RVZ 2015). Ehealth concerns websites and applications to support clients. Because they can expect some or all of the contact with healthcare professionals, it is expected that cost savings will be possible (Rademakers 2016).

Conditions to be met are:

- Attention to the competence development of professionals and citizens
- Revision of guidelines
- Data standardization
- Acceleration of transparency of outcomes
- Investments in technology that can take over care and support
- Higher first-line organization degree
- More control and attention to upscaling
- Pooling of Zvw, Wmo and Wlz
- Right incentives
- Multi-year agenda

Meeting these preconditions leads to clients who are empowered to take on a greater role and cooperation between professionals based on trust and a cross-domain vision of health.

The use of various aspects of ehealth such as online viewing, video calling, apps, telemonitoring and other IT applications requires that these applications are well anchored in the (integrated) care processes (Nictiz and Nivel 2019; RIVM 2018; Vilans 2018). It is striking that the supply is greater than the use. Although professionals are predominantly positive, the applications are still insufficiently embedded in healthcare practice. What is needed are preconditions that make ehealth applications work optimally. Healthcare processes are being redesigned based on the added value of ehealth applications.

Agility

This new way of working focused on showing how you can work better as a professional with the new digital tools; how to strengthen collaboration; how to solve and adjust the digital (work) environment on the basis of daily work problems. The same applies for the client, who can more easily access information and forms of service.

Agility is decisive for competitiveness and has four main building blocks: look outside, good examples are followed (connecting leadership), self-organizing units and modelling and generation: flexible processes and IT. Developing agility requires, among other things: insight into customer behaviour, process-oriented management, dynamic competence, networks and sensemaking (Veuger 2017, 5). This implies a change strategy focused on working with clients and professionals to achieve awareness of the added value of this new working method (Ten Have, Ten Have and Janssen 2009). Without that awareness, and thereby resolving one's own bottlenecks, effective implementation remains hardly possible. Bisognano: 'Getting the triple aim of better health, better care, and lower per capita costs will require new designs and models of care. This can only be achieved by real co-production of care, with patients and families as drivers' (KPMG 2016).

Points for attention (KPMG 2016, 4) are:

- Vision to introduce new methods; technology is supportive not leading;
- System design is needed to provide solutions to the problems that clients and professionals have.

Medical technology is defined as all technology aimed at improving the quality of care for patients/clients. By digitizing healthcare close to the client, healthcare becomes more personalized, leading to higher-quality healthcare for individuals. Technology is therefore seen as an important impulse to grow outpatient care. The medical technology market in the Netherlands in the home situation is estimated at € 2.3 billion (KPMG 2017). A number of conclusions:

- Therapy and treatment are shifting to prevention (stimulated by ehealth solutions and smart apps).
- Care is becoming increasingly personalized, and medical technology is more focused on a specific patient.
- A shift from inpatient care (hospital/nursing home) to care in the home situation is stimulated by developments in medical technology (Internet of Things).

Value and outcome must be at the top of the agenda (KPMG 2014). It is about personalized care.

Digital Health Management

In this way, an element in stimulating digital health management is an expected contribution to the scarcity of health care professionals: it is not only about values such as autonomy but also about the cost-effective organization of health care (Niezen and Verhoef 2018). The establishment of a data value chain means that based on data and its analysis, interventions in the lives of citizens can be achieved.

Healthcare has specific values with regard to governance issues, for example that there must be support for the content of care and for the way in which that care is provided (Berenschot 2019). The use of blockchain technology means, among other things, autonomously regulating the integrity and quality of the provision of information and validating automated chain processes. At present, there are no large-scale applications in health care in the Netherlands (Berenschot 2019).The National Science Agenda does, however, offer a framework for further interpretation of technological developments and their impact on, for example, healthcare (Ministry of Economic Affairs and Climate 2018).

Deciding together is about the process of shared decision making. The RVS (2017) does not advocate an evidence-based approach, but a context-based practice. It is essential to keep track of the specific context of a client and to connect and deploy the available knowledge accordingly. Healthcare professionals must insert shared decision making practice in the context of a client. It is not so much about the dissemination of information but about listening to the client (RVS 2017).

The client has the relevant and objective information about the care process, and the care professional is aware of the preferences of the client. It is precisely outcome information (value-driven care) that could further support healthcare professionals and clients in making the right assessment (Equalis 2019). Deciding together works best if it fits in with existing healthcare practice. Healthcare professionals use this methodology if they can integrate it into their own working method and professional identity.

When a healthcare professional gives information to a client, it is important to provide support with interpretation, sketching the right context and bringing together wishes and goals of clients with the available information (Equalis 2019). The caregiver becomes a guide who provides the client with relevant information and explores the values and preferences of a client. The point is that clients are involved in their own care and the choices they have and that they are given room for reflection on what is important in their own lives (Equalis 2019).

Consumer Driven Care

A form in which this takes place is Consumer Driven Care (CDC). CDC is both a philosophy and an orientation towards the provision of care services to clients in which they choose and determine which they purchase (KPMG 2014). This is a model developed in Australia. ‘CDC is a way of delivering services that allows consumers to have greater control over their own lives by allowing them to make choices about the types of care and services they access and the delivery of those services, including who will deliver services and when.

Under a CDC approach consumers are encouraged to identify goals, which could include independence, wellness and re-ablement. The consumer decides the level of involvement they wish to have in managing their care. Through the introduction of an individualised budget, CDC provides greater transparency to the consumer about what funding is available under the package and how those funds are spent' (2014, 7).

To achieve shared decision-making, other skills of healthcare professionals are needed, such as coaching and open conversation techniques. It is about translating professional jargon and thinking into the environment and context of clients (Huijsman 2013, 41). This is not self- evident because, just as in health care in general, little attention is paid to the world of the elderly in elderly care (Luijkx 2014, 3). In designing the care process, it is not self-evident that the goals and needs of clients and care professionals run parallel (Zwakhalen 2018).

Sensemaking of data should take place in the conversation between caregiver and patient about what is currently good care for this patient; in a process of shared decision-making, in which decisions are made about care and treatment. The effects of such a process are still unclear: whether there is a more efficient use of care is unclear (Delnoij 2019).

Determining and involving the preferences of the patient in decision-making leads to a fundamental change in the interaction between client and care professional, but it is also problematic because it has not been properly realized for many care professionals. Healthcare professionals have a strong tendency to direct, while in many cases, the autonomy of the client can be much more central (Ubbink 2018).

Personalized care is about respecting the individuality of the care recipient, whereby the care professional recognizes the client as an individual and guarantees autonomy and independence for the person as well as possible. The quality of care, the relationship with the client and the environment contribute to the client's independence. It is therefore about an individualized care philosophy (KPMG 2014).

Provision of Information

The client's story is essential to achieve compassion. Compassion translates into seven dimensions (Van der Cingel 2012): attention, active listening, dialogue, involvement, helping, presence and correct understanding of the other. Care and compassion take the subjective story of the client as a starting point. The practical wishes presented by the elderly do not necessarily translate into survival, a lower percentage of readmissions or a reduced decline in independence and are often not reflected in validated questionnaires that measure the quality of life. They are matters that are difficult to make tangible and objectify and that have to do with the feeling of safety, with fear of the consequences of deterioration and of loss of control and self-respect (2015, 12).

Because information is available, professionals can independently come to: distribution of (shared) resources, accountability of own resources, mapping effectiveness and efficiency and elaboration of operational plans. The RVZ (2014b) advised on structuring the provision of information about the patient. First, give the patient (also the insured or citizen) insight into his or her health information. This must be extended to a personal health record 'PGD'. This PGD (PGO) contains (digital) copies of electronic medical records of healthcare providers and data that the patient adds to this. The patient decides whether he wants a PGD and who manages it.

Information Standards

Recently, developments in the Netherlands in the field of digital information exchange in healthcare have accelerated. Nictiz is a Dutch knowledge organization that is committed to digital information exchange in healthcare. Together with the healthcare field, this organization develops and manages information standards that are necessary for the proper exchange of information. Examples include information standards for nursing transfer, for the exchange of data in acute care, in maternity care, the exchange of data from laboratories, medication safety and care for people with chronic diseases. Examples include information standards for nursing transmission, for the exchange of data in acute care, in obstetric care, the exchange of data from laboratories, medication safety and care for people with chronic diseases.

An information standard is a collection of agreements designed to ensure that care information can be recorded, retrieved, shared, exchanged and transmitted with the right quality. Examples of care information include blood pressure, discharge date, diagnosis and weight but also civil status, gender and name. Because the healthcare field is too complex to describe in a single information standard, Nictiz develops information standards together with the healthcare field for specific and well-defined situations in which healthcare professionals exchange information, with each other and with their patients (use cases). The information standards are infrastructure-neutral.

An information standard forms the basis for the functional and technical requirements imposed on the applications such as the electronic patient file (EPD) and the infrastructure. The dataset is a crucial part of an information standard. This contains the specification of all data (clinical concepts) that are recorded or exchanged within the context of a specific care process and the use-case(s) defined thereby (https://www.nictiz.nl/rapporten/informatiestandaarden-basis-voor-gegevensuitwisseling-in-de-zorg/). Simply put, the dataset describes which data is involved.

Datasets are built up as much as possible on the basis of healthcare information building blocks (zibs). Zibs are small information blocks that you can use to easily and unambiguously describe what the dataset of an information standard consists of. Zibs specify clinical and other terms relevant to healthcare, such as body weight, medication or alcohol consumption. Figure 4.1 shows the relationship between the information standard, dataset and zib. The Basic Care Data Set ('Basisgevensset Zorg'; BgZ) is a collection of zibs. The BgZ is a 'patient summary' of (medical) data that healthcare providers have determined to be important for continuity of care. In the Dutch context, it has been agreed that the BgZ is the national standard. Nictiz plays a central and facilitating role in the development of information standards and zibs in the Netherlands.

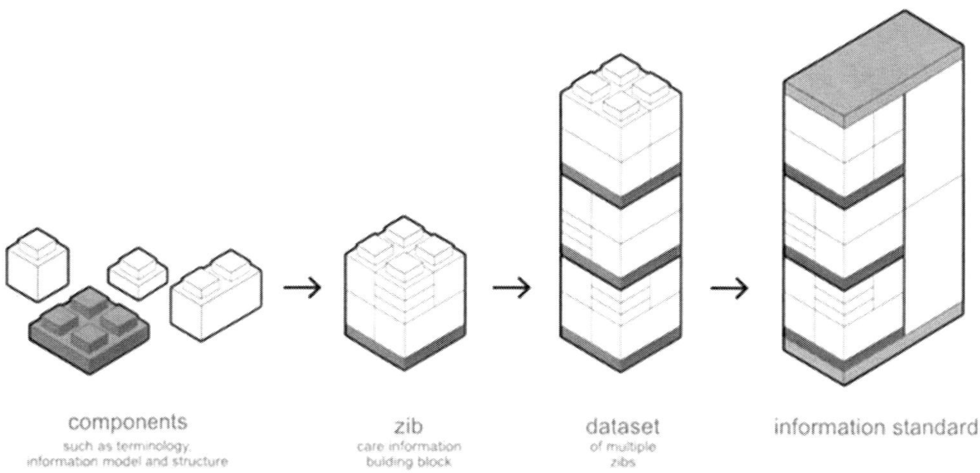

Figure 6. Personal health environment.

Starting 1 July 2020, citizens must be able to view their own data digitally (online inspection: Personal Health Environment). Both clinical and patient-reported information are available within a personal health environment. For feedback, information at the level of the client is compared with information from comparable clients (patients like me) (Zorginstituut 2018a). Experience with the use of outcome information is still limited (Jeninga and Woldendorp 2019).

It is not clear whether the date of July 1, 2020 will be met. Digital support is essential in the director's role of clients:

- Insight into lifestyle consequences
- Personalization of health and care
- Possibility of prevention

Blockchain will have a major influence on how we share information and execute transactions. Blockchain technology is the ability to create and exchange unique digital records without requiring a centralized, trusted party (Schwab 2018: 87). Blockchain requires a network: this not only means a change in one's own business model, but also in that of the partners. Blockchain is a shared and unchanging management of facts and transactions where calculation rules replace the original supervisor to ensure the correctness of the data (Broncker and Veuger 2018: 126).

Anyone who wants to can have their own health data in one place in his or her personal health environment (PGO). This concerns medical data from files at (BIG-registered) healthcare providers, but also health data collected from gyms or smartphones for example. All that data can be aggregated in a PGO. The Ministry of Health, Welfare and Sport: 'The working methods of health care professionals will also change with the emergence of Personal Health Environments (PGO): the directorship of patients and citizens over their own health data will therefore increase' (VWS 2018, 17). How you deal with the choice of certain outcome measures and indicators derived from them is never just a methodological exercise. Indicators are about more than measuring; they lead to certain effects and can therefore be used for managing (Delnoij 2019).

The central question when choosing indicators is who asks for certain information and what the underlying question is. Is it about an effective care process or the choice of a specific care professional? (Delnoij 2019, 25). That is why the process of sensemaking with data must take place between the client and the healthcare professional (shared decision making).

Setting up a PGO is therefore only effective if it is done jointly. Patients choose a personal health environment (PGO) based on privacy, functionalities, ease of use, accessibility and costs. This is according to research by the Patiëntenfederatie ('Patient federation'). Participants in the Patiëntenfederatie study considered a medication overview and a summary of the medical file as the most important functions of a PGO. Online management of appointments, requesting repeat prescriptions and requesting an e-consult also score high. The general practitioner is considered to be the most important source of medical information. The hospital is in second place, and the pharmacy, in third place.

A personal health environment is therefore broader than a client portal. A client portal is linked to a specific care provider system, for example the HIS of the general practitioner. A PGO is not just for healthcare (provision). A PGO is focused on autonomy (direction and self-reliance and co-sufficiency), better quality and safety of life and lower costs for the person. That is why a PGO integrates facilities that are broader than care: living, well-being/ relaxation, education/work/daily activities, neighbourhoods, municipalities, health insurers.

The idea is that a PGO allows a patient to view data from multiple healthcare provider systems at the same time. The exact data that a patient can view differs per PGO. The NHG and the Patiëntenfederatie of the Netherlands have jointly drawn up a guideline for access to the file. This sets out which set of basic data must be available for online viewing by the patient. The personal work notes of the general practitioner are always excluded from inspection by the patient.

With a PGO, patients are given the opportunity to gain more insight into their health data, which can support them in managing their health. From 2020, patients have the right to (free) electronic access to their own file. In addition, patients must be able to indicate which data may or may not be viewed by which (categories of) healthcare providers with whom there is a treatment relationship. A PGO can be a method for the patient to get that electronic view.

Two parties are needed to exchange health data:

- The patient with an app or website in which he wants to collect and use health data (personal health environment).
- A healthcare information system from the healthcare provider in which the patient's data is stored.

A PGO reinforces the network aspect in healthcare: data from the outside in, meaningful functionality and a network structure. The client becomes a digital player in healthcare. This strengthens the interaction between client and professional. A PGO can also forward information. A PGO is a lifelong digital tool in which the owner collects, manages and shares his or her health data from various healthcare providers. The patient/client therefore has control over his own (healthcare) data. With PGOs, the technical intervention in the IT infrastructure is aimed at extracting information from the source system of the healthcare provider and passing it on to the PGO of the client/patient and vice versa.

At the time of information transfer, the patient is responsible for the data, the path this information travels and with whom it is shared. The management of the medical data lies with the owner of the PGO. The healthcare provider is responsible for the quality of the information provided. MedMij is responsible for a personal health environment in which the healthcare information systems of healthcare providers can communicate with each other not only in a secure but also in a clear way.

Quli wants to operate as a citizen platform. The platform is set up within the framework of the MedMij standards. It is about a safe exchange between clients and care professionals (VIPP scheme). A number of information standards have since been developed: basic healthcare data (hospital care); medication; GP data (upload measurement values); Ggz (municipal mental health).

Patients Know Best (PKB)

In the UK, Patients Know Best (PKB) (www.patientsknowbest.com) is available for 12 million (in the near future 20 million) clients. CarePoint Nederland has concluded an agreement with PKB for implementation in the Netherlands and Germany. PKB has four main domains: General, Social, Sexual and Mental Health.

In order to adequately set up information provision, it is essential for CarePoint to start with the question of what goal must be achieved. The point is to get a good picture of that. In practice, this question is skipped, making implementation insufficiently manageable. The aim of PKB is to optimize the interaction between the healthcare professional and the client through a new structuring and sharing of information. It is about improving the quality of communication and interaction.

COVID-19 has acted as a catalyst in achieving this goal. In the English context, the number of users increased by 77% between March 2020 and September 2020. An important reason was that patients and clients did not want to come to the care provider. Just as in the Netherlands, for example, there was a large drop in demand in hospitals and in the home situation. The need for an alternative was enormous.

There was also a major change in the thinking of healthcare professionals. Figures from the English hospitals show that medical specialists found prior to COVID-19 that 80% of patient contacts had to take place face to face and 20% could take place via digital devices. This is reversed after six months: 80% of patient contacts take place via digital devices and 20% face to face. A calculation by CarePoint at a large Dutch hospital showed that such an implementation led to a saving of €1 million (less space, less parking space and less CO2 etc.).

An essential precondition for digitization of care is that new technology should lead to a fundamental reorganization of work processes. If it is used to adapt existing work processes, this only leads to higher costs in practice. This means that technological and social innovation must take place together. This is a requirement of CarePoint to introduce PKB. When digitizing healthcare, organizations and healthcare professionals are therefore faced with a strategic choice to shape their current work processes completely differently.

The introduction of PKB has led to better capacity utilization in England for COVID-19. Because a large number of clients in elderly care are now connected to PKB; it is easy for general practitioners to do early diagnosis via questionnaires. It is possible to serve 100,000 clients per day. The introduction of PKB makes 'symptom tracking' possible: by establishing a number of criteria for COVID-19, a filter is laid over a large number of people, which focuses the available capacity on that part of the total that may have COVID-19. As a result, testing facilities can operate much more effectively. In addition, this way of working leads to simple contact between a client and a healthcare professional, which in turn reduces anxiety and fear among clients.

The introduction of PKB is a fundamental change: information is already shared before an interaction between client and healthcare professional takes place. This strengthens communication and the interaction based on it in terms of quality. That leads in turn to a more effective treatment process. Collaboration and coordination between healthcare professionals is greatly improved. For example, in chronic care where clients usually deal with multiple healthcare professionals, the English context shows that significant cost savings and quality gains are achieved.

There is also much to be gained for informal care. In the process of sharing information, informal care becomes an integral part of the treatment process. This positioning results in a better recognition of one's own position.

The introduction of a PGO does not in itself solve the problem of illiteracy. However, PKB is designed in such a way that visualization and speech technology are built in.

The organization of PKB also ensures that fragmentation of information is prevented. CarePoint expects many apps to be too limited to be future-proof. A better solution is full integration into the PGO. The PKB information architecture is fully geared towards this.

The application of the possibilities of artificial intelligence also makes it possible to use PKB as an early warning system. By bringing vital values together, it is possible to detect deterioration of a patient much earlier.

It is essential that linking to other systems is easy to achieve. An important development in this regard is the link between the health care domain and the social domain. More and more healthcare professionals are choosing an independent role. The connection between PKB and the VmZ platform contributes to this. The role of the district nurse is strengthened by having access to the care information about a particular client.

The impact of COVID-19 is that there is a different way of thinking among healthcare professionals. In the current context, the continuation of existing forms of interaction is not future-proof. In addition to the fact that the position of a client is strengthened (control over one's own data), it is necessary to closely involve the healthcare professionals in the design of the information provision. Technological innovation always goes hand in hand with social innovation in the area of work processes, professional cooperation and the design of interactions with clients.

Strengthening Position Professionals

Entrepreneurship

Different definitions of reality can be used simultaneously within care processes. The reality of organizing as we perceive it, we cast through organizational theories and organizational models in an explainable form. It is therefore proposed to introduce the model of a start-up when stimulating entrepreneurial behaviour within organizations or upon starting as an entrepreneur (Van Gaal 2012). The (French) word entrepreneur (dictionary 1723) means someone who organizes a company by taking a financial risk. The term entrepreneurialism can be translated as both entrepreneurship and being entrepreneurial.

Entrepreneurship is mainly about its metaphorical use: it is mainly about activating action (Engel 2015). For professionals, self-organization is about connections with other professionals and with clients. Entrepreneurship is about being able to cope with increasing variety and the (possible) uncertainty that goes with it (Eijssen 2016). Minderhoud (2017) describes entrepreneurship as the ability and willingness to develop, organize and manage a business venture to make a profit. Entrepreneurship is simultaneously an organizational form, a competence and a property (Blom 2002). Entrepreneurship among clients and healthcare professionals is about giving substance to the interaction based on a self-reliant position of the client.

A specific form of entrepreneurship is a start-up: a starting company that tries to make a new idea successful in circumstances of high uncertainty (Kawasaki 2015). Start-up thinking helps to break through the resistance to change because the existing mindset is broken (Ries 2011). A start-up can handle the need for faster change and agility. A professional should be constantly experimenting and adapting to accommodate to the effects of digitalization and technology. Start-ups are often seen as digital role models (Kane, Phillips, Copulsky and Andrus 2019: 25).

A start-up is a temporary organization that is looking for a scalable and repeatable business model (Blank 2013). Its characteristics are: speed, scalability, disruption, continuous willingness to improve and using digitalization (Hoogveld 2017). Start-ups are by definition focused on learning (Razeghi 2014). Hoffman (2013) states that the entrepreneurial strategy that successful start-ups use is comparable to the career strategy that successful professionals use.

Research by Anne Annink (2017) shows that entrepreneurs who start because they see opportunities (and are not necessarily self-employed) are more satisfied with their work- life balance. Independent entrepreneurs have the following characteristics (Annink, 2017): customer focus, innovation, motivation (business) phase. Her research shows that there is a positive relationship between the motivation to be an independent entrepreneur based on opportunities and the work-life balance. There is a negative relationship between excessive stress and customer focus and satisfaction with the work-life balance. She concludes her research with the conclusion that independent entrepreneurs, compared to employees, are relatively satisfied with their work-life balance and well-being, even though they also experience tension between autonomy and financial uncertainty.

Entrepreneurship appears to be hereditary. However, predicting entrepreneurship based on genetic data is not possible. Entrepreneurship is most likely the result of hundreds if not thousands of genes, each with a very small effect. You can say that some genes apparently lead to entrepreneurship, but you cannot say which genes they are (Loos 2013). The most important aspect of entrepreneurship is: how can you as a company develop products and services that customers really want? (Apello 2011).

Entrepreneurial Professionals

Kwakman (2011; 2012; 2015) has worked out various aspects of entrepreneurial professionals. Being good in your profession is no longer enough. You are constantly challenged to reinvent yourself. You must be able to handle higher demands from customers, more competition, new business models and digitalization. A professional who makes a difference in this market and is successful for his customers, organization and himself has the following characteristics: he or she has a personal mission, has a unique offer, dares to approach new customers, deepens the relationship with existing customers, is part of a community, is proactive in his or her business and keeps his or her body and mind vital. In addition, it is about being proud of one's own profession (Jansen, Van den Brink and Kok 2009).

Van Delden (1992) indicates which four quality factors apply to professionals: using professional knowledge, developing methods, improving services and personal quality. For professionals, it is increasingly the case that team skills and great flexibility towards situations and clients are essential. In fact, there must also be the core motivation to fulfil this function, i.e., the tireless response to changing situations (De Jonge 2015; Maister 1997). It is about connecting and complementary action in a group that is put together on a case- by-case basis (group of sole proprietors). Professionals increasingly work together in teams and function within networks: this applies to doctors, nurses, notaries, accountants, psychotherapists, architects etc. It is therefore about being able to communicate with others: talking with clients, consulting with colleagues, coordinating with other professional groups, being able to propagate new ideas (Van de Water 2017).

In short, the young professional has a keen eye for the changing world of his or her clients and is authentic and inspired in his or her ambition to be significant. He or she has a vision, but is also practical, and therefore knows how to inspire the environment.

Blom (2001): entrepreneur is in fact a profession for which you should study. People always think: you will learn that in practice. You can teach eighty percent of entrepreneurship through courses in management or entrepreneurship. It is necessary to have a digital mindset .It is not about what they can do today but about what they will be able to do tomorrow, based on their mindset and their ability to learn and to grow (Kane, Phillips, Copulsky and Andus 2019: 115).

Van Brussel (2012) distinguishes four ways to develop entrepreneurship, whereby the degree of entrepreneurship increases:

- Floater: you leave the development of your career mainly to the environment and fate and your hitchhike, as it were, for possible opportunities. You are hereby clearly depend on your environment.
- Opportunity Taker: you move flexibly with your environment and use opportunities that come along to realize personal goals. You are a scanner and

therefore interested in developments, but you wait and do not look seek them out yourself.

- Surveyer: you are open to what the future brings, you know who you are and what you can do, and in this way you discover opportunities for your career. In addition to scanning opportunities, you also know how to pick up other signals and link them to your personal goals.
- Shaper: You know what you want with your future and you set concrete goals for your career from an orientation towards yourself. You create more yourself and take matters into your own hands, and you opt for self-management instead of dependence on your environment.

Rotmans (2012; 2014; 2017) indicates that the current transitions (period of revolution) are shaped by experimenting from below. The digital working environment makes it increasingly difficult to find the right balance between work and private life. To get out of this, at least more room to manoeuvre is needed for professionals. There is therefore also an increase in (social) entrepreneurship, professionals who choose to become self-employed, citizens who want to direct themselves in their neighbourhood. This is partly due to own choices, and partly due to necessity. A growing group of people can and want to do many things themselves, and also no longer wants to be dependent on the government or existing institutions.

Thomas Davenport and Julia Kirby (2016) state that people can help shape their future in a digital world. They see three developments: people who improve their ability to deal with a digital work environment, people who organize that digital work environment (super specialists) and people who further develop the digital work environment and ensure innovations.

Start-Up Approach

Flexibility

The start-up approach offers an approach that focuses on flexibility, dealing with uncertainty and resilience (Brack 2017; Blank 2013; Hoogveld 2017; Ries 2011, 2017). The scale for new developments in healthcare is not fixed in advance (Postma 2015).

Start-ups have a number of characteristics:

- Scalability: Can you grow quickly?
- Searching: constantly testing and validating whether your product or service is scalable;
- Focus on technology;
- Entrepreneurial mentality.

A start-up is a starting company that tries to make a new idea successful in circumstances of high uncertainty. Start-up thinking helps to break through the resistance to change because the existing mindset is broken (Ries 2011). A start-up is a temporary organization that is looking for a scalable and repeatable business model (Blank 2013). Its characteristics are: speed, scalability, disruption, continuous willingness to improve and using digitalization (Hoogveld 2017).

Start-ups are known for their entrepreneurship, adaptability and vitality (Woldendorp and Woldendorp 2019). Starting businesses are often characterized by individual entrepreneurship. They are thus able to operate quickly, flexibly and decisively, so that they can work efficiently and in a customer-oriented way and easily notice new opportunities. The essence is that employees of a start-up behave like an individual company (Brack 2017).

Characteristics of start-ups are: they solve a problem, they show that what is conceived also works, they invest in networks, they are agile, and they ensure that they are visible. Ries talks about a start-up state of mind (2011). Ries defines the term 'start-up' broadly: everyone who tries to set up something new with an uncertain outcome is working on a start-up. Characteristic is that you do something from the start and learn by doing what works and what does not. Ries 2017: identify the leading assumptions that must be true for the start-up to succeed. Have an experiment in which the assumptions can be tested quickly and cheaply. Use each experiment as an opportunity to learn what works and what does not (Kolb 1984). Use your learning ability to start a new experiment and start again. Periodically determine whether you will work with a pivotal approach (change of strategy without change of vision).

Learning

Start-ups are by definition focused on learning (Razeghi 2014). The start-up approach forms a form of life with its own language game. This form of life initiates activities of entrepreneurs who, from the start of their work, are focused on testing their own ideas. A form of life applies as a complex of coherent rules.

Love (2016) has developed a J curve for start-ups:

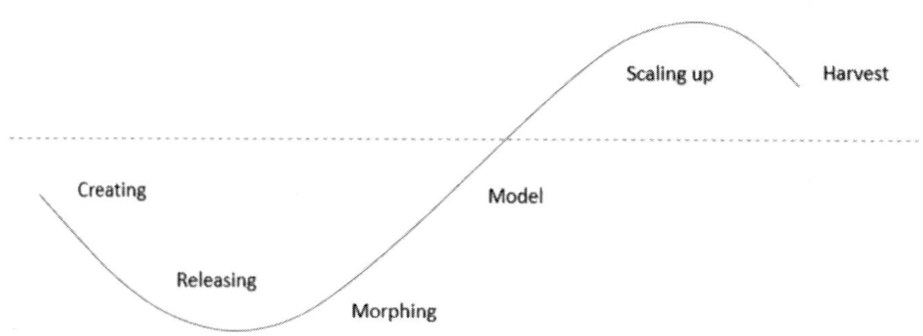

Figure 7. J curve (Love 2016).

The model works as follows. In the first phase, the creative phase, it is all about the idea. In the release phase, it is about being able to deal with disappointments. In the model phase, we determine what costs we want to (or can) incur to get the idea onto the market.

Morphing is about adaptation, also at a fundamental level. The market determines what a success is; adapting is therefore following that market and not the original idea. It concerns questions such as: What opinion do customers have? What attracts customers? Scaling up also involves three components: Can we find the right people? Do we have enough money? And do we keep work processes in order? By harvesting we can 'cash in'.

Every business model has three components: provide the product or service; care for a customer; ensure the revenues are higher than the costs. In start-up jargon, it is about the release of an MVP (Minimum Viable Product): what is sufficient to find out if it works. Make sure you really know what your customers think and organize feedback. By quickly making a minimum testable variant (MVP: Minimum Viable Product) of the product or service, it is possible to quickly test whether the concept appeals to the target group and where it needs to be adjusted. Tips are: do not assume who your (future) clients or customers are too quickly; consider in advance what important measuring points are for success; there is an overlap between the needs of providers and buyers.

Success

Schevernels (2015) elaborates seven essential aspects for successful start-ups: ambition, new developments, quality, culture, talent, focus and funding. It is essential to arrive at a coherent approach:

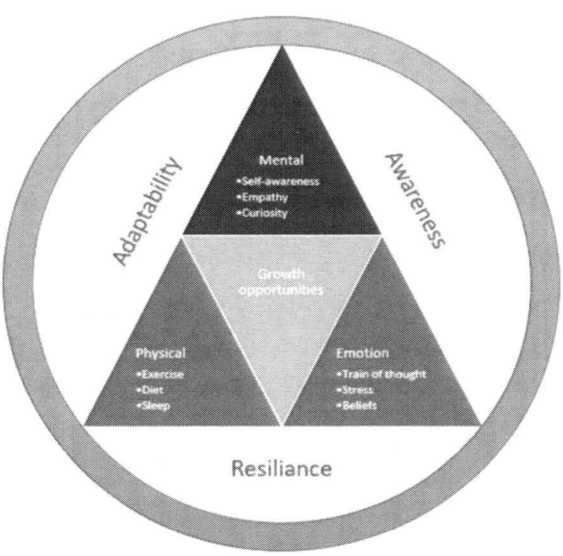

Figure 8. Aspects of successful start-up (Schevernels 2015).

Ries (2017) defines the term 'start-up' broadly: everyone who tries to set up something new with an uncertain outcome is working on a start-up. Characteristic is that you do something from the start and learn by doing what works and what does not.

PERSPECTIVES IN HEALTHCARE

Future-Proof Care

A large number of national umbrella organizations issued a manifesto in March 2021 on the organization of future-proof care for the elderly (Tien uitgangspunten voor toekomstige ouderenzorg; 'Ten principles for future care for the elderly'). The bottlenecks include:

- With unchanged policies: the number of elderly care jobs must grow from 350,000 in 2016 to 700,000 in 2040
- Increasing pressure on informal care
- Growth in nursing homes: from 135,000 in 2019 to 261,000 in 2040

In the short term:

- Strengthening primary care
- Complexity of regulation makes appropriate care difficult to arrange
- Growing waiting lists
- Lack of qualified personnel
- Insufficient valuing of healthcare professionals

The manifesto is a call to politicians to address 10 principles:

- Focus on the needs of the elderly and space for informal care and local initiatives: establishment of networks covering all areas of life
- Greater simplicity, coherence and cooperation
- Eye for prevention in the elderly person's own living environment: strengthening personal control
- Direction of the government towards realizing reliable and structured exchange of client data
- Sufficient diversity of forms of housing

- Sufficient employability of professionals
- Opportunities in healthcare
- Debate over quality
- Extensive scaling up of innovations and digital care
- Radical stripe through bureaucracy

The essence is that elaboration of the principles leads to a transformation of elderly care. This involves shaping technological innovation, professional behaviour and connection with clients in a coherent manner. Within the VmZ platform, for example, we have set this up with our own Electronic Client File and a Client Portal for each client. In this way, professional action and personal control are connected. Our CuraeVitel Balie living concept (https://www. youtube.com/watch?v=_vtSJ6JEYC8) brings together technology, care, comfort and living.

Smart Home technology ensures that the elderly can continue living at home longer. With this technology, it is also ensured that residents feel less lonely. They can continue living, for example, in their familiar surroundings. PlatformVmZ works with Loxone (www.loxone.com) within the CuraeVitel Balie client portal.

By using smart home technology, the independence and autonomy of a resident are supported as long as possible. As a result, the quality of life for those living independently is promoted. Research has shown that the elderly experience the loss of their independene and privacy as extremely serious. In contrast to camera surveillance or active monitoring devices, the smart home technology monitors passively by checking habitual patterns via sensors.

Falls usually occur during the activities of daily living. The goal of the Ambient Assisted Living, developed by Loxone, is to improve the quality of life for the elderly and to ensure that they can continue living independently at home for as long as possible with the help of technical solutions, even if they have a physical and/or mental handicap. The needs and wishes of the elderly and their caregivers are the starting point on which certain solutions such as fall detection are integrated.

Thanks to the intelligent automation, passive monitoring can be realized, potential risks can be identified and managed, visual and/or acoustic messages can be given and lifestyle monitoring can be integrated. Above all, this all happens automatically, so that the elderly resident does not have to do anything.

In this chapter is elaborated how the interaction between client and professional is shaped in five perspective. The interaction between client and healthcare professional takes place in a certain context. Depending on that context, one or a combination of the perspectives has added value.

Narrative Perspective: De Hoven VVT Institution

De Hoven is a VVT institution in North Groningen, and its mission is that elderly people in North Groningen should be able to continue living in their own way, even if they become very vulnerable, need home care, rehabilitation or live protected at De Hoven. Well-being is central because they can continue to follow their own habits. De Hoven has approximately 920 employees and around 500 volunteers. The policy is based on the principle that professional conduct is always interpreted from the perspective of whether it is important for residents. This perspective has been developed in collaboration with professor Slaets (Leyden Academy on Vitality and Aging). Central to this is what older people themselves find important. In addition, it is about meaningful life: being able to live one's own life despite increasing vulnerability. Finally, it is about connection between generations.

Since 2017, De Hoven has been working with the Leyden Academy on the development of a life enjoyment plan. Working with a life enjoyment plan makes a narrative perspective possible. Within De Hoven, a mix of perspectives is used: every client situation must be re-examined. In addition, systems can be a hindrance to self-thinking capacity. The Health and Youth Inspectorate (IGJ) still works too much from a closed system. (You can break through that by involving relatives).

The awareness of the situation is important. By understanding your own paradigms, you are more open to other approaches. That is why there is a personal leadership program aimed at looking through the eyes of the other. The narrative perspective is methodical. This methodology shifts the focus from doing to 'being there'. The story is fragmented: these fragments are (statistically) converted into values that are expressed in feelings. In any case, it leads to increasing variety. Accounting for one's own behaviour has two dimensions: via guidelines and testing by IGJ (externally). By conviction (internally). It is about value-driven organizing and acting.

The narrative perspective is therefore part of the care. In addition, there are still guidelines (for example washing hands). The core is a better-living client and not a better-living professional. With personal directorship, it is about conducting a dialogue in which trust and equality are central. Bravery is needed to change the system. This applies to all levels: including the Supervisory Board (which must be composed on shared values) (Interview with manager at De Hoven). Within De Hoven, the personalized approach is used:

- Clients are involved in all decisions concerning healthcare.
- There is the possibility of valuing risks: some decisions made by clients can entail a certain risk.
- Professionals are autonomous in taking decisions.

- Care is regenerative: a focus on restoring or maintaining functions in vulnerable circumstances.

The starting point for employees is to enter into a daily dialogue with clients and their families about how to shape the support in such a way that life retains the meaning that the elderly person and his or her family want to give it. The individual quality of life is therefore the guideline of the professionals' actions.The target group of De Hoven can only give a very limited interpretation to a directing function. The aim is to connect closely with the living environment of residents based on this. There is an attempt to gain insight into the values that a client uses by entering into conversations as openly as possible.

The VVT institution De Hoven is one of the institutions that participated in the low-control care experiment. Two central insights emerged from the evaluation of institutions with low control (Eindevaluatie 2016):

- Value-driven work promotes the quality of care: starting with good care for the client changes the way the organization works (at all levels) and how this work is experienced by professionals.
- By focusing on the care relationship between client and professional, it became clear which rules are an obstacle to making good care central.

The client and the professional are the centre of the care process. The starting point of the experiments was to reshape care based on this relationship. Clients gain more control, and professionals facilitate clients retaining as much control as possible over their own lives (2016, 9). This way of working requires reflection on one's own professional actions. However, that is not easy for a number of levels within healthcare. In addition to cognitively focused reflection methods, it is also important to develop other forms of reflection.

The narrative perspective is central in this context (Slaets 2017). In practice, narrative stands for telling, using the conversation as a bridge to the other. A conversation is an exchange of narrative, personal and relational. It requires being present, a presence. This framework requires two-way traffic and an open and investigative attitude. An important aspect of this is the realization that granting people directorship does not mean that everyone can do something with it. Many residents cannot arrange their own lives. It is precisely this fact that makes it important that effort is made to direct one's own life.

In that sense, the conversation and the narrative are essential for the quality of life and therefore also for the quality of care. This framework is not about needs but about desires, about positive well-being. The desire is not told and heard when completing questionnaires but becomes known and tangible in the relationship (Slaets 2017). A point of attention in the organization of care and, in particular, the accountability thereof, is that this open approach in terms of governance is often difficult to implement.

It is difficult to translate conversations with residents/family into results of quality of care, for the professionals and for the supporting administrative processes. No suitable narrative accountability tool has been developed for this framework. Because De Hoven wants to be able to account for the quality of care internally and externally, De Hoven has included stories in the quarterly accounting. In addition, De Hoven has hired a practicing researcher who, based on conversations and observations, draws up reflections on (professional) action.

For the professionals, it is not about entrepreneurial behaviour but especially about professional maturity. It is important that they can direct their own professional skills. De Hoven has therefore also hired a philosopher who, based on conversations and observations, draws up reflections on (professional) action. A Hoven-wide plan has been drawn up to strengthen working on well-being, using the Groningen Well-being Indicator (GWI). Well-being is measured with the Groningen Well- being Indicator consisting of 8 areas: enjoying eating and drinking; good sleep and rest; pleasant relationships and contacts; being active; caring for yourself; being yourself; feeling healthy in body and mind; enjoyable living. The central question is: What do you enjoy? It is also asked which of the above 8 areas the elderly person finds important and then how satisfied he or she is with this. Scores: number of areas important (0-8); positive and negative sources of well-being; ratio of number of areas satisfied to number of areas important (0-1).

Based on this, De Hoven's philosophy is that it is visible in the care plans (GWI/goals/care agreements/evaluation based on conversations) that care is arranged in consultation with the resident. Policy-wise, under the title Working on Well-being, it is worked out what it means to take the well-being of clients as a starting point in their own actions. On the basis of this questionnaire, there is discussion with the client/family about the wishes in terms of daily life and care. These conversations are then held regularly.

Building on GWI, we work with the method of the Life enjoyment plan. As a result, caregivers get to know the residents better and know what their life gives colour; they can better meet the personal wishes and desires of the residents in their daily rhythm and activities. The subjects that are mentioned do not count as a checklist, but as subjects that can be discussed in an interview. For all parts of the narrative approach, it is about avoiding instrumental thinking and acting as much as possible.

By giving residents freedom, however, events (such as traps) also arise that are perceived as incidents by healthcare supervisors. From the narrative approach, however, it is about parts of the life story. The basic principles of the narrative approach are of great importance to De Hoven. The terminology around the life enjoyment plan does not really do justice to the problems of residents. Acceptance of vulnerability and the suffering that goes with it is essential (Coolen 2015). Preconditions for quality of life lie in this acceptance. Given the problems of residents, the outcome of the life course within De Hoven is inevitably dying.

De Hoven is indirectly involved in the further development of the narrative approach. The Leyden Academy and other organizations are actively continuing with the introduction of the life enjoyment plan, organization-wide. A narrative accountability tool is also being developed. De Hoven remains involved. De Hoven uses the previous experiences to come to a methodical elaboration throughout the organization. The core of this is the interpretation of 'the good conversation'.

Technology only makes sense if the residents and professionals understand and can use the added value. Within De Hoven, use is made of an e-learning module developed by Slaets. In this way, the development of a professional learning curve is accessible to everyone, but the way of thinking is often difficult for professionals. It appears that they fall back on the traditional way of working. The Central Client Council is positive about the focus on good conversation and narrative accountability.

The aim is to use the resources of Waardigheid en Trots and the quality funds in such a way that the directing role of residents is strengthened. It is striking that the accounting for those funds in the context of the quality report is an obstacle to a narrative approach. De Hoven has collaborated for many years on the development of a narrative accounting method with Dr Slaets. The GWI, as applied by De Hoven, provides a discussion at an individual level about the quality of care and what needs to change in view of the development of the resident and his or her wishes in his or her phase in life. Because the GWI does not lead to a good narrative accountability for the quality of care, a start was made with training in the 'doodle me' technique: attention for the client, getting the life story visible, asking the question behind the question and converting it in a Life Enjoyment Plan.

The narrative approach is not about universal principles, autonomy, but about:

- a contextually coordinated concern ('caring about')
- responsibility for care ('taking care of')
- the care itself: the technical and moral components ('care giving').
- recognition and acknowledgement of the differences: care for difference.

The current set of quality instruments (quality plan) forces standards that have insufficient connection with the life plan of residents. It is therefore always important to consider how the individuality of the client remains visible in the consultation between professional and client.

The core is that De Hoven and the family come to good agreements based on respect for that individuality. In the practice of care, these are often difficult considerations and that is why the moral concept of 'responsiveness' is so important. We must constantly observe what happens to the other person as a result of our behaviour and adjust that if necessary. A reflective attitude is important. Vulnerability is central to the interaction.

The starting point of the Life Enjoyment Plan is that nurses and carers get to know the residents better: What is their story? Who is important to them? What gives their life colour? Through intensive contact with the resident, the care staff goes in search of what is of value to that person and what matters. A kind of mind map is made of all information with photos, pictures, drawings and names. The Doodle me method helps with conversations and gives the resident and caregiver a personal handle to conduct conversations and to discuss topics that matter to the resident.

Self-Managing Perspective: Buurtzorg

The transition program (2009) already established 10 years ago that a great improvement can be made in the district nursing by redefining the desired care and services and starting from the self-management of professionals in result-responsible units (Lindberg, Nash and Lindberg 2008). The Buurtzorg model is in line with this. The added value of self-managing teams is mainly seen in the light of the success of Buurtzorg.

At Buurtzorg, the management of care lies with the teams. The team consists of a mix of level 3 personal healthcare assistants, level 4, and 1 to 2 at level 5). The district nurse is not by definition in charge. Part of self-management is that everything is done in consensus, with all levels having the same level of control. The care is organized in small teams (around 12 professionals), close to the client with authority and space to act for care providers. The success of Buurtzorg translates into a large number of studies (De Blok 2010; De Blok et al. 2015; Van Dalen 2010; Van Dalen 2012; Green 2016; Nandram 2015; Pool 2011). These studies have been used in this elaboration.

Buurtzorg, for example, is not based on a care vision but on a human vision. They have set up their system in such a way that self-reliance and independence from care are central. Together with their clients, they look for a solution that matches their experience and wishes. This requires flexibility in the way of working, exchange of knowledge and an eye for the local context (Van Dalen 2010).

Buurtzorg uses the principle that the content of the care can only be put at the centre when the person providing the care also has directorship and control over the way in which the work is organized. Self-management at Buurtzorg therefore requires self-organizing: by trial and error; diversity and overlap; learn to handle load and boundaries; joint solving of individual problems at work; every team has its own learning process; further detailing the vision is an ongoing process; every team has its own ideal mix of commitment, plans and flexibility (Van Dalen 2010).

Freedom is also connected with autonomy. According to De Blok (2010), professionals within healthcare organizations have few opportunities to be relieved of the limitations that the organization imposes on them. 'At Buurtzorg these obstacles are missing, and there is great reliance on the personal capacity to act "from within."'

The starting point of Buurtzorg is a human vision and not a healthcare vision (Van Dalen 2010). This human vision applies broadly in healthcare: holistic, social context, trust, autonomy and self-esteem. The distinguishing feature is the translation into practice-related practice and the rules that are applied. Buurtzorg has a number of leading organizational principles:

- The starting point for organizing is the content of the care.
- Care is based on self-organization.
- Supporting/coaching instead of managing.
- Organizing as a continuous process.

Clients have confidence in the care professionals of Buurtzorg (De Veer 2008). Sufficient time is set aside for the care and the treatment and professionalism are very good. The quality of care is experienced as above average. Buurtzorg has the following objectives: the client has one permanent well-trained care provider for coordinating all care with as few different hands as possible at the bedside; healthcare professionals have professional freedom to provide generalist care; GPs work together with the care providers at Buurtzorg. The core concept is that there is trust in and familiarity with Buurtzorg employees. The healthcare professionals easily adapt to the situation of clients. The information transfer is good. Shared Decision Making (SDM) translates at Buurtzorg into:

- Personal attention to the client
- Involving caregivers and loved ones
- Relationship between client and care provider: the course of care is determined together with client and informal care (Van Meijeren 2014).

A small number of clients state that they are asked about their wishes with regard to care. If they have wishes, these will be listened to and then carried out satisfactorily or followed up (De Veer 2008, 25). The practice looks different: planning, times, frameworks etc. Care is used that does not always correspond to the wishes of the client.

Understanding and designing systems and knowing the system principles is a key competence for current organizations (Huguenin and Van Gestel 2007; Kay 2015; Lockwood 2010). An important function is the control function. This is not visible, but the presence (or absence) can be derived from the behaviour of the system. To bring a system under control, the control system needs as much variety as the system itself. The structure of the system gives shape to control.

It is therefore about the organization finding a balance between autonomy and control that fits with its own environmental variety. The added value of self-managing teams is mainly seen in the light of the success of Buurtzorg. Buurtzorg uses the principle that the content of the care can only be put at the centre when the person providing the care also has directorship and control over the way in which the work is organized.

Buurtzorg is valued because it puts people first. It focuses on how you closely connect team members (example: team members look for an office themselves and design the interior, within the framework of Buurtzorg). This can lead to much consultation. The technology is supportive to achieve better mutual coordination (Heimans 2018).

Freedom is also connected with autonomy. According to De Blok (De Blok and Pool 2010), professionals within healthcare organizations have few opportunities to be relieved of the limitations that the organization imposes on them. 'At Buurtzorg, these obstacles are missing, and there is great reliance on the personal capacity to act "from within."' Buurtzorg now also has a number of frameworks that can act as a hindrance from the original vision.

Characteristic of this form of management is that there is room for employees to interact with each other in their own way. There are opportunities to meet each other, talk to each other, work with each other, define performance with each other. This means that professionals have the necessary resources (information, technology, powers) available. This relates to:

- Quality
- Service provision
- Costs
- Innovation
- Promoting autonomy
- Dividing systems into smaller parts and broadening perspectives (thinking from the client).

Healthcare professionals can operate independently and autonomously. The organization is set up to support the interaction between client and healthcare provider. The client's situation is leading. Buurtzorg is based on the needs, possibilities, wishes and preferences of the client (demand for care) and on the professionalism, direction and autonomy of the care professionals who work together in the team. The balance between responsibilities and authorities is (TNO 2012):

- Top-down control is minimal.
- Powers, responsibilities and tasks are specified at the team level; employees coordinate with each other.
- Teams are integrally responsible: result, operation and HR.
- No covenants at administrative level; local collaboration relationship has primacy.
- Each team has a procurement budget, the use of which it can determine for itself.

The accountability for the content of the work goes through team compass. The most important indicator is client satisfaction. The registration of care provided supports practice. A regional coach looks at what the team could do, but ultimately the decisions are made by the neighbourhood team. Management control is in fact carried out by personnel control: the recruitment of higher educated people (Groen 2016). Healthcare is aimed at empowering the client to become more independent as quickly as possible.

The method is divided on the basis of a number of building blocks (Transitieprogramma 2009). The start is the needs indication (indication based on what needs are living and the way in which they can provide supportive, supplementary or replacement care and welfare services). The informal client network plays an active role in this: 'first neighbourhoods then care'. There is a comprehensive formal network. High-quality and responsible care is provided.

Key concepts in the provision of care are: equality, dialogue, reciprocity, adaptability and autonomy. This translates into adaptive help from experience-oriented care. Unburdening is achieved by working on care independence, self-reliance and client-friendliness within the system. To what extent is there consultation between the client and the professional?

The management approach is based on the recursivity model described earlier: 'higher organizational levels only intervene in the event of non-performance or if the integrity of the organization as a whole is at stake. This principle gives every lower level the freedom and responsibility to act in the spirit of the vision and goals of the organization' (Van Dalen 2012, 260).

The holistic approach makes it more complicated for healthcare professionals because they are dealing with more information; for the client, however, it is a simplification (Nandram 2015).

Entrepreneurship plays a role in developing ideas and taking initiative. Buurtzorg is distinguished by a coherent vision based on (Nandram 2015, 135):

- Focus on clients
- Professionalism
- Intrapreneurship

- Pragmatic IT solutions
- Following the higher goal.

The IT infrastructure facilitates that healthcare professionals are focused on phasing out the care. A number of indicators have been developed for this (Nandram 2015, 101):

- Duration of the average care process
- Client satisfaction
- Employee satisfaction
- Team productivity and benchmark with the other teams
- Client hours versus contract hours
- Extent of monthly client hours and specification for certain client groups
- Average size of client hours.

Characteristic of this form of management is that there is room for employees to interact with each other in their own way. There are opportunities to meet each other, talk to each other, work with each other, define performance with each other. This means that professionals have the necessary resources (information, technology, powers) available. You concentrate on quality, services, costs and innovation. It is about: promoting autonomy, putting emphasis on doing and experiencing, making the organization design more playful, dividing systems into smaller parts and broadening perspectives (thinking from the client's point of view).

Within Buurtzorg, work is done with virtual platforms that facilitate planning, a forum for sharing experiences and contributing to innovative solutions (Nandram 2015).

The framework that Buurtzorg uses is aimed at clients, but is strongly substantiated from its own professional (human-centred) vision.

Network Perspective: Network Structures

Networks form a central component in the organization of healthcare in the Netherlands. Dutch society is developing in the direction of a network society (Rotmans 2012; Rotmans 2014; Rotmans 2017).The transition of Dutch society is the centre of 'The eye of the hurricane' (Rotmans 2012). Society is driven less top-down: networks and decentralized communities increasingly determine what happens. According to him, there is increasing interest in cooperatives, social importance and solidarity. The 21st century is described as a network world. Everything is connected to everything: interaction is central. Because events are connected, the likelihood that they will happen is also connected.

It was stated earlier that professionals are expected to be able to operate in network structures (network care). More and more care is also taking place in network structures. This means that the role of management, professional (multidisciplinarity) and client (coordination issue) needs to be redefined. There is no generally defined definition of healthcare networks (Verver, Merten and Wagner 2016). Based on this research, a network is defined as a form of cooperation that leads to better solutions for clients. The description mainly looks at how networks organize themselves. In the context of this research, no statements are made about the results achieved within the networks. It is specifically about how the interaction within a platform is designed.

The mapping of relationship networks leads to the discovery or clarification of boundaries in system terms. Borders are important connectors. A network has boundaries: these vary in fluidity. It concerns boundaries at the organizational level and within professional domains. Networks are structure and process. One part of the process is the relationships and the community that create a network structure. A degree of consistency of interaction is required. In the start-up phase, a network is a project (team). When networks shift to activities, they develop a shared identity. This is followed by the phase of self-organization: there are shared skills and a sense of legitimacy. The last phase is when activities repeat themselves: it becomes a network of practice (Pomeroy 2018). How a network is designed depends mainly on how information flows through the organizations concerned (Aalbers 2015: 8). The success of a network is determined by the organization of horizontal and vertical relationships and how the organization and professional boundaries are handled (Aalbers 2015: 143).

Chain care fits within care if there is good collaboration between care providers within the same funding basis. Network care is aimed at setting up an integrated care demand where the different foundations (Social Support Act, Health Insurance Act, Long-term Care Act) are worked around and over (Fabrricotti 2007). Due to its integrated nature, network care has a high degree of complexity with a high degree of management demand (Malby and Anderson-Wallace 2016).

As indicated in this book, clients increasingly have a role to play in monitoring their health, but there are also people who have difficulty with this. Clients increasingly receive customized care at home in their own environment. In that context, they manage as much as possible themselves. All these developments require care that goes beyond the boundaries of individual care providers, disciplines and sectors: network care (IGJ 2018). Effective network care requires a number of preconditions (Kremer 2018):

- Attention to values that motivate people from within
- Balance between trust and clear agreements
- Creativity from all participants

A network is a collaboration between individuals, organizations or small associations that bind themselves temporarily and equally, around a task, a theme or a challenge (Willems, Linck and Kaats 2018). The development of healthcare in care networks yields new questions, such as: What can be expected of healthcare and care providers in the cooperation in healthcare networks? Where do the responsibilities lie? When is coordination necessary? What is the role of the client and the role of the informal caregiver? Who is responsible for the coordination? Collaboration requires the fulfilment of 5 conditions: shared ambition, clear interests, a good relationship, an appropriate organization and a well-running process. Investing in collaboration skills leads to more successful partnerships (Boonstra 2007).

Care networks are becoming increasingly common around clients. Elderly people who live at home often have to deal with different care and assistance providers. Together with informal care, they form the 'network' around the elderly. It is important for the patient that this care network works well together, certainly when a patient can no longer take good care of themselves. Care networks therefore fall into two main groups: organized networks of care providers (chain care and network care) and personal care networks around clients (care networks). Organized networks usually involve agreements with regard to target groups or within regions. A personal care network concerns all professional care professionals around a client.

However, little is known about underlying collaboration processes under integrated care (Valentijn 2015). This research shows that relational collaboration mechanisms (interests and relationships) are more important than management collaboration mechanisms (process management) in the development of integrated primary healthcare projects. To achieve integrated primary healthcare, a multi-perspective approach is needed: people-oriented, population-oriented and value-driven. Mirella Minkman (2020) describes five factors to arrive at the appropriate scale:

- Scale and volume (large volumes can lead to a local scale; what (specialist) knowledge is required)
- Opportunities for digitization (what can be far and what must be close)
- Region governance: what and who can bear responsibility
- Balance between inclusiveness and efficiency
- Experience and history of and within a region

Networks of people are ecosystems. When there is 'vital space', people coordinate their efforts. Each individual gives up freedoms in exchange for what results from the collaboration. The interaction in the network moves between the poles of the I and the we. The path to vitality and co-creation is only open if they want to investigate the effect of their actions. In the course of its development, a vital network acquires emergent properties (Wielinga and Robijn 2018).

Chains and networks must be designed depending on the characteristics of the client and their problems. This also involves new, integrated organizational forms around target groups based on their clinical picture, with disease management. With multimorbidity and vulnerability, the care and support process is characterized by variety. Customization is therefore required here (Nies 2012).

The research of the Healthcare and Youth Inspectorate (IGJ 2018) into care networks shows the most important risks:

- insufficient collaboration
- non-coordinated care
- insufficient transfer of care.

The design of the interaction between client and professional is therefore a central element in the design of network structures. Pressure on the formation of a network may be the relationship between cooperating parties as well as within parties (Batterink 2004). A network determines and justifies its own area of responsibility. The starting point is the complexity and reality of the specific needs and questions of the target group within this area of responsibility. Healthcare professionals can be active in multiple networks. A network provides insight into the blind spots with regard to the care and support of people with a complex, long-term care demand (Van den Heuvel 2014).

Kreijveld (2012) works out how individuals are connected via the internet and work together in networks. Through the internet, society will be more co-creative and take on more tasks itself (Rifkin 2014). The internet and social media have made it easier to collaborate and develop new ideas (Robertson 2015). On the other hand, the use of the internet also entails risks, for example in the area of privacy (Bridle 2018).

Network structures in healthcare are defined as partnerships between autonomous care providers (including sole proprietors) with a common goal, joint risks, costs and revenues and joint decision-making. Bloem (Gepersonaliseerde zorg; speech 2012) described it as care circuits: all those providers who look for people and use them to do something about their health. It often turns out to be a search. Incidentally, there are many guides (health insurers; commercial parties (Lekker Leven; Leefstijlgids); municipalities (Wmo desk); care organizations (member associations) and private initiatives (care cooperatives)) involved in the search. New forms of network structures are initiatives from citizens who organize the care themselves: half-line care (Nies 2012).

Zegveld (2018): when studying a network, it is important to have a clear picture of the limits. Network analysis is a means to describe reality (at an abstract level). The network approach is based on the idea that patterns in the relationships between actors in the network have important consequences for these actors (Zegveld 2018, 45). Social networks determine the possibilities and impossibilities to which individuals and groups are entitled.

Network participants each have their own goals, resources, priorities, vision, target group and culture (Van den Else 2017). Within most, (technological) product innovations are developed and process innovation is to a lesser extent (2017, 10). By placing responsibility with professionals, organizational forms can arise around work processes (chains) that transcend the boundaries of one's own organization (Homan 2005). Because information is available, professionals can independently come to: distribution of (shared) resources, accountability of own resources, mapping effectiveness and efficiency and elaboration of operational plans.

At the network level, physical and data connections also come together. Collaboration via (data) platforms is becoming increasingly common. A healthcare network consists of healthcare providers from various organizations. The exchange of information is therefore of great importance (ParkinsonNet 2019).

In this perspective, a future-oriented healthcare company will be characterized as a network organization where people work who feel addressed by a common vision that is in line with their own values (Roobeek 2005). This is possible within existing organizations, but also by starting a healthcare company yourself.

Evaluation of networks can be done on the basis of four levels of outcome indicators:

- Individual: impact on individuals within the participating organizations and on individual clients. Indicators are: quality of life of clients or customer satisfaction
- Organizational: impact on participating organizations (referrals, financial health, name recognition)
- Network: evaluation of the network itself: how active are participants
- Community: contribution of the network to the population it serves (local employment, healthcare costs, accessibility of care) (2017, 2013)

Within care organizations, the process of care and service provision is focused on a client-friendly meeting of client demand, which determines the organizational design.

Responsibilities and authorities with regard to the primary care process are positioned as low as possible in the organization (self-organization; self-management).

In practice, there appears to be no formal 'care networks' around vulnerable elderly people living independently. The directorship of care and assistance is primarily the responsibility of the elderly themselves. Although attention is paid to the importance of cooperation between care providers, the lack of preconditions seems to stand in the way of development: financing that makes (intensive) cooperation possible and agreements on data exchange and privacy.

Verver (Verver, Merten en Wagner 2016: 9) presents a number of recommendations regarding healthcare practice:

- Awareness that care and care providers are part of a (care) network around elderly people living independently, ensuring that they are familiar with the existing guidelines and standards in the field of cooperation in care and support and the social map of relevant region
- Agreeing on how control is monitored within the (care) network and agreements on actions to be taken when loss of control occurs
- Identifying vulnerable clients, their degree of control, make an inventory of the (care) network (both formal and informal) and seek coordination and exchange information.

Bloem (KPMG 2014) has worked out this as follows within ParkinsonNet:

- Ensure that active patients can manage their care themselves and are involved in important decisions.
- Determine what value-driven care should look from the patient's perspective.
- Change the way healthcare professionals work: they become patients' partners.
- Provide a network of experts.
- Connect all this with IT tools.

The question of how care organizations and professionals have shaped the management role in the care network shows that there is hardly any care coordinator, that in about one-third of the cases, agreements are made about the point of contact regarding care, that the identification lies mainly with the elderly themselves and that in most cases the care providers leave the directing role to the client. Research from 2017 (Gijzel 2017: 12) shows that the term self-reliance is hardly used by clients or healthcare professionals. They mainly use the term personal directorship, and healthcare professionals sometimes also use quality of life. Most healthcare professionals, clients and informal caregivers are not or are only to a limited extent familiar with the term and function 'independent client support'. According to healthcare professionals, care plan discussion, involvement of the social network and the use of volunteers contribute to the quality of life of the client. However, clients themselves indicate that they are still not sufficiently involved in their own plan (Gijzel 2017: 126).

Collaboration with family and informal care around healthcare and support are becoming increasingly important in elderly care. When setting up network structures between professional care and informal care, there are four roles that an informal caregiver can play: as a colleague, expert, client and neighbor. Which role is most prominent may differ, for example, due to the phase of the disease or the living situation of a patient. The emphasis on collaboration is different for each role. A lot of attention is paid to digital systems to support the collaboration. Platform technology reinforces the role of the informal caregiver (RIVM 2014).

Time and again it appears to be difficult to find the right balance in a network between the self-management of participating institutions or care professionals and the management needed to turn a chain into a logistically coherent process (Hardjono 2010). The frequently stated management role of health insurer or municipality also appears to have insufficient consequences for the success or failure of a chain. This often concerns the tension between substantive considerations and control options. By making use of an information model based on platform technology, that dilemma can be partially solved.

In such a complex system, it depends on the context in a certain area or for the benefit of a certain patient category to what extent chain formation is more or less successful. A lot of (administrative) consultation appears to be necessary in order to connect patients (clients), care providers, resources and knowledge.

By combining data from the integrated information system into reports, supervision of the results from operations is facilitated and guaranteed. This facilitates supervision and makes it possible to assess the business results on the basis of current data in current events and to make timely adjustments where necessary.

The question is always: how does adequate information management promote the work of professionals. The point is that the results that the introduction of an information system delivers to healthcare organizations lead to involvement, insight, coherence, connection, simplicity, cost savings, ease of use, completeness, reliability and timeliness. This means that with digital developments the professional (and therefore also the client's question) is central.

The perspective of clients and professionals increasingly forms the basis for the structuring of the organization. Professionals are trained to perform complex tasks. However, complexity requires a certain degree of autonomy in a decision-making sense. This autonomy enables the professional to respond quickly to new (complex) developments.

Autonomy translates organizationally into self-organization. Visser et al. (2012): quality improvement and cost reduction can be achieved by involving clients more in professional decisions. The client will increasingly determine where, when and how care is given.

Professionals will increasingly focus on each other and less and less on their own organization. With many care organizations (not all) you see that professionals focus on their own team and their 'own' clients. Self-organization promotes strong mutual solidarity. Within organizational forms (networks or care organizations), there is freedom to innovate by, for example, re-writing rules. This is where entrepreneurship of healthcare professionals comes into the spotlight (Koudstaal 2016). Because information is easily and horizontally distributed, it is easy for (new) preferences, ideas and experiences to be disseminated (Ahlers 2016).

Jeurissen (2016) states that there are large variations in the practice of care, both care focused on healing and the nursing and care of people. In itself, self-regulation and self-ordering are mechanisms for managing complex subjects. It is necessary to disclose existing knowledge in combination with real-life implementation. Real life means that existing interests and existing instruments must be taken into account (2016, 39).

Poor communication between primary care and the hospitals leads to fragmentation of care. The core of the care is: higher expectations of clients, new technologies and treatments, rise in the chronic sick and multi-morbidity, new providers. The supply thus determines the type of questions (KPMG 2014, primary care paradox). This brings the ability to deal with variety increasingly to the centre of attention.

The relationship with the client is central. It is thus not primarily about a service; it is about the relationship between people (Van der Lans 2008). Important characteristics of that relationship are (should be): accessibility, recognition of professional expertise, mutual trust, reciprocity, proximity, goal and solution orientation. To be successful, the following points for attention for participants must be worked out in a recognizable way (Minkman): client-oriented, chain management and logistics, result management, optimal care, result-oriented learning, interprofessional cooperation, role and task distribution, chain commitment and transparent entrepreneurship.

Tonkes has formulated three 'framing rules' around the organization of informal care (Tonkes, Van den Broeke and Hoytink 2008) that determine how informal care is viewed. Moral framing rules relate to what you see as your duty. Historical framing rules relate to our own history. ('We used to take better care of each other.') Pragmatic framing rules relate to what is available in the eyes of those involved. ('Everyone has a mobility scooter. Why do I have to wait so long?') Framing rules are largely determined by the organization of care in a country (2008, 14).

In a system of market forces, different framing rules apply than when the government is primarily responsible. Framing rules determine what we think we can demand and how we experience our situation. They thereby determine our 'feeling rules' about which we experience angry, disappointed etc. The combination of framing rules and feeling rules determines the life form in which care is provided.

Professionals often have a coordinating role in professional networks. In that situation, informal caregivers have less control over the way in which care is provided. Informal caregivers have more influence in mixed networks (Tonkes, Van den Broeke and Hoytink 2008). Tonkes (2008) distinguishes 5 types of networks:

- Mixed network: balanced combination of professionals, volunteers and informal caregivers. The division of tasks between informal carers and clients is often not clear in advance.
- Family networks. Care is mainly given by (mostly female) active family members. Are supplementary.
- Professional network. Informal caregivers are additional here.
- Isolated pivotal care network. Limited number of people active.

- Disappointed pivotal care network. Disappointment about the deployment of professionals.

Working in networks makes it possible to scale up healthcare. This concerns: broad services, emphasis on area-specific care, investment in IT and increasing career opportunities. With networking, the aim is to make the patient a participant in the care. There is a considerable difference in the degree of control when someone is asked to respond to something that a healthcare professional has already written or when an open conversation is conducted first. As a rule, the care plan is not immediately accessible to most clients, which means they may have an information deficit. Attention to the client's personal directorship and the provision of customized work by the healthcare professional has developed further in recent years and continues (130).

Quality in healthcare is not only about issues of individual citizens, but also about systems. In addition, it is about the position of clients (Van Leeuwen 2007). More and more consumers are going to do product innovation. This involves improving, innovating and customizing existing products and developing new products and services. Marketing is no longer aimed at customers, but is produced by them (Downes 2014). Different connections between consumers and producers are emerging: consumers are increasingly doing more on their own. It is therefore desirable that organizations look fundamentally at their own work organization (Ten Have 2011).

In the Vision Document Medical Specialist 2025, the ambition, expectations and goals for medical specialist care in 2025 are elaborated. I will discuss the possible consequences for elderly care. The provision of information within healthcare in 2025 is as follows: there is digital registration at the source (point of departure: more information and less registration). A distinction is made between three forms of information:

- 'hard' quality criteria, such as morbidity and mortality, or measurements from national registrations
- 'soft' quality criteria, such as patient responses, service measurements and individual or team assessments
- efficiency information: costs per intervention or treatment process, request or prescribing behaviour

(Elderly) care is directed towards the development of care networks of care professionals, both physically and digitally. A care network takes the needs of the client as a starting point; different players in the network can add value at different times (Van der Krogt 1995). In this way, a network of various professional expertise and informal contacts is created around a client, contributing to the care process and the quality of life.

Digital developments play an important role in this. The medical specialist plays an active role in the development, assessment and implementation of technological innovations that actually add value for the patient. That is why the patient is explicitly involved in the development, adoption and implementation of innovations. For the nurse and care professionals (Peters 2014), this means:

- More severe clients, more multi-morbidity, more complex care situations (inpatient and outpatient)
- Focus on your own health and behaviour, on participation, on what the client (with the help of social network) can still do
- More focus on prevention (prevention of deterioration)
- From caring for to ensuring that: self-reliance, self-management and self-management
- Collaboration with informal caregivers
- More ambulatory work (cross-sector teams)
- More flexibility required, more autonomy
- Working with care technology
- Digital communication and digital recording of data
- Broad deployment: different target groups, living/day care
- Working in care paths, specialized, less generic
- Increase in nursing duties, including taking over duties from doctors

The role of the nurse is therefore more focused on directing the network. High-quality and efficient care requires location and time-independent exchange and availability of information: for both care professionals and the patient and his or her caregivers. Within healthcare provision, a professional or an organization is seldom seen in isolation. Although the client regards the relationship with a professional (caretaker, nurse, doctor etc.) as central, the professional depends on the input of others. Of course, the way in which clients experience the service is important. For professionals, it is about core values and working environment being interconnected.

Between 2008 and 2011, there was a platform called Palliatieve Zorg (Poortvliet 2011). The purpose of the platform was to realize the action points in the palliative care action plan, to monitor progress and to evaluate the action plan. The platform did not opt for a focus on the primary process (healthcare provider, professional, volunteer and patient) but for a policy focus.

Poortvliet: 'As a result, projects were somewhat more abstract and not directly applicable in practice. That is why the benefits are not immediately noticeable in practice but mainly concern an indirect effect' (2011: 22). The bottleneck was identified as the fact that half of the platform members lacked a coherent and shared vision of palliative care (2011: 26). The platform had added value in the network function and for the agenda setting.

The deployment of volunteers is mainly based on standards and values that fit in to mean something to the other (Rossen 2012). Preconditions for volunteer organizations concern the provision of appreciation, satisfaction and scope for self-determination.

The elderly are entitled to driven professionals who respect their own position and role. A vision must convince clients rather than persuade them (Geursen 1996; Geursen 2000). The way of working should be organized around the problem of clients. The core values form the foundation for the decision-making process and determine how management, professionals and clients interact (Older people 2004).

Identity relates, among other things, to concepts such as (recognizable and experienced) vision, core values and motives. One of the cases studied is the 'Netwerk patiënt onderzoeksvragen' ('Network patient research questions'). The relationship between professionals and patients can be described as asymmetrical due to the difference in social status and the added value to the knowledge of both groups. Elberse (2012) therefore advocates the application of inclusion strategies. He distinguishes three categories:

- Circumstances: precautions related to preparation and organization (creating basic conditions)
- Behaviour
- Verbal interaction.

People are often unaware that they exclude others through verbal and non-verbal communication. A network offers opportunities to ensure that people feel that they are part of a group. Strategies to improve partnerships between patients and researchers should focus on training in the necessary competencies (awareness of patient participation, a positive attitude, skills and knowledge) and building a strong network structure.

Client Perspective: Platform Structures

This chapter describes a number of platforms that have been designed from a client perspective:

- 'Humanisering van de ouderenzorg' platform
- 'Nieuwe zorg' platform
- 'De Academische Werkplaats Ouderenzorg' platform
- Stichting Digitale Zorg
- Samenwerkende Academische Netwerken Ouderenzorg

- OZO Verbindzorg
- Zorgplatform ouderen
- Nationaal Programma Ouderenzorg
- BeterOud
- IkWoonLeefZorg.nl

There is a wide variety of platforms. In the context of this research, platforms were sought that provide insight into how clients are involved in the design of the services. The description mainly looks at how networks organize themselves. In the context of this research, no statements are made about the results achieved within the networks. It is specifically about how the interaction within a platform is designed.

The technology that makes remote monitoring and care possible will be increasingly used. This further strengthens self-direction (self-management) for clients. The IT infrastructure (electronic client file) supports both caregivers and professionals (Kool, Verhoef and Kremer 2014). This makes the care around the client and his or her network much more person-oriented. When determining what a client needs, the client and his or her social network become the starting point (Noddings 2002).Research into client platforms shows that clients can learn a great deal from each other. The care is in line with what the client needs and what the client's own network cannot handle (Poortvliet, Vennekens en Heine 2011).

How will platform technology strengthen the position of clients (and professionals)? Parker (2016): a platform is a business based on value-creating interactions between producers and consumers. A platform is the common basis of technologies, technological, economic and social rules and agreements (such as standards) on which multiple players can jointly develop additional technologies, products or services (Kreijveld, Deuten and Van Est 2014).

Organizations always revolve around regulating or utilizing supply and demand friction in one way or another (Strikwerda 2014). For example, a hospital organizes the demand-supply friction between people who are sick and people who can heal. Platform friction eliminates those frictions. We are thus going from organizations to organizing (Aslander (2010; 2015): occasional partnerships). IT and platforms are increasingly becoming the critical success factor for organizations. That also applies to professionals: by using platforms, you maintain your knowledge. Organizations can create access to the latest technology through their own innovation, partnerships or technology investments.

Platforms build totally new business models at a very low cost that destroy old markets. An important element is the impact of freely accessible information. Organizations are increasingly being designed as platforms (organizing). Platform technology reinforces the position of clients (and professionals). Parker: a platform is a business based on value-creating interactions between producers and consumers. Kreijveld, Van Deuten and Van Est (2014): a platform is the common basis of technologies, technological, economic and social rules and agreements (such as standards) on which multiple players can jointly develop additional technologies, products or services.

An important element is the information that is available for a client (and healthcare professionals). A personal health environment or personal health record is a website or app that gives a patient access to his own health data. This concerns data stored by, for example, the general practitioner or medical specialist in the hospital. The patient can use this data in the personal health environment and also record his or her own data.

A platform is the common basis of technologies, technological, economic and social rules and agreements (such as standards) on which multiple players can jointly develop additional technologies, products or services. For the organization of healthcare processes, this involves organizing flexible capacity, starting from the wishes and schedules of clients, providing value-driven health care (for clients) and identifying and resolving obstacles (Rummler and Brache 2013).

This leads to a completely different approach to the interaction between client and professional. Professionals play the central role in (starting to) work with the client as director. In addition to the appropriate competences and skills, they need more professional space for this and a corresponding organizational structure (network structure) (De Laat 2012).

A platform focuses, among other things, on organizational forms such as cooperatives that contribute to the elderly maintaining directorship over their lives and local collaborations. Social technology supports the ability to continue living independently. In addition, models for transmural care, early detection and prevention are being developed. In healthcare, you see an increase in apps to support the healthcare process.

Andries Baart (2013: 25) indicates that the deployment of vulnerable people must first and foremost come from themselves and then from caregivers and close neighbours. Only then will professional help and care providers get involved. On this basis, the role of citizens (citizens' initiatives) becomes increasingly important. For the organization of healthcare processes, this involves organizing flexible capacity, starting from the wishes and schedules of clients, providing value-driven health care (for clients), identifying and resolving obstacles and monitoring quality.

More and more citizens are organizing their own care or setting up platforms for their own neighbourhood: mijnbuurtje.nl, buuv.nl, burenetwerkwerk.nl, voordebuurt.nl. There will be insight into one's own health via the Medical Internet of Everything model. This is, for example, advice to preventively improve one's own lifestyle. If treatment is required, the platform helps to make choices. Healthcare providers can then offer services themselves.

It has already been established that the Dutch health care system is on its way to an environment that has (more) dynamics and customers who 'will pay and determine (more) themselves' (Boer and Croon 2011).

By introducing a platform strategy, personal directorship and control is increased. This concerns the principle of 'open' innovations (Chesbrough). In addition, it is not only about developing innovations, but more about how the invented innovations are organized (Elsen 2017). Key words here are: self-organization, close social networks and cooperation with customers. It is about virtualizing organizations: professionals develop in the conversation with clients.

Zohar (2017) indicates that new organizational concepts are based on: trust in people and in the system; building relationships and teams; remaining flexible and in dialogue with changing circumstances; being open and ready for all kinds of possible future scenarios (Harari 2016). It also means more emphasis on meaning, vision and values, in particular the value of service. Especially the conversation (and being able to listen) between client and professional is essential.

Professionals play a role in understanding client needs, being able to collaborate with other professionals on the basis of self-organization, room for experimentation and being able to give account. Partly due to the tight labour market for elderly care, interest in remote care is increasing. An example of ehealth is the 'Alfred' programme of the European Commission. Apps and sensors are being developed that make speech commands easier and transmit signals to professionals and caregivers.

Care processes are organized differently under the influence of digitalization. Sensor technology ('guiding environment') works as a memory aid for a resident with early dementia. An example is care organization Siza, which has developed tailored homes for people with disabilities. The home has smart apps and applications.

An effective organization model is aimed at an adequate implementation of a care process in which various products and expertise are set up in conjunction. The criteria used for this are: matching clients' wishes (demand-driven), efficient and effective access to healthcare, adequate information provision, creating connections between professionals, defining the funding basis and determining the management model of healthcare.

There is a growing number of platforms in elderly care. The *platform 'Humanisering van de ouderenzorg' ('Humanization of elderly care')* focuses on clarifying (through lectures) what good elderly care is and how you create space for sensemaking questions. Through the Ouderenzorg platform, researchers from the University for Humanistics share their knowledge and expertise about elderly care with professionals and volunteers. The platform is coordinated by the professor of Care Ethical Aspects of Informal Care and the special professor of Empowerment of Vulnerable Elderly Persons.

The platform *'Nieuwe zorg'* ('New Healthcare') organizes, among other things, the healthcare debate in which politicians, healthcare providers, patient organizations and healthcare insurers enter into discussions with each other about elderly care. Stichting Digitale zorg (digital care platform) is an initiative for and by people who are active in the field of care, IT and innovation. The aim is to contribute to the successful development and implementation of ZorgICT initiatives and innovation. To realize this, knowledge and news from inside and outside the Netherlands (EU) are collected, knowledge is shared and activities are developed.

The platform 'De Academische Werkplaats Ouderenzorg' ('The Academic Workplace for Elderly Care'; AWO) is a virtual workplace in Limburg. The work is being done at various locations within the various organizations. Maastricht University plays an intermediary role and creates the connection between research, practice and policy. A senior researcher from Maastricht University is associated with each healthcare institution involved.

The six *'Samenwerkende Academische Netwerken Ouderenzorg'* ('Cooperating Academic Networks for Elderly Care'; SANO) now have structural funding. The additional structural financing, which is implemented by ZonMw, provides new knowledge about, for example, the effects of innovations in the organization of care for the elderly, smart connections to the labour market and further improvement of the quality of nursing home care. This new knowledge becomes available nationwide for all nursing homes in the Netherlands.

OZO *Verbindzorg* is a digital platform for healthcare providers in the western part of the Achterhoek, driven by patients themselves. The various care providers, such as the general practitioner, home help and caregiver, will soon be able to contact each other via the platform. The client decides which of the aid providers can access the platform. When the client himself is unable to manage the platform, this task can be placed in the hands of a family member or caregiver after consultation. However, the client always remains leading. OZOverbindzorg stands for collaboration and sharing of care. All parties (informal caregivers, family and care providers) involved in the care and welfare of a client are brought together. A network is formed around the client, where the client decides who will participate.

'Zorgplatform ouderen' offers knowledge and expertise with regard to care for vulnerable elderly people. It is about offering instruments, guides for practice nurses and practice assistants. The platform is an initiative of V&VN Praktijkverpleegkundigen.

The Nationaal Programma Ouderenzorg ran from 2008 to 2016 (125 care projects). It concerned innovative projects to organize care and support differently. The 1st phase of the national programme Ouderenzorg ran from 2008 to 2013 and had a budget of 80 million euros. From this, 75 transition experiments, research projects and implementation projects, and 8 regional networks were funded. This programme was about improving care for the elderly with complex requests for help; the elderly were explicitly involved themselves (Bussemaker 2019).

Many experiments are about the different organization of care and welfare based on the demand of the elderly. Many projects are about the timely detection of problems in the elderly, the preparation of a care plan and proper alignment and coordination. The second phase ran from 2014 to 2016 and had a budget of 9 million euros. This money is intended to further disseminate and guarantee the results. The BeterOud platform and the 8 regional networks ensure this.

The *BeterOud* platform was developed by Movisie and Vilans. It is made possible by ZonMw. There is collaboration with and it comes from the 'Nationaal Programma Ouderenzorg' ('National Programme for Elderly Care'; NPO). There is collaboration with Habion, Movisie, KBO-PCOB, NVOG/KNVG, ROS network, Social Work Netherlands and Vilans. In addition, the Laego and Pharos organizations are closely involved. BeterOud focuses on coming up with and developing new initiatives.

Rabobank has set up *IkWoonLeefZorg.nl*. Here, information is collected about longer independent living (technical and digital support), care and assistance, finances and social activities. Woonz.nl offers information about senior housing-related services. The ikwordzzp'er platform focuses on information for starting sole proprietors.

The wide variety of platforms makes it difficult to get a clear picture. On the one hand (OZOverbindzorg), there is an explicit choice for a central positive of clients. A number of other platforms are aimed at giving substance to the renewal of elderly care from the professional domain. The issue of elderly care is taken as the point of departure.

Care Technology Perspective: Platformvmz

Platform Verbinden-met-Zorg ('Connect-with-Care'; PlatformVmZ) is set up as an infrastructure for care professionals (self-employed professionals), care institutions and clients so that they are facilitated as optimally as possible and was co-founded by me. Since January 1, 2017, PlatformVmZ has focused on district nursing and in particular on non-contracted independent care professionals (self-employed professionals) and (smaller) care institutions. The infrastructure is set up in accordance with the nationally applicable conditions and standards. At the moment, there are approximately 1300 sole proprietors affiliated with PlatformVmZ as well as 100 (smaller) care institutions.

In addition, a client portal has been set up (CuraeVitel Balie) that, in addition to care services, also offers living and comfort services for the elderly who want to continue living independently at home for as long as possible. The elderly also receive support in navigating through the care system.

Platform technology creates new ecosystems that connect clients, partners and providers (Evans 2016). This leads to a more integrated approach and ensures that quality is improved and costs are reduced. A platform is the common basis of technologies, technological, economic and social rules and agreements (such as standards) on which multiple players can jointly develop additional technologies, products or services (Parker 2016). For the organization of healthcare processes, this involves organizing flexible capacity, starting from the wishes and schedules of clients, providing value-driven health care (for clients) and identifying and resolving obstacles (Kuiper, Van Amelsfoort and Kramer 2010).

The platform for entrepreneurs in the healthcare sector was launched in 2017 (www.platformVmZ.nl). A client portal (www.CuraeVitelBalie.nl) was set up in 2018 so that clients can arrange care themselves online. In 2019, a subsidy was granted under the subsidy scheme Stimulering E-Health Thuis (Stimulation of E-Health at Home; SET) to make the client portal accessible to a broad group of clients.

The PlatformVmZ has network relationships with health insurers, health care institutions, interest groups in health care, general practitioners, hospitals and the Ministry of Health, Welfare and Sport. From CuraeVitel Balie, there are network contacts with general practitioners, hospitals, health insurers, patient associations, Per Saldo and municipalities.

Digitalization makes the relationship between clients and healthcare providers fundamentally different. Clients are increasingly gaining insight into their own limitations and the behaviour of professionals. This development will lead to the strengthening of self-management for clients. The information management of a care organization must be adjusted accordingly. In addition, there is an increasingly precise form of (material) control.

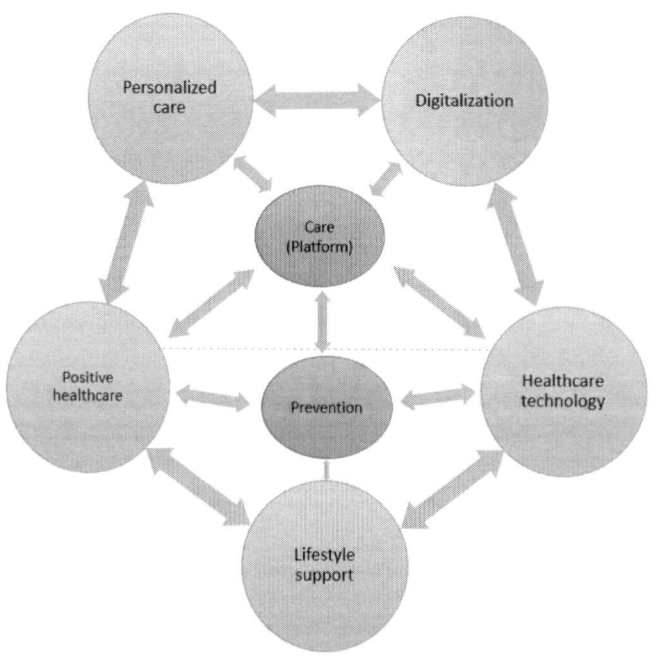

Figure 9. Care platform (prepared by Thomas Woldendorp).

Small healthcare institutions will increasingly come into the picture if their (administrative) accountability is not in order. For large healthcare institutions, more and more attention is being paid to monitoring and protecting data. The approach is based on an (integrated) connection between care content, organizational form and IT infrastructure.The PlatformVmZ was established to shape healthcare much more from this perspective.

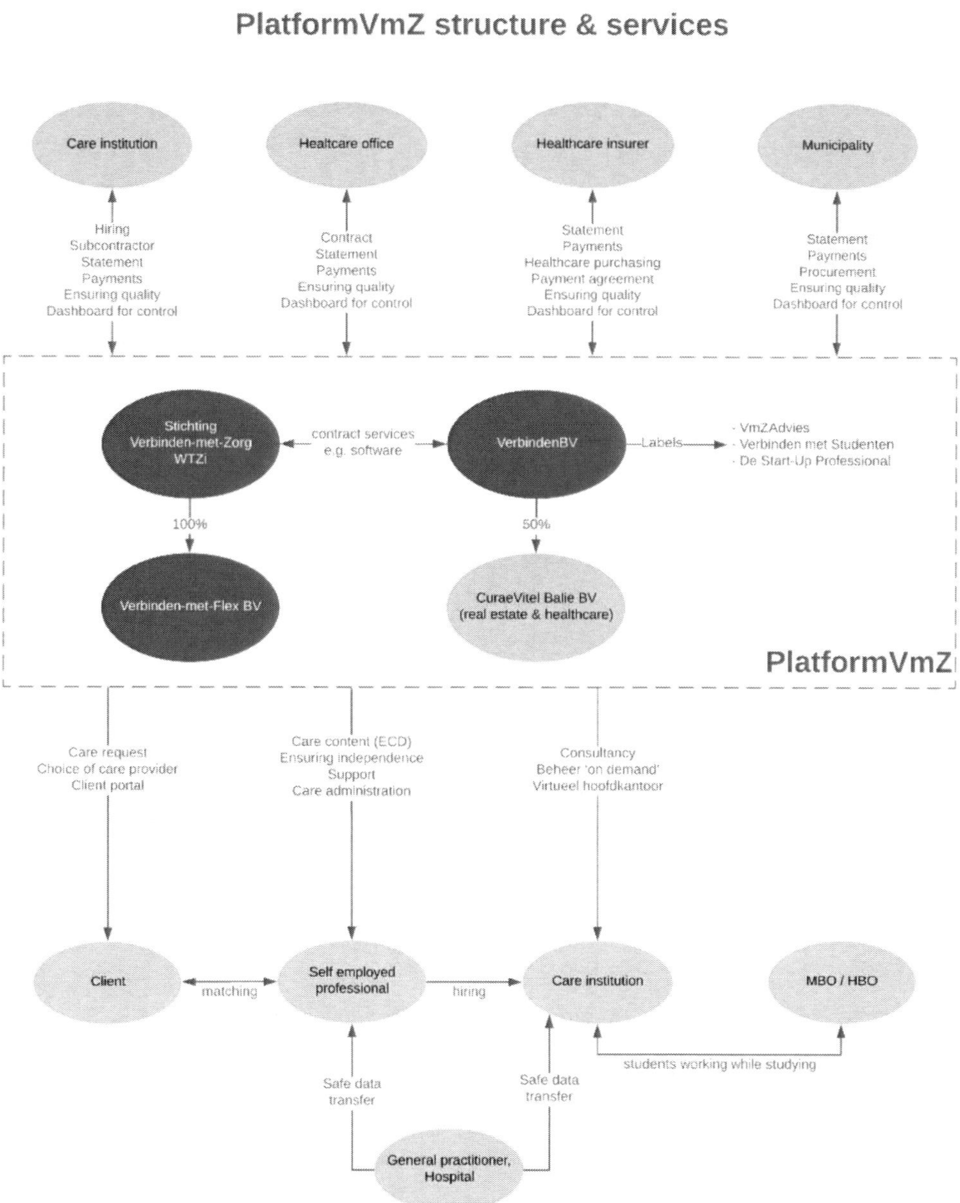

Figure 10. Structure of PlatformVmZ (prepared by Sander Duindam).

Bloem argues for personalized care: care contributes to the person's own perception of health benefits. This is possible if the care is transparent: What is the effectiveness, quality and cost of care? The PlatformVmZ is of the opinion that the steering role is very important in this: How do I keep a grip on what is happening around me? That is why a personal client portal (CuraeVitel Balie) has been developed that makes it possible for care recipients to follow (and determine) what should happen around them. The PlatformVmZ is designed to take the individual diversity (variety) of clients as a starting point. The PlatformVmZ therefore has a private client portal so that clients themselves can act as the 'head office'. Clients are supported with access to care (Wme, Zvw and Wlz). Clients have insight into profiles of healthcare professionals who match their healthcare needs. The choice for certain healthcare professionals lies with the client. Clients have insight into the balance between the indicated care and the care provided. They (or the authorized network) have insight into the care plan and the communication between care professionals.

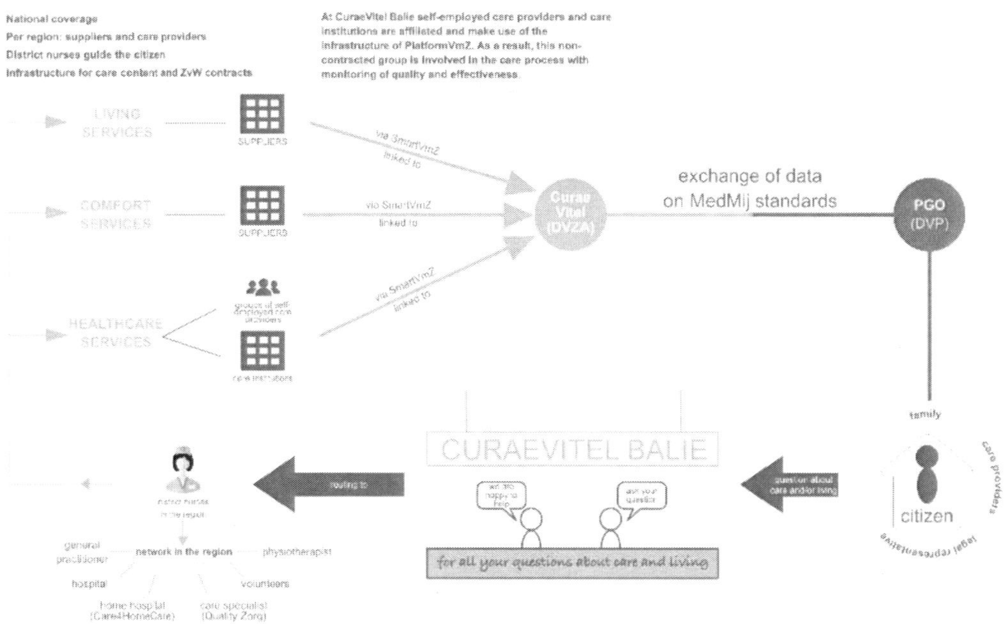

Figure 11. CuraeVitel Balie, prepared by Sander Duindam.

By introducing a platform strategy, personal directorship and control is increased. As a professional, you can achieve the high-quality realization of your profession from the platform technology. Thanks to the platform technology, the clients are directly at the wheel. Next to a platform for self-employed professionals, a client portal for the elderly has been set up. At CuraeVitel Balie, it is all about living and care that adds value for the citizen.

The CureaVitel Balie is also set up as a helpdesk to which all citizens in the Netherlands can address questions about the use of care or living or comfort services at home. The citizen is guided by the Personal Digital Assistant with these questions. In this way, access to health care (Zvw, Wmo, Wlz) becomes much easier for citizens.

The IGJ (Inspection of Healthcare and Youth) has issued a new assessment framework for inpatient care. The wishes and desires of the client are the starting point for providing care. Characteristics of the relationship between professional and client are:

- Professional knows the client (history; what is important etc.)
- Relationship is balanced and respectful
- Listening ear for client and his or her loved ones
- Client is in control.

At the end of 2016, this framework was established for networks of professionals who provide care to vulnerable clients who live at home. The most important starting points are:

- Client perspective: contribution of care to his or her adaptability and personal directorship;
- Networks: working in conjunction between professional care providers, informal caregivers and volunteers;
- Vulnerable clients: testing specifically against citizens with the greatest risks;
- Standards: from the client's perspective;
- Role of IGJ: quality of care.

This assessment framework has the following themes:

- Client-centred: need for care established in consultation with client; client has insight into care process; strengthening self-reliance and directorship;
- Integrated care: the client experiences that professionals have mutual contact and that the care is coordinated;
- Informal care: caregivers can count on professionals taking their capabilities into account;
- Safety: risks in the area of the home/living situation, medication safety, domestic violence reporting code, medical aids and medical technology are signalled in time by the care provider.

Through the platform, care providers (and clients) become involved with the aforementioned themes. For example, it is possible to identify early and monitor where any deviations from the testing standards occur. Healthcare professionals are supported on all aspects of an independent fulfilment of their role: assessment, preparation of care plan, planning, registration hours, invoicing and invoicing, guaranteeing independence and support for professionalism. This applies to the (recursion) level of individual interpretation, team and healthcare company (for example, healthcare cooperative).

There is currently clear growth in the number of independently working care professionals (currently around 121,000 self-employed professionals work in care, 10% of the total; Trouw). In view of the various developments, PlatformVmZ is focused in this phase on supporting healthcare professionals who want to work as an entrepreneur (individually or collectively) within the healthcare sector. To be able to guarantee independence, the affiliated self-employed professionals are fully autonomous in their actions. There is monitoring of the applicable laws and regulations, and the district nursing standards framework applies.

In view of the analyses from the past year and a half, PlatformVmZ has obtained a good picture of how non-contracted independent care providers (self-employed professionals) act:

- Knowledge of legislation and regulations with regard to healthcare (administration and content) is moderate;
- Moderate knowledge of conditions for (non-) contracted care;
- Little intervision, peer evaluation and other promotion of expertise;
- Money driven (would rather deliver care to a client who needs a high number of hours of care than many clients with a low need for care);
- A group of independent district nurses has as its core business the setting of indications.

In these cases, these district nurses also provide a great many indications (> 200 on an annual basis). As a result, the care process is under pressure, less time for coordination, monitoring, more frequent evaluation within six months and no involvement with clients.

PlatformVmZ is set up as an infrastructure. This means that self-employed professionals and organizations in the care sector make use of the services with which they can function at a high level in legal, care-related and care-administration areas. The VMZ platform has its own model agreements that guarantee independence in outpatient care and inpatient care.

The client has insight into and management of the care providers, can determine the planning himself, has insight into the budget (with PGB) and the course of the care process. Because this information is collected in a client portal, the family can also follow what is happening and make adjustments (remotely). To promote efficiency, the aim is to reduce (minimize) the existing practice variation in the area of indication. This is done by standardizing (and digitally supporting) the indication process.

The infrastructure that PlatformVmZ has set up not only involves a digital platform (ECD) or the (online) matching of care providers to care questions/assignments, agreements are also concluded by PlatformVmZ with care providers and health insurers. In addition, partnerships are entered into with companies that offer new opportunities for (independent) care providers.

Within the Platform VmZ, the Electronic Client Dossier (ECD) is set up on the basis of the work processes as carried out by a healthcare professional. In addition to the ECD, the platform also has its own matching software with which services (care requests) and availability of care professionals are brought together in a simple manner. The demand for care is related to a profile (expertise level, experience, reserved procedures, travel distance, etc.). Balance is thus achieved in a simple way.

The PlatformVmZ is designed in such a way that the model of person-bound funding and a personal health environment can be easily arranged. The client is aware of the care to be used during the entire care process and is in direct contact with the self-employed professionals. The client portal developed by PlatformVmZ is based on a number of assumptions: the client is optimally in control of healthcare; the client has full insight and management of their own data/file; the client must be able to determine who has access to what data (informal caregiver, family, GP); the client must be able to participate actively in the care process, for example by recording data themselves (reporting, measuring, social contacts, communication, agreements etc.); client has full access to their own data such as care plan, agreements, agenda/planning, documents; digitally sign care plans, agreements, deployment of care; The client must be able to communicate easily regarding the quality and deployment of care.

Our partner Deladus Healthcare Systems Group argues that all over the world, healthcare providers are data rich but poor on insights, mainly due to siloed applications, legacy data models, shadow IT and lack of budget to gain value from the vast amount of data they already have.

Patient data integration across providers, processes (clinical, administrative, public health and clinical research) and IT systems is the cornerstone of digitalization. With an "intelligent" data integration platform, integration is not only regarded as data aggregation, but also as the ability to integrate different stakeholders across the care continuum, as well as existing vendors in an application architecture ecosystem.

The call is to empower healthcare stakeholders to engage more effectively and realize value-based and consumer-driven healthcare. The focus is on supporting patient and client experiences by enabling new digital capabilities, operational efficiencies and enhanced levels of (clinical) effectiveness.

Healthcare can be provided by platforms that benefit patients with more convenience, personalization and value. A digital health platform can create the scenario needed to better integrate traditional and next-generational interoperability services for analytical and operational workloads that leverage historical data (i.e., patient records, clinical research, reimbursements) and data streams (from medical devices, logistics systems, wearables, etc.) to assemble new information bridges and streams. The ensuing information fabric can better support real-time decision making and intelligently driven workflows while empowering organizations to gain elastic infrastructure properties that make future gains towards better levels of business agility.

Cloud-based digital health platforms can lay down the foundations for that transition and digitally transform the identity of healthcare organizations from traditional to next-generational innovation. To make an integrated healthy outcomes ecosystem a reality, it's necessary to have a platform that leverages industry standards, such as Fast Healthcare Interoperability Resources (FHIR), to allow the exchange of data.

For Dedalus Healthcare Systems and PlatformVmZ digitalization is not about technology for the sake of technology, but about leveraging it to offer all stakeholders (the patients, most importantly) a seamless care experience across the healthcare journey:

Our partner Deladus Healthcare Systems Group argues that all over the world, healthcare providers are data rich but poor on insights, mainly due to siloed applications, legacy data models, shadow IT and lack of budget to gain value from the vast amount of data they already have.

Patient data integration across providers, processes (clinical, administrative, public health and clinical research) and IT systems is the cornerstone of digitalization. With an "intelligent" data integration platform, integration is not only regarded as data aggregation, but also as the ability to integrate different stakeholders across the care continuum, as well as existing vendors in an application architecture ecosystem.

The call is to empower healthcare stakeholders to engage more effectively and realize value-based and consumer-driven healthcare. The focus is on supporting patient and client experiences by enabling new digital capabilities, operational efficiencies and enhanced levels of (clinical) effectiveness.

Healthcare can be provided by platforms that benefit patients with more convenience, personalization and value. A digital health platform can create the scenario needed to better integrate traditional and next-generational interoperability services for analytical and operational workloads that leverage historical data (i.e., patient records, clinical research, reimbursements) and data streams (from medical devices, logistics systems, wearables, etc.) to assemble new information bridges and streams. The ensuing information fabric can better support real-time decision making and intelligently driven workflows while empowering organizations to gain elastic infrastructure properties that make future gains towards better levels of business agility.

Cloud-based digital health platforms can lay down the foundations for that transition and digitally transform the identity of healthcare organizations from traditional to next-generational innovation. To make an integrated healthy outcomes ecosystem a reality, it's necessary to have a platform that leverages industry standards, such as Fast Healthcare Interoperability Resources (FHIR), to allow the exchange of data.

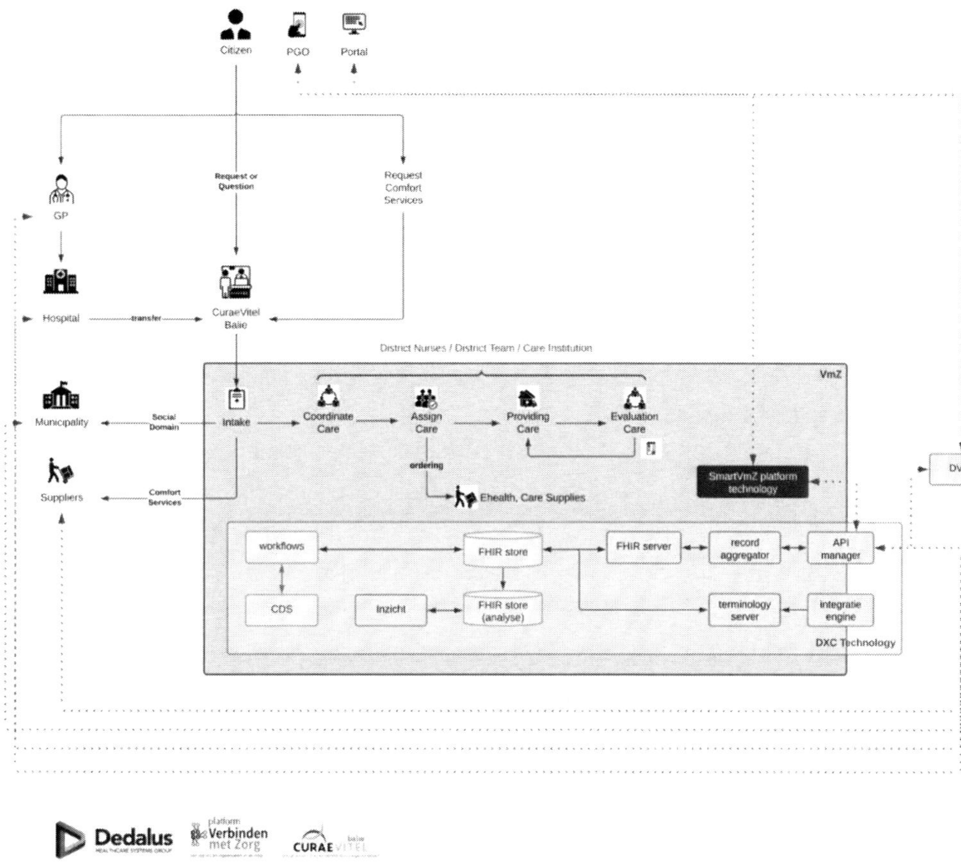

Figure 12. Prepared by Remco van Kralingen en Sander Duindam.

For Dedalus Healthcare Systems and PlatformVmZ digitalization is not about technology for the sake of technology, but about leveraging it to offer all stakeholders (the patients, most importantly) a seamless care experience across the healthcare journey.

Conclusion

There is much talk about demand management, but little actual demand management is implemented. This also applies to putting clients at the centre: some of the clients do not so much need direction, but rather that care be available. Many clients like that they do not have to arrange the care themselves. There is often limited assertiveness. On the other hand, clients who do want that directorship to have to deal with obstacles with healthcare professionals and healthcare organizations. The question is whether the current system design is not too restrictive. This is apparent, for example, from how complex the application for a Person-Bound Budget (PGB) is. The role of the Social Insurance Bank is purely focused on checking accountability. There is no interaction about substantive considerations.

The professional practice of care professionals shows that work processes are the main focus, not the client. Residents have power in one of De Hoven's locations (narrative perspective). This leads to a completely different organization of work processes.

Changes will only occur through a fundamental shift in the influence position of clients. In addition, changes to the financing and the structure of the health care system (position of insured persons) are necessary to achieve this. The impact of technology on the labour market problem is much greater than is currently thought. This means that care provisioncan be carried out with fewer care professionals. Practice shows that the innovative capacity of healthcare professionals is actually present in every system.

Partly due to the development of citizens' initiatives and care cooperatives, there is a movement towards a stronger position for clients. Good care starts with a home environment that makes self-reliance possible. That is why the connection between living and care is essential. In addition, a shift in the influence position is feasible for a proportion of the elderly; however, 30% are unable to fulfil such a role. In addition, there is also a great deal of demand shyness. It is precisely through citizens' initiatives that a certain degree of equivalence is created. A role for healthcare professionals is to make personal directorship possible.

Demand management: It is important to be clear what equality means. It is not about equality (healthcare professional has unique expertise) but about the structuring of the interaction. Much is determined by the conceptual system that clients and professionals use. That is why it is important to make explicit what is meant by personal directorship. One aspect of that definition is clarification about the difference between willing and able.

This is a core task for policymakers (administrators): ensuring that clients and professionals do not suffer from the (alleged) bureaucracy.

Technology impact: testing grounds, however, show that large effects can already be achieved with the help of technology in the home situation. However, the turning point to a broad commitment has not yet been reached. Knowledge of the technological possibilities is essential to achieve them. Technology also requires the skills to cope with it. Broad application leads to other forms of individual care provision.

Personal directorship: starts with citizens themselves. A citizen must be capable of actually fulfilling that director's role. Then a new dynamic is created between client and healthcare professional. Choices become easier if information about healthcare is easily accessible. In the current system design, it is difficult that an immediate policy framework often arises in the event of an incident.

Personal directorship can also mean that a conscious decision is made not to want to have directorship. Professionals have long been trained within the perspective that 'they know better'. This proves difficult to let go of in practice. Through more ownership with clients, the system design will develop more dynamically. Precisely by giving direction, the interaction between client and professional changes. The network around a client also offers the opportunity to introduce new perspectives.

Quality can be defined as care provision that matches the demand a client has. Here, too, language is essential: quality of life leads to different considerations than quality of care. Much attention is already being paid to reflection within the study programme. However, it appears to be very difficult to find enough space and time to devote to reflection in work practice. The work practice is characterized by a 'do-it-yourself' culture. From the study programme, it is therefore desirable to pay more attention to how reflection forms an integral part of work practice. From within the organization, it is important to give space to reflective practice in the work processes. Attention to the financing system is important. Health insurers are already developing forms of joint financing (partly with the client). With regard to forms of personal funding or forms of population funding, mutual trust is the core theme. The point is that a new funding system is based on the individuality of the client in relation to the healthcare provider.

Working with a Personal Health Environment (PGO) has a high degree of future-proofing, provided that the client can handle his or her own information in a user-friendly manner.

SUMMARY

The interaction between client and professional is about insight into self-organization:

For clients, strengthening the director's role means less variety: the client gets (more or less) what he or she asks for. For the professional, the variety increases from this perspective. The system theory provides a framework for the interpretation of variety.

The word system is loaded in healthcare: the system world is set against the (intended) living world. A system is defined from the system theory:

- A system is a collection of relationships between elements.
- A system is determined by an observer.
- A system is what it does.

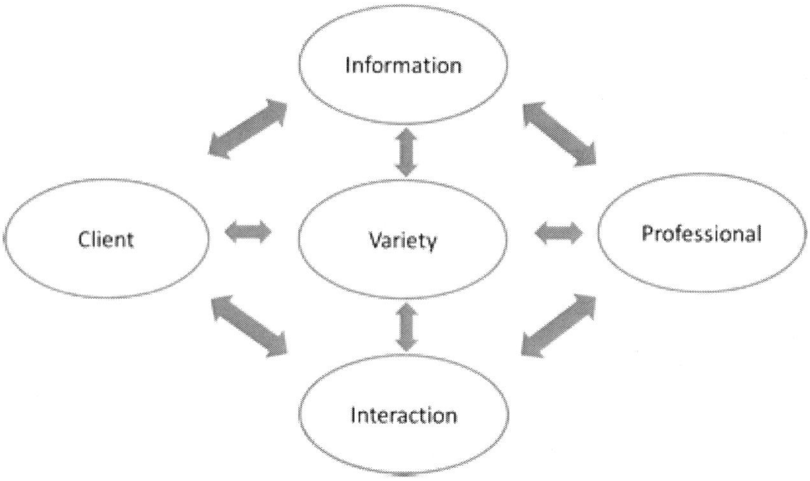

Figure 13. Model of self-organization (prepared by Thomas Woldendorp).

The interaction between client and healthcare professional is a system. Implementing 'Back to the intention' (Hart 2012) is a system. The core is to strengthen the autonomy and management role of the client and to support and thereby strengthen the entrepreneurship (entrepreneurial behaviour) of professionals. We started with the explanation that the roles will shift. This shift leads to two forms of variety:

- For the client, variety decreases when the individuality of the client is central.
- For the professional, the variety increases because the individuality of each client is central to the interaction

This means that new forms of interaction between client and professional are needed. The underlying principle is that there is clarity (back and forth) about the assumptions underlying the interaction. In addition, the role of the care recipient is different from that of the care provider. There is asymmetry in the roles: the person requiring care is dependent. However, there is equality in the relationship: both care recipient and care provider bring their own person (identity). This has been worked out in detail in presence-based theory (Baart 2011).

The interaction takes place in a context that is rapidly transforming. New forms of care provision are emerging through technology and digitalization. This may involve predictive care, but also clients who organize themselves via, for example, a platform in order to gain more influence on the care process. This is about the connection between technological innovation and social innovation. Technological innovation has various components: Home, Garden and Kitchen Technology, but also the application possibilities of artificial intelligence. Social innovation is reflected in, for example, healthcare cooperatives.

Social innovation is expressed in various ways to achieve more autonomy. An important part is that clients have access to their own health information. In terms of policy, it is about interpreting demand-driven management: the organization of care on the basis of an equal position between client and care professional, whereby the client has the relevant health information available. Interacting with each other in a certain way creates a form of life however, it can also be interpreted differently. for both, it is about finding meaning in which the unequal roles lead to equal people. Important elements are:

- Understanding of each other's position
- Reflection on the own position
- Provision of information that matches the client's wishes and approach of the care professional
- Information provision that meets the needs of informal caregivers
- Funding model that facilitates equivalence
- Space for professionals to handle variety (innovation of regulatory space)

Preconditions as a result of digitalization are:

- Digitalization leads to predictive and precision medicine. Interaction must be designed on the basis of newly available information. Possibilities of self-management for clients are increasing; healthcare professional is expected to respond to client preferences. The client shifts from being a consumer to a prosumer.
- The way in which information provision is arranged determines interaction: involve clients in the establishment of a Personal Health Environment (PGO).
- Regulatory space for professionals is increased; new organizational concepts are needed that are founded on the system concepts of variety, balance and recursion.

The added value of this approach is strengthening the position of clients). To achieve this, the added value of five perspectives was examined:

- Narrative perspective: attention and respect for the life story
- Self-managing perspective: attention and respect for the professional role
- Network perspective: trying to give substance to an integrated approach
- Client perspective: trying to give substance to the positioning of clients in the care process
- Care technology perspective: giving substance to a digital living and working practice

In these perspectives, the way in which the interaction between the client and the healthcare professional is designed is differentiated. The starting point is the extent to which the client can manage. Here, too, it applies that no single one of these perspectives is decisive, but that a mix of approaches is always sought depending on the context. That context is the position and preference of the client. Translated to the five perspectives:

- Narrative perspective: Stories are central to the interaction. One challenge is the translation into working practice.
- Self-managing perspective: The autonomy of professionals is central. A challenge is to sufficiently involve the client perspective in the interaction as well. At Buurtzorg, there can be a closed ideology that hinders reflection.
- Network perspective: Interaction is shaped by creating cohesion. The challenge for many networks is organizational hassle that actually impedes interaction.
- Client perspective: Client preference and needs are central. The challenge is to link these preferences to management of the care process.
- Care technology perspective: Preference, information and management are linked. The challenge is to let clients navigate in the care system.

From the system approach, it has been indicated that the interaction must be completed from an open system perspective. It is not the case that one of these perspectives is decisive. Depending on the context, a mix of perspectives provides added value. Perspectives cannot be taken for granted. It is about creating coherence around individual questions where one's own lifestyle remains central. In addition, this approach also states that not everyone can come along: there are also clients with limited self-reliance.

The relationship between language and reality requires insight (reflection) into one's own standards. This insight makes new ways of acting (enactment) possible. Shared meaning is essential for effective interaction between client and healthcare professional. Sensemaking involves underlying (often unclear) assumptions under the interaction. A meaningful dialogue is about insight and respect for the meaning of the client and that of the healthcare professional.

Although there is a need for a clear conceptual framework, words and concepts are context-dependent. A translation issue arises here. The interaction is effective if the position of the other can be understood. The story of a client is often translated by the healthcare professional into their own professional domain. This translation removes the variety from that story and thus impedes sensemaking. Interaction by definition takes place in a certain context. Healthcare often starts with a biased view of the patient. There is often categorization where someone with an illness or disability is seen as that disability. That is precisely why this chapter focuses on empowerment: disease and management come together in balance. A multiple perspective is created.

If the position of the client is strengthened, the variety (of the offering) decreases for the client: there is a connection to his own needs and not that these needs have to fit into a certain offer. The opposite applies to healthcare professionals: recognition and acknowledgement of the uniqueness of a client leads to an increase in variety in care provision. It becomes necessary to be able to provide a new interpretation of the interaction from a system perspective.

To do justice to the uniqueness of every client situation, attention is needed to the context and a broad perspective. This can be achieved by giving clients a role in the design of the care process, whereby digitalization and technology are a precondition. By working from an integral approach (preventive, care and wellness) and principles of self-management, the positive aspects of the client are strengthened, and new opportunities for participation are created. For clients, technological possibilities will increase. However, this requires clients to keep abreast of technological developments, digital skills and their own interpretation of data (Morgens 2019). Digital skills are also needed for care professionals (www.digivaardigindezorg.nl). Vulnerable groups such as the elderly are often less able to find and use ehealth applications. This can lead to greater inequality in healthcare (Bolman 2019).

Participation requires a context in which self-organization is central. Within society, there is increasing pressure on individual responsibility and self-reliance of citizens. This applies to both clients and informal caregivers. Personal care offers a quality model that is focused on the client perspective. Directorship requires a form of activating action. However, client situations are also characterized by vulnerability. There are complex healthcare issues that require a broad perspective from the healthcare professional. In that context, a clear role of the client is essential. Care can be made suitable through better insight into the life story of a client.

The model of person-focused care consists of the following three core elements: the care relationship, the context in which care is provided and the results. Daily care is provided in the interaction between client and healthcare professional. The point is that care professionals pay attention to each individual elderly person (Emmelot 2019).

The context in which care is provided is designed in such a way that personal care is the starting point. The results of personal care are the core element; what matters is the effect on clients. The client experiences his or her own competence when the healthcare professionals see them as individuals and act accordingly. Then the values do not have to be the same. The complexity of elderly care can be felt by both clients and healthcare professionals. To ensure that innovations work for the elderly in a positive way, it is important to take the living environment of the elderly (their preferences, wishes, experiences and their meaning) as a starting point for changes (Luijkx 2014, 19).

Complex problems do not require a simplifying approach but a broad diagnosis (Buurman 2018, 8). It is essential to involve clients with a complex demand for care in improving care and using technology (Buurman 2018; Zwakhalen 2018). This means:

- Client experiences must be actively used to achieve improvements in healthcare.
- Justice must be done to the complexity of the demand for care.
- Healthcare professionals and healthcare organizations are jointly responsible for the outcomes of healthcare.
- Healthcare professionals are facilitated by the training of competencies (Buurman 2018, 9).

Self-management determines the quality of life and is increasingly emphasized by the chronically ill and (vulnerable) elderly. Self-management is about 'the capacity and skills of a person to experience a certain degree of balance and well-being even in old age despite age-related losses, with the aim of maintaining or achieving the best possible quality of life' (Vilans 2007). The core of the interaction is that the client and the care professional find a way of working that best suits the client and his situation.

What is needed is for professionals to increase their learning capacity. This requires an innovative working environment and a learning model that is focused on results. The increasing complexity of care requires that the logic of the professional and the logic of the client become aligned. The starting point for this is acting on the basis of trust and accountability. Personal functioning is central.

Regulatory space can be filled in from entrepreneurial action. Here action, responsibility and accountability are central. The competencies and skills that are expected from a healthcare professional fit well with personal entrepreneurship. A model that allows reflection on this personal entrepreneurship is the start-up method. This is about being able to deal with uncertainty and being able to show resilience and courage.

Central are the concepts of professional, personal entrepreneurship and start-up approach. The above-described increase in variety in the care process requires, according to the elaborated system principles, two approaches: damping the variety through standardization of care and strengthening the variety by increasing professionals' room to manoeuvre.

We see a struggle to deal with this in care organizations: on the one hand, forms of self- management and self-organization are chosen; on the other hand, those forms are being phased out.

What is needed is for professionals to increase their learning capacity. This requires an innovative working environment and a learning model that is focused on results. The increasing complexity of care requires that the logic of the professional and the logic of the client become aligned. The starting point for this is acting on the basis of trust and accountability. Personal functioning is central.

In the interaction with the client, insight is always needed into the specific context in which that client is located. A better digital and technological working environment can support the professional in the organization of care. Digitalization and healthcare technology only work effectively if it is a normal part of healthcare practice. Directing one's own life is difficult if that life is vulnerable. Personal directorship means: the ability to arrange your own life and necessary support and the practical ability to be self-sufficient in physical, social and psychological terms. If a healthcare professional has a certain perspective on the dependence of the elderly, that usually determines what is seen and how we will behave. Healthcare interventions stem from professional practice. These interventions must be in balance with the perspective of a client.

The key is that by strengthening the position of the client, the variety for the client decreases, and for the healthcare professional, it increases. Because the needs of the client are central, the variety for a healthcare professional increases. After all, every client has his or her own context. For organizations, this must lead to regulatory space for professionals. For clients, the variety decreases. The client receives what is needed in the right way.

Due to the described increasing complexity, open systems are needed. This requires a different role interpretation of healthcare professionals. Central to the interaction with the preferences of clients is reflection on their own actions. The system approach makes it possible to interpret these various aspects of the interaction cohesively and to act on the basis of that interpretation. The healthcare professional can work effectively in a healthcare practice of increasing complexity (caused by variety) if the self-regulatory capacity (learning, agility, adaptation) is strengthened. The healthcare professional determines the extent to which the variety is dampened or strengthened:

- Make sure in the interaction that both the perspective of clients and the perspective of professionals can be reflected;
- Make more use of the narrative approach and the presentation theory to maintain a view of the individual identity of the client (dealing with variety);
- Ensure an information management system that supports clients' own management (user-friendly);
- Work out a funding model based on the individuality of the client.

There are no certainties in advance in the interaction between client and professional. Handling variety is the core of the interaction between client and healthcare professional. Because the client can have more self-management (decrease in variety), the healthcare professional has to handle more variety due to the individual diversity. A system is viable if it can handle variety. This always requires a search for balance and reinforcement of the adaptive capacity: the healthcare professional is able to deal with the various individual contexts. Quality, effectiveness and efficiency take place in interaction. The client has a central role in that: it is about how the client experiences the various interventions and what possibilities they have for management. For the professional, it is about creating a working environment that guarantees quality of care (and offers opportunities for improvement), for optimal digital support (reduction of administrative burden and possibility of feedback on one's own professional actions) and for a method of organization where self-organization is paramount.

A meaningful dialogue is only possible if there is respect for the views of the client and the healthcare professional. It is precisely about equality. A reality is constructed every time in the interaction between the client and the healthcare professional. The narrative approach has added value here.Baart shows that, at the moment, there is a big difference between the position of the client and the care professional. This pattern is broken by the effects of digitalization and more insight into processes of sensemaking. It is about balancing understanding of the professional conceptual apparatus and understanding of the other person. The process of providing healthcare is always about shared understanding (agreement, consensus) between two or more people about suitable procedures, interpretations and actions with regard to a care demand. This leads to the following preconditions for meaningful interaction:

- Awareness of professional dominance in the interaction (expert knowledge; authority as a professional; anchored in regulations)
- Understanding the position of the other: awareness of the individuality of experiences
- Developing new (inclusive) mental models: interaction always needs a shared balance
- Developing common meaning: recognition of one's own history and the attendant opinions

How to achieve a more equal interaction between client and professional, is:

- Insight into sensemaking
- Sensitivity to sensemaking
- Insight into the context in which the interaction takes place Elaboration of sub-questions:

Knowledge and work practices arise in social interaction, whereby solutions to problems are found through action. Weick therefore calls organizing 'negotiating verbs'. By observing a discourse (language game), an observed reality is interpreted. That reality comes about through language and through action. The interaction is ultimately realized by assigning meaning to it. This leads to the following preconditions for meaningful interaction:

- Realization of implicit assumptions in professional language

Language and behaviour of a client stem from their own life story. Without insight into that life story, effective interaction is not possible. Personal directorship requires coherence between one's own network (informal care), person-oriented care and care technology. It is about creating coherence around individual questions where the client's life is central. This cohesion is designed as an open system. This creates the possibility for the client's management role. Clients can only be themselves. A professional offer is then about recognizing that integrality.

With personal directorship, it is about a psychology of possibilities. Clients must have the opportunity to participate in the decision-making process. A model to implement this is value-driven care: this way the entire care process is organized around the needs and possibilities of the client.

Based on this book the following preconditions for an interaction based on client autonomy emerge:

- Create an activating environment for interaction in which the client's own capabilities are central;
- Ensure a coherent care process in which the social network, personal care and care technology come together in a coherent way;
- Ensure that care technology and digitalization are part of the primary process;
- Make sure in the interaction that both the perspective of clients and the perspective of professionals can be reflected;
- Make more use of the narrative approach and the presentation theory to maintain a view of the individual identity of the client (dealing with variety);
- Ensure an information management system that supports clients' own management (user-friendly);
- Work out a funding model based on the individuality of the client.

To guarantee autonomy, it is essential that (continuation of) one's own life is central to the interaction between client and healthcare professional. Within care for the elderly there are six models in which the values of clients are increasingly central:

- Integrated care
- Personal care
- Value-driven care
- Positive healthcare
- Narrative approach
- Presence approach

A mix of such approaches per context is effective for strengthening the autonomy of clients. This can also be achieved by giving clients a position in policy-making and implementation. The core of the presence-based theory is that the healthcare professional starts from the other person and not only from your own good intentions. The practice of healthcare is extremely complex and requires complex thinking. Professional acting is about handling variety. That can lead to a higher degree of uncertainty in your own actions. An entrepreneurial attitude makes it possible to handle that uncertainty. The increased variety due to preferences of clients requires new organizational concepts.

For professionals to handle variety, regulatory space is essential. This means that the care must be organized on the basis of principles of self-organization. In the educational programme, therefore, attention must be paid to professional competences based on this.

To guarantee autonomy, it is essential that a professional has sufficient self-regulating capacity to focus on the client's own life in the interaction between client and care professional. This is required because the strengthening of the position of clients will increase the variety within their own care practice. The effects of healthcare technology and digitalization also require an agile approach.

The role of the healthcare professional is fulfilled out of personal entrepreneurship. The choice to work as an entrepreneur is independent of this. It is about the interpretation of the professional actions. What is essential here is what contribution is made to the client's request for care. The start-up methodology is introduced as a language game. This makes it possible to handle variety and to be helpful. Personal entrepreneurship is not so much about operating as an entrepreneur as about being entrepreneurial. In addition to being able to conduct a dialogue, this also translates into the capacity to use digital work forms. In addition, it is necessary to be able to innovate.

A logical model for a healthcare professional to deal with variety is personal entrepreneurship. Personal entrepreneurship focuses on regulatory space (autonomy), agility, flexibility and innovation. A workable model for this is the start-up approach.

The redesign of the interaction is about striking a good balance between the client perspective and the professional perspective. The core objective is to arrive at an equal positioning in an asymmetrical relation. The realization of an effective dialogue thus comes to the centre of the interaction. This leads to the following preconditions for meaningful interaction:

- Awareness of professional dominance in the interaction (expert knowledge; authority as a professional; anchored in regulations)
- Understanding the position of the other: awareness of the individuality of experiences
- Developing new (inclusive) mental models: interaction always needs a shared balance

- Developing common meaning: recognition of one's own history and the attendant opinions
- Realization of implicit assumptions in professional language

Based on this book the following preconditions for an interaction based on client autonomy emerge:

- Create an activating environment for interaction in which the client's own capabilities are central;
- Ensure a coherent care process in which the social network, personal care and care technology come together in a coherent way;
- Ensure that care technology and digitalization are part of the primary process;
- Make sure in the interaction that both the perspective of clients and the perspective of professionals can be reflected;
- Make more use of the narrative approach and the presentation theory to maintain a view of the individual identity of the client (dealing with variety);
- Ensure an information management system that supports clients' own management (user-friendly);
- Work out a funding model based on the individuality of the client.
- Support for the use of digital technologies

Based on this book the following preconditions come to the fore for an interaction based on autonomy of the professional:

- Create an environment for interaction in which the self-regulating capacity of the professional is central;
- Ensure a coherent care process in which the role of the professional is to reach a solution within the professional standards from the perspective of the client;
- When choosing your own actions, use the start-up method to increase your manoeuvrability;
- Position the professional domain from the perspective of interaction (organizing) and not from an organizational interest;
- Support for working with digital technologies;
- Insight into changes in role as coach

In summary the following actions will lead to a more effective interaction between client and professional.

Client perspective	Interaction	Professional perspective
Decrease in variety	Establish effective dialogue	Increase in variety
Central is own life story (narrative approach)	Professional domain is based on interaction	Working in network structures
Self-insight into own capacities	Understanding of others	Increasing self-regulatory capacity (work and learning environment)
Perspective of client is in focus	Development of new (inclusive) mental models	Awareness of implicit assumptions
Designing user-friendly information management (directorship)	Development of common sensemaking	Awareness of professional dominance
Funding model based on person-bound funding (target group approach)	Sensitivity to sensemaking	Insight into the context in which the interaction takes place Insight into changes in role as coach
	Establishing a coherent care process (social network, care technology, digitalization)	Using a mix of care models Insight into outcomes of care
	Application of platform technology	Personal entrepreneurship (application of start-up methodology) increasing agility

Figure 14. Summary of findings.

REFERENCES

Aa, A. van der en T. Konijn. (2001). *Ketens, ketenregisseurs en ketenontwikkeling. Het ontwikkelen van transparante en flexibele samenwerkingsverbanden in netwerken.* Utrecht: Lemma. [*Chains, chain directors and chain development. Developing transparent and flexible partnerships in networks*.]

Aalbers, R. en W. Dolfsma. (2015). *Innovation networks. Managing the networked organization.* London: Routledge.

Achterbergh, J. and D. Vriens (2010). *Organizations. Social systems conducting experiments.* Second revised edition. Berlin: Springer Verlag.

Ackoff, R. L. (1999). *Ackoff's best. His classic writing on management.* Chichester, England: John Wiley & Sons Ltd.

Adler, R. and R. Mehta (2014). *Catalyzing technology to support family caregiving.* National Alliance for Caregiving.

Ahlers, J. and R. C. W. Boender (2016). *Generatie Z en de vierde (industriële) revolutie.* Haarlem: Bertram en De Leeuw Uitgevers. [*Generation Z and the fourth (industrial) revolution.*]

Akkermans, J. (2013). *Well begun is half done. Investigating the work and career of the young workforces.* (PhD thesis, Universiteit Utrecht).

Allen, D. (2015). *The invisible work of nurses: hospitals, organization and healthcare.* London: Routledge.

Almekinders, M. (2006). *Teams beter thuis in thuiszorg? Resultaatverbetering in thuiszorg met behulp van sociotechnische organisatievernieuwing.* (PhD thesis, Radboud University). [*Teams better at home in home care? Result improvement in home care with the help of sociotechnical organizational innovation.*]

Anderson, G., K. Dunlap, J. Rademacher and N. McMenamy. (2009). *Metaplan: a mutual methodology for interdisciplinary research.* SoTL Commons Conference. 104.

Angronison, M. (2007). *Doing ethnographic and observational research.* Thousand Oaks, CA: Sage.

Annink, A. (2017). *Busyness around the Business - A cross-national comparative research of the work-life balance of self-employed workers.* (PhD thesis, Erasmus University Rotterdam).

Appello, J. (2011). *Management 3.0 Leading agile developers, developing agile leaders.* Addison-Wesley.

Ardon, A. (2011). *Doorbreek de cirkel. Hoe managers onbewust verandering blokkeren.* Amsterdam: Business contact. [*Break the circle. How managers unconsciously block change.*]

Arets, J., V. Heijnen and C. Jennings (2015). 702010. Naar 100% performance. Sutler Media Argyris, C. and D. A. Schön (1977). *Theory in practice. Increasing professional effectiveness.* San Francisco: Jossey-Bass.

Ashby, W. R. (1956). An introduction to cybernetics. London, England: Chapman & Hall Ltd. Aslander, M. and E. Witteveen. (2010). *Easycratie. De toekomst van werken en organiseren.* The Hague: Academic Service. [*Easycracy. The future of work and organisation*]

Aslander, M. and E. Witteveen (2015). *Nooit af (Permanente Beta). Een nieuwe kijk op de fundamenten van ons leven: werk, school, zorg, overheid en management.* Amsterdam: Business Contact. [*Never Finished (Permanent Beta). A new look at the foundations of our lives: work, school, care, government and management*]

Aukes, L. C. and H. Woldendorp (1994). *Organisatieverandering: een punt van orde. Principes van verandermanagement.* Deventer: Kluwer. [Organizational change: a point of order. *Principles of change management*]

Baan, C. (2015). *Integrale gezondheidszorg. Meer dan de som der delen.* Oratie. Tilburg: Universiteit Tilburg. [*Integrated healthcare. More than the sum of its parts.*]

Baarends, E. en F. Simon. (2017). *Over validering van praktijkgericht onderzoek.* Kwalon, 22, no 3, 5 – 13. [*About validation of practice-oriented research*]

Baart, A. (2011). *Een theorie van de presentie.* The Hague: Boom. [*A theory of presence*]

Baart, A. (2016). *Over de nieuwe regels, gehoorzaamheid en verstandigheid.* Utrecht: Stichting Presentie. [*About the new rules, obedience and prudence.*]

Baart, A. (2018). *De ontdekking van kwaliteit. Theorie en praktijk van relationeel zorg geven.* Amsterdam: Uitgeverij SWP. [*The discovery of quality. Theory and practice of relational care.*]

Baart, A. and C. Carbo (2013). *De zorgval.* Amsterdam: Thoeris Uitgeverij. [*The care trap.*]

Baets, W. R. J. (2002). *Wie orde zaait, zal chaos oogsten. Een vertoog over de lerende mens.* Assen: Van Gorcum. [*He who sows order will reap chaos. A discourse about the learning person*]

Bahlmann, J. P. and B. A. C. Meesters (1998). *De organisatie die nooit bestond. Een zoektocht naar vormen van organiseren.* Schoonhoven: Academic Service. [*The organization that never existed. A search for forms of organizing*]

Bakas, A. (2017). *Ziel in de zorg. Hoe technologische revoluties en nieuw burgerschap leiden tot een vernieuwde zorgbranche.* Bakas Books. [*Soul in care. How technological revolutions and new citizenship lead to a renewed healthcare industry*]

Baldwin, R. (2019). *The globotics upheaval. Globalization, robotics, and the future of work.* London: Weidenfeld & Nicolson.

Barabási, A. L. (2003). *Linked. How everything is connected to everything else and what it means for business, science and everyday life.* New York: Plume.

Barrett, R. (1998). Liberating the corporate soul. Building a visionary organization. Butterworth. Bateson, G. (1972). *Steps to an ecology of the mind.* St. Albans: Paladin.

Becker, H. (1992). *Generaties en hun kansen.* Amsterdam: Meulenhoff. [*Generations and their chances*]

Becker, H. M. (2011). Hands off not an option! *The reminiscence museurm mirror of a humanistic care philosophy.* Delft: Eburon.

Beckford, J. (2016). *The intelligent organization. Realizing the value of information.* London/New York: Routledge.

Beek, J. W. van and R. Huizenga (2017). *Voorbij de start-up mania. Succesvol innoveren op eigen kracht.* Amsterdam: Business contact. [*Beyond the start-up mania. Successfully innovate under your own steam.*]

Beer, S. (1978). *Platform for change.* Chichester, John Wiley and Sons.

Beer, S. (1979). *The heart of the enterprise.* Chichester, England: John Wiley & Sons Ltd. Beer, S. (1981). Brain of the firm, 2nd edition. Chichester, England: John Wiley & Sons.

Beer, S. (1985). *Diagnosing the system for organizations.* Chichester, England: John Wiley & Sons Ltd.

Begemann, D. (2008). *Natuurlijk veranderen. Principes voor zelforganisatie in veranderprocessen.* Assen: Van Gorcum. [*Change of course. Principles for self-organization in change processes*]

Begun, J. W., B. Zimmerman and K. Dooley (2003). Health care organizations as complex adaptive system'. In S. M. Mick & M. Wyttenbach (Eds.), *Advances in health care organization theory* (pp. 253-288). San Francisco: Jossey-Bass.

Bijl, R. V. (1991). *Constructie van toekomstscenario's: beleidsgericht scenario-onderzoek toegepast op het gebied van de geestelijke volksgezondheid.* Proefschrift. Utrecht: Universiteit Utrecht. [*Construction of future scenarios: policy-oriented scenario research applied to the field of mental health.*]

Binkhorst, T., E. Posma and S. Lobenstein, eds. (2009). *Patiënten betrekken bij de zorg in het ziekenhuis. Een handboek.* Kwaliteitsinstituut voor Gezondheidszorg CBO. [*Involving patients in hospital care. A handbook.*]

Birkinshaw, J. (2010). *Reinventing management.* Smarter choices for getting things done. Jossey-Bass.

Bisschop Boele, E. (2017). *Op zoek naar de betekenis van cultuurparticipatie.* Oratie. Rotterdam: Erasmus University Rotterdam. [*In search of the meaning of cultural participation.*]

Bisschop Boele, E. (2018). Etnografisch onderzoek: het perspectief van de ander. *Cultuur + Educatie*, 17, no.50, 85-93. [*Culture + Education*]

Bisognano, M. and C. Kenney (2012). *Pursuing the triple aim: seven innovators show the way to better care, better health, and lower costs.* San Francisco: Jossey-Bass.

Blank, S. (2013). *The four steps to epiphany. Successful strategies for products that win.* K&S Ranch Consulting.

Blijham, G. en H. Hillen. (2019). Interne geneeskunde, terugblik en toekomstvisie. *Interne Geneeskunde*, no. 3, vol. 10, 24 – 27. [Internal medicine, retrospect and vision for the future. *Internal Medicine*]

Blok, J. de and A. Pool. (2010). *Buurtzorg: menselijkheid boven bureaucratie.* The Hague: Boom Lemma Uitgevers. [*Neighborhood care: humanity over bureaucracy*]

Blok, J. de, H. Suichies, L. Vogelpoel and T. Jansen. (2015). *Het alternatief voor de zorg. Humaniteit boven bureaucratie.* Amsterdam: Uitgeverij Boom. [*The alternative to healthcare. Humanity over bureaucracy*]

Bloem, S. (2012). *Gepersonaliseerde zorg. De juiste richting.* (Speech, Nyenrode Business Universiteit). [*Personalized care. The right direction*]

Blok, A. (1976). *Wittgenstein en Elias. Een methodische richtlijn voor de antropologie.* Amsterdam: Polak en Van Gennep, 1. [*Wittgenstein and Elias. A methodical guideline for anthropology.*]

Blok, J. de and A. Pool (2010). *Buurtzorg: menselijkheid boven bureaucratie.* The Hague: Boom Lemma. [*Neighborhood care: humanity over bureaucracy.*]

Blom, R. J. (2002). *Startend ondernemerschap in de praktijk.* Amsterdam: Graydon. [*Start-up entrepreneurship in practice.*]

Blommaert, D. E. (2014). *The role of the nurse in practising benificence in palliative care.* (Master thesis. Utrecht Universiteit voor Humanistiek).

Blumer, H. (1969). *Symbolic interactionism. Perspective and method.* Englewood Cliffs: Prentice-Hall.

Boer, F. (2011). *De Grounded Theory Approach: een update. Kwalon. Tijdschrift voor kwalitatief onderzoek*, vol. 16, no. 1, 25-33. [The Grounded Theory Approach: An Update. Qualon. *Journal of qualitative research*]

Boer, N. de and A. van Diepen. (2013). *Swingen met lokale kracht. Overheden en de netwerksamenleving.* The Hague: Raad voor Maatschappelijke Ontwikkeling. [*Swinging with local power. Governments and the network society.*]

Boer & Croon. (2011). *Een goed gesprek over vernieuwen van de zorg.* Amsterdam. [*A good conversation about innovation in healthcare.*]

Boeije, H. (2014). *Analyseren in kwalitatief onderzoek. Denken en doen.* Amsterdam: Boom. [*Analyzing in qualitative research. Thinking and doing.*]

Bolman, C. (2019). *eHealth toepassingen bij kwetsbare groepen: een uitdaging.* Oratie. Heerlen: Open Universiteit. [*eHealth applications in vulnerable groups: a challenge.*]

Bommerez, J. (2007). *Door de bomen het bos zien. Ontdek de eenvoud onder de complexiteit in relaties en organisaties.* United Media Company. [*Seeing the forest through the trees. Discover the simplicity beneath the complexity in relationships and organizations*]

Bommerez, J. and K. van Zijtveld (2001). *Kun je een rups leren vliegen. Over de noodzakelijke kwantumsprong van veranderingsmanagement naar transformationeel leiderschap.* Eemnes: Uitgeverij Nieuwe Dimensies. [*Can you teach a caterpillar to fly? About the necessary quantum leap from change management to transformational leadership*]

Bontekoning, A. (2014). *Nieuwe generaties in vergrijzende organisaties.* Amsterdam: Mediawerf Uitgevers. [*New generations in aging organizations.*]

Boonekamp, L. and H. Woldendorp (2006). 'Een strategisch model voor de ouderenzorg', *Zorgspecial*, 2006, no. 7, 4- 11. ['A strategic model for elderly care']

Boonstra, J. J. (2000). *Lopen over water. Over dynamiek van organiseren, vernieuwen en leren.* Oratie. Amsterdam: Universiteit van Amsterdam. [*Walk on water. About dynamics of organising, innovation and learning*]

Boonstra, J. ed. (2007). *Ondernemen in allianties en netwerken. Een multidisciplinair perspectief.* Deventer: Kluwer. [*Doing business in alliances and networks. A multidisciplinary perspective.*]

Boonstra, J. J. (2013). *Verandermanagement in 28 lessen.* Amsterdam: Business Contact. [*Change management in 28 lessons*]

Boonstra, J. (2014). *Leiding in cultuurverandering. Een praktische gids voor strategische en culturele veranderingen in organisaties.* Assen: Koninklijke Van Gorcum. [*Leadership in culture change. A practical guide to strategic and cultural change in organizations*]

Bones, C., J. Hammersley and N. Shaw. (2019). *Optimizing digital strategy. How to make informed, tactical decisions that deliver growth.* London: KoganPage.

Bos, R. ten (2000). *Fashion and utopia in management thinking*. Amsterdam: John Benjamins Publishing Company.

Bos, R. ten (2001). *Strategisch denken. Op zoek naar nieuwe helden.* Zaltbommel: Uitgeverij Thema. [*Thinking strategically. Looking for new heroes.*]

Boschma, J. and I. Groen (2010). *Generatie Einstein 3.0. Slimmer, sneller en volwassener.* Amsterdam: A.W. Bruna Uitgevers. [*Generation Einstein 3.0. Smarter, faster and more mature*.]

Bosma, H. and C. van Haaften. (2013). *Klaar voor de toekomst? Passende werkmodellen voor VVT organisaties in het nieuwe krachtenveld.* PhD thesis. Rotterdam: Erasmus Universiteit Rotterdam). [*Ready for the future? Appropriate working models for VVT organizations in the new force field*.]

Bovenkamp, H. M. van de. (2010). *The limits of patient power. Examining active citizenship in Dutch healthcare.* PhD thesis. Rotterdam: Erasmus Universiteit Rotterdam).

Bovenkamp. H. van de, A. Stoopendaal. M. van Bochove, H. Hoogendijk and R. Bal (2017). *Persoonsgerichte zorg, regeldruk en regelruimte: van regelreflex naar spiegelreflex*. Rotterdam: Erasmus School of health policy and management. [*Person-oriented care, regulatory pressure and regulatory space: from regulatory reflex to SLR*]

Brack, A. (2017). *De verborgen dimensie van leiderschap. Evolutie van macht naar kracht.* Zaltbommel: Thema. [*The hidden dimension of leadership. Evolution from power to power.*]

Brafman, O. and R. A. Beckstrom (2010). *De zeester en de spin. De onstuitbare kracht van organisaties zonder leider*. Utrecht: Bruna Uitgevers BV. [*The starfish and the spider. The unstoppable power of organizations without a leader*]

Brandenburg, C. (2008). *A transaction cost analysis of Dutch hospital care.* PhD thesis. Rotterdam: Erasmus Universiteit Rotterdam).

Bree, T. de. (2017). *Kan het vliegen? Van idee tot succesvolle start-up.* Culemborg: Van Duuren Management. [*Can it fly? From idea to successful start-up*.]

Breedveld, E. J. (2003). *Thuiszorg in bedrijf: herstructurering van de thuiszorgbranche tussen 1987 en 1997*, Tilburg: IVA Tilburg. [*Home care in operation: restructuring of the home care industry between 1987 and 1997*]

Brentes, M. (1999). *De organisatie als netwerk. Hoe mensen organisaties veranderen en organisaties mensen.* Alphen a.d. Rijn. [*The organization as a network. How people change organizations and organizations change people*.]

Bridle, J. (2018). *New dark age. Technology and the end of future.* London: Verso.

Broek, A. van den, C. van Campen, J. de Haan, A. Roeters, M. Turkenburg and L. Vermeij, eds. (2016). *De toekomst tegemoet. Leren, werken, zorgen, samenleven en consumeren in het Nederland van later.* The Hague: Sociaal en Cultureel Planbureau. [*Towards the future. Learning, working, caring, living together and consuming in the Netherlands of the future.*]

Broese van Groenou, M. (2015). *Digitale communicatie in zorgnetwerken van kwetsbare ouderen. Evaluatie van de implementatie van een digitale tool in de thuiszorg om de communicatie met mantelzorg te verbeteren.* Amsterdam: Vrije Universiteit. [*Digital communication in care networks of frail elderly. Evaluation of the implementation of a digital tool in home care to improve communication with informal care.*]

Broncker, J. and J. Veuger. (2018). Blockchain: technology lookin for a problem? Vision on the application of blockchain technology in real estate. Grum, J. and J. Veuger, eds. *Cirre 2018 3th conference of interdisciplinary research on real estate* (pp 124 - 130). Groningen.

Browne, J. (2019). *Make, think, imagine. Engineering the future of civilization.* New York: Pegasus Books.

Brunsson, N. (1987). *The irrational organization. Irrationality as a basis for organizational action and change.* Chichester: John Wiley & Sons.

Brunsson, N. (1989). *The organization of hypocrisy. Talk, decisions and actions in organizations.* Chicester: John Wiley & Sons.

Brussel, G. van (2012). *De creatie van Ruimte met Stijl: de ontwikkeling van intrapreneurship als een loopbaanperspectief voor senior professionals.* (PhD thesis, Open Universiteit). [*The creation of Space with Style: the development of intrapreneurship as a career perspective for senior professionals*]

Bruijn, H. de, H. van der Voort, H. Warmelink, R.v.W. de Joode and N. Willems (2014). Nieuwerwets organiseren. Assen: Van Gorcum.

Bryant, a. and K. Charmaz, eds. (2007). *The Sage handbook of Grounded Theory.* Los Angeles: Sage Publications.

Buitendam, A. (2001). Een open architectuur voor arbeid en organisatie. Assen, Van Gorcum. Bulck, A. van den. (2017). *Nieuw bekostiging wijkverpleging: kennis als basis. Tijdschrift. Maatschappij en Gezondheid*, vol. 17., n 4, 8-9. [An open architecture for work and organization. Assen, VanGorcum. Bulck, A. van den. (2017). *New funding for district nursing: knowledge as a basis. magazine.*]

Burns, L. R., ed. (2005) *The business of healthcare innovation.* Cambridge University Press.

Burrell, G. and G. Morgan (1985). *Sociological paradigms and organizational analysis. Elements of the sociology of corporate life.* Hants: Gower, 1985.

Buurman, B. (2018). *Van symptoombestrijding naar duurzame acute ouderenzorg.* Oratie. Amsterdam: Universiteit van Amsterdam. [*From symptom control to sustainable acute care for the elderly.*]

Buuse, S. van den, L. Vermeulen en M. Smit. (2017). *'Het ligt in onze handen': zelfstandig werken in de zorg bevorderen. Een evaluatieonderzoek naar cultuurprogramma 'De werkvloer centraal'.* Amsterdam: Universiteit van Amsterdam. [*'It is in our hands': promoting independent work in healthcare. An evaluation study into the culture program 'The workplace is central'.]*

Bussemaker, J. (2019). *Zorg als sociale kwestie.* Oratie. Leiden: Universiteit van Leiden. [*Care as a social issue.*]

Bussemaker, J. (2020). *Samen beslissen als ontwerpprincipe voor het tweede decennium.* Speech. Den Haag: Raad voor Volksgezondheid en Samenleving. [*Deciding together as a design principle for the second decade.*]

Cabrera, D. A. (2006). *Systems thinking* (PhD thesis, Cornell University, 2006). Dissertation Abstracts International-A, 67, 303.

Calman, L. (2006). *What is grounded theory?* Presentation. Manchester: University of Manchester.

Campen, C. van, J. Iedema, M. Broese van Groenou and D. Deeg. (2017). *Langer zelfstandig. Ouder worden met hulpbronnen, ondersteuning en zorg.* The Hague: Sociaal en Cultureel Planbureau. [*Longer independent. Aging with Resources, Support and Care*]

Caris, J. (2013). *De organisatie van professionele zorg.* Tilburg: Universiteit, oratie. [*The organization of professional care*]

Caris, J., T. Poiesz en F. Lapré. (2019). *Complexe sociale vraagstukken vragen om een Integraal Analyse Model.* Neer: Kloosterhof. [*Complex social issues require an Integral Analysis Model.*]

Chapman, B. (2015) *Everybody matters. The extraordinary power of caring for your people like family.* London: Penguin Books Ltd.

Charmaz, K. (2006). *Constructing grounded theory. A practical guide through qualitative analysis.* London: Sage.

Charmaz, K. (2008). Constructionism and the Grounded Theory. In: J. A. S. Holstein and J. F. Gubrium, eds. *Handbook of constructionist Research*, 397 – 412. New York: The Guilford Press.

Charmaz, K. (2010). *Constructing grounded theory: a practical guide through qualitative analysis.* Thousand Oaks, CA: Sage.

Choy, Y. W. (2005). *De vraag op het antwoord. Systemische interventies voor conflicten in organisaties.* Santpoort: NISTO publicaties. [*The question to the answer. Systemic interventions for conflict in organizations*]

Christakis, N. and J. Fowler. (2010). *Connected. The amazing power of social networks and how they shape our lives.* Harper Press, 2010.

Christensen, C. M., J. H. Grossman and J. Hwang (2009). *The innovator's prescription. A disruptive solution for health care.* New York: MCGraw Hill.

Cingel, C. J. M. van der. (2012). *Compassie in de verpleegkundige praktijk. Een leidend principe voor goede zorg.* PhD thesis. Rotterdam: Erasmus Universiteit Rotterdam. [*Compassion in Nursing Practice. A guiding principle for good care*]

Clark, T., A. Osterwalder and Y. Peigneur. (2012). *Business Model You. A one-page method for reinventing your career.* Hoboken, NJ: John Wiley and Sons.

Clarke, K. E. (2005). *Situational analysis. Grounded theory after the postmodern turn.* Thousand Oaks, CA: Sage.

Coole, M. de and T. Verlaan, ed. (2009). *Ouderenzorg met toekomst. Visies en voorbeelden van een nieuwe aanpak.* Amsterdam: SWP. [*Elderly care with a future. Visions and examples of a new approach.*]

Coolen, J. (2008). *Ouderen in zorghuizen: broze mensen en leefplezier.* Waardigheid en trots. [*Elderly people in care homes: frail people and enjoyment of life.*]

Cooper, R. (1987). Information, communication and organisation: a post-structural revision, *The Journal of Mind and Behavior,* vol. 8, no. 3, 395-416.

Cooper, R. and S. Fox (1989). Two modes of organization. R. Mansfield, ed. *Frontiers of management.* London: Routledge and Kegan Paul, 247-261.

Cooperrider, D. L., D. Whitney and J. M. Stavros (2005). *Appreciative Inquiry Handbook. For Leaders of Change.* San Francisco: Berrett-Koehler Publishers.

Corbin, J. and A. Strauss. (2008). *Basics of qualitative research: grounded theory, procedures and techniques.* 3rd edition. Newbury Park: Sage.

Cornelis, A. (1990). *Logica van het Gevoel. Filosofie van de stabiliteitslagen in de cultuur als nesteling der emoties.* Amsterdam: Boom. [*Logic of Feeling. Philosophy of the stability layers in culture as the nesting of emotions.*]

Cornelis, A. (2000). *De Vertraagde Tijd. Revanche van de geest als filosofie van de toekomst.* Amsterdam: Boom. [*The Delayed Time. Revenge of the mind as philosophy of the future.*]

Covey, S. R. (1997). *De zeven eigenschappen van effectief leiderschap.* Contact. [*The Seven Habits of Effective Leadership.*]

Cozijnsen, A. J. (2001). *Anders veranderen. De nieuwe balans tussen mens en technologie.* Oratie. Amsterdam: Vrije Universiteit). [*Change differently. The new balance between people and technology.*]

Cozijnsen, A., P. van Dun and E. Kimman, *Het theater van verandering. Regie en rolverdeling bij veranderprocessen.* Prentice Hall, 2009. [*The theater of change. Direction and division of roles in change processes*]

Creswell, J. W. (2009). *Research design. Qualitative, quantitative, and mixed method approaches.* Los Angeles: Sage.

Czarniawsky-Joerges, B (1992). *Exploring complex organizations. A cultural perspective.* Newsbury Park: Sage.

Dalen, A van. (2010). *Uit de schaduw van het zorgsysteem. Hoe buurtzorg Nederland zorg organiseert.* Boom Lemma, 2010. [*Out of the shadows of the healthcare system. How neighborhood care in the Netherlands organizes care*]

Dalen, van, A. (2012). *Zorgvernieuwing. Over anders besturen en organiseren.* The Hague: Boom Lemma. [*Healthcare innovation. About managing and organizing differently.*]

Dautzenberg, M., E. Curfs and D. de Bakker. (2013). *Zorgnetwerken van ouderen met een complexe zorgvraag. Onderzoek naar fragmentatie en integratie in de eerstelijnszorg voor thuiswonende ouderen.* Heerlen: Open Universiteit. [*Care networks of elderly people with complex care needs. Research on fragmentation and integration in primary care for community-dwelling elderly people.*]

Davenport, T. H. and J. Kirby. (2016). *Only humans need apply. Winners and losers in the age of smart machines*. New York: Haper Business.

Davenport, T. H. (2019). *The AI advantage. How to put the artificial intelligence revolution to work*. Cambridge, Mass.: The MIT Press

Delden, P. no 22, 53-65 (1992). *Professionals. Kwaliteit van het beroep.* Amsterdam: Contact. [*Quality of the profession.*]

Delden, P. van. (2009). *Sterke netwerken. Ketensamenwerking in de publieke dienstverlening.* Van Gennep. [*Strong networks. Chain collaboration in public services.*]

Delnoij, D. (2019). *Samen beslissen. Via uitkomstinformatie naar patiëntgerichte zorg?* Oratie. Rotterdam: Erasmus Universiteit Rotterdam. [*Decide together. Via outcome information to patient-oriented care?*]

Diamandis, P. H. en S. Kotler. (2020). *The future is faster than you think. How converging technologies are transforming business, industries and our lives.* New York: Simon & Schuster.

Dierendonck, J. H. van. (2015). *Oud of wijs: ervaringsdeskundige maakt het verschil in onderzoek naar de ouderenzorg.* Utrecht: Nederlandse Federatie van Universitair Medische Centra. [*Old or wise: an experience expert makes the difference in research into elderly care.*]

Dijck, J. van, T. Poell and M. de Waal (2016). *De platformsamenleving. Strijd om publieke waarden in een online wereld.* Amsterdam University Press. [*The platform society. Battle for public values in an online world*]

Dijk, A. van and H. Woldendorp. (1993). Sturen in complexe organisaties: organisatiekundige modellen. In: A. van Dijk, G. Smid and H. Woldendorp, ed. *Sturen in complexe organisaties. Theorie en praktijk in het hoger onderwijs*. Assen: Van Gorcum, p.11-22. [Managing in complex organizations: organizational models. In: A. van Dijk, G. Smid and H. Woldendorp, ed. *Management in complex organizations. Theory and practice in higher education.*]

Dijk, N. M. H. (1989). Een methodische strategie van organisatieverandering. Delft: Eburon Dijkstra, L. en J. D. van der Bij. (1991). *Ordinale meetschalen in bedrijfskundig onderzoek.* Eindhoven: Technische Universiteit Eindhoven. [A methodical strategy of organizational change. Delft: Eburon Dijkstra, L. and J.D. van der Bij. (1991). *Ordinal measurement scales in business research.*]

Dinten, W. L. van. (2002) *van, Met gevoel voor realiteit. Over herkennen van betekenis bij organiseren.* Delft: Eburon. [*of, With a sense of reality. About recognizing meaning in organizing*]

Dinten, W. L. van en I. F. M. Schouten (2008). *Zijn zij gek of ben ik het? Hoe je oriëntaties gebruikt bij organiseren.* Delft: Eburon. [*Are they crazy or is it me? How to use orientations in organizing.*]

Dinten, W. L. van, en I. F. M. Schouten. (2015), *Voorbij het vanzelfsprekende- op safari in de wildernis van betekenisgeving.* Delft: Eburon. [*Beyond the obvious - on safari in the wilderness of meaning.*]

Douglas, M. (1987). *How institutions think.* Londen: Routledge and Kegan Paul.

Downes, L. and P. Nunes. (2014). *Big bang disruption. Strategy in the age of devastating innovation.* New York: Penguin Putnam.

Drucker, P. F. (2017). *Innovation and entrepreneurship. Practice and principles.* London: Routledge.

Duin, P. van der. (2006). *Qualitative future research for innovation.* Delft: Eburon.

Edwards, T. (2015). *Management by initiatives. A new paradigm for executing business strategy and achieving meaningful business results.* Philadelphia: TMBE.

Ehrenhard, M. L., B. Kijl and L. J. M. Nieuwenhuis. (2014). *Barrières in marktadoptie van domotica. Slimme technologie voor zorg, veiligheid, energiebesparing en comfort.* Research report. Enschede: Universiteit Twente). [*Barriers to market adoption of home automation. Smart technology for care, safety, energy savings and comfort*]

Eilenberger, W. (2018). *Het tijdperk van de tovenaars. Het grote decennium van de filosofie, 1919 – 1929.* Amsterdam: De Bezige Bij. [*The Age of Wizards. The Great Decade of Philosophy, 1919 – 1929.*]

Eijkenaar, F. (2013). *Pay-for-performance for healthcare providers. Design, performance measurement, and (unintended) effects.* PhD thesis. Rotterdam: Erasmus Universiteit Rotterdam).

Eindevaluatie experiment regelarme instelling. (ERAI). (2016). Den Haag: Ministerie van VWS. [*Final evaluation experiment with a controlled setting*]

Eisenhardt, K. M. and M. Graebner (2007). Theory building from cases: opportunities and challenges. *Academy of Management Journal,* vol. 50, no. 1, 25 -32.

Elberse, J. (2012). *Changing the health research system. Patient participation in health research.* PhD thesis. Amsterdam: Vrije Universiteit Amsterdam).

Ellinor, L. and G. Gerard. (1998). *Dialogue: rediscovering the transforming power of conversation.* John Wiley.

Elsinga, B. (2014). *De jonge professional. Hulpmiddelen voor richting en groei.* Zwaag: Vior Webmedia. [*The young professional. Tools for direction and growth.*]

Elsen, T. van den. (2017). *Analyse innovatienetwerken in de zorg. Ervaringen uit de praktijk: de meerwaarde, kansen en uitdagingen.* Utrecht: Vilans. [*Analysis of innovation networks in healthcare. Experiences from practice: the added value, opportunities and challenges.*]

Emmelot-Vonk, M.E. (2019) *Klinische geriatrie: de gouden herfst.* Utrecht: Universiteit van Utrecht. [*Clinical geriatrics: the golden autumn.*]

Engel, Y. (2015). *Venturing into the unknown, but not for the first time. An examination of firm- founders' careers and entrepreneurial decision-making under uncertainty.* (PhD thesis, Vrije Universiteit).

Ertel, C. and L. K. Solomon. (2014). *Moments of impact. Hoe je strategische conversaties ontwerpt die verandering versnellen.* Deventer: Vakmedianet. [*How to design strategic conversations that accelerate change.*]

Eijkenaar,F. and E. Schut. (2015). *Uitkomstbekostiging in de zorg: een (on) begaanbare weg?* Rotterdam: Erasmus Universiteit: iBMG. [*Outcome funding in healthcare: an (im)passable road?*]

Eijssen, D. H. (2016). *De juiste balans tussen ondernemen en professionaliseren vanuit een stevige basis.* Blog, 1 January 2016. [*The right balance between entrepreneurship and professionalization from a solid foundation.*]

Eisenhardt, K. M. and M. E. Graebner (2007). Theory building from casrs: opportunities and challenges. *Academy of Mangement Journal,* vol. 50, no. 1 p. 25 -32.

Es, R. van. (2008). *Veranderdiagnose. De onderstroom van organiseren.* Deventer: Kluwer. [*Change diagnosis. The undercurrent of organizing.*]

Evans, D.S. and R. Schmalensee. (2016). *Matchmakers. The new economics of multisided platforms.* Boston, MA: Harvard Business Review Press.

Fabbricotti, I. N. (2007). *Zorgen voor zorgketens. Integratie en fragmentatie in de ontwikkeling van zorgketens.* (PhD thesis, Erasmus Universiteit Rotterdam). [*Taking care of care chains. Integration and fragmentation in the development of care chains*]

Fairclough, N. (1992). *Discourse and social change.* Cambridge: Polity Press, 1992.

Feenstra, H. and W. P. M. Wansink (2009). *Zo gaat het in de zorg. De burger als klant, speelbal of koning, mondig of monddood.* Amsterdam, Nederland: Atlas-Contact. [*That's how it works in healthcare. The citizen as customer, plaything or king, empowered or silenced.*]

Foerster, H. von. (1981). *Observing systems.* Seaside, CA, Intersystem Publications, 1981.

Foerster, von H. (1984). On constructing a reality. In: P. Watzlawick, ed., *The invented reality. How do we know what we believe we know?* Contributions to constructivism. New York: Norton p. 41-63.

Ford, M. (2015). *Rise of the robots. Technology and the threat of a jobless future.* New York: Basic Books.

Ford, M. (2018). *Architects of intelligence. The truth about AI from the people building it.* Birmingham: Packt Publishing.

Frankl, V. E. (1978). *De zin van het bestaan.* Donker. [*The meaning of existence.*]

Freedman, L. (2013). *Strategy. A history.* Oxford: Oxford University Press.

Freeman, Jr. S. (2018). Utilizing multi-grounded theory in a dissertation: reflections and insights. *The Qualitative Report*, vol. 23, no. 1, 1160 -1175.

Gaal, A. van. (2012). *Ambitie. Adviezen van een ondernemer.* Amsterdam: Nieuw Amsterdam Uitgevers. [*Ambition. Advice from an entrepreneur.*]

Garwin, D. A. (2000). *Learning in action. A guide to putting the learning organization to work.* Boston, MA: Harvard Business School Press.

Geertz, C. (1983). *Local knowledge. Further essays on interpretive anthropology.* New York: Basic Books.

Geisler, E. ed. (2003). *Technology, health care and management in the hospital of the future.* Praeger.

Gemert-Pijnen van. (2015). *Persuasieve gezondheidstechnologie. Synergie door verbindingen.* Oratie. Enschede: Universiteit Twente. [*Persuasive health technology. Synergy through connections.*]

Gemmel, P. and L. de Raedt (2008). *De gezondheidszorg als complex adapatief systeem. Een ander perspectief op innovatie.* Obtained from the Flanders DC website: http://www. flandersdc.be/ sites/default/files/gezondheid_incl_cover.pdf. [*Healthcare as a complex adaptive system. A different perspective on innovation*]

Gershenson, G. (2007). *Design and control of self-organizing systems.* PhD thesis. Brussel: Vrije Universiteit Brussel).

Geursen, G. (1996) *Virtuele tomaten en conceptuele pindakaas. Hoe interactiviteit, zelforganisatie en bewustzijnsverruiming de marketing op z'n kop zetten.* Deventer: Kluwer. [*Virtual tomatoes and conceptual peanut butter. How interactivity, self-organization and awareness-raising turn marketing upside down.*]

Geursen, G. (2000) *Wie zijn ik? De magie van drijvende en verbindende krachten in organisaties.* Alphen a.d. Rijn: Samson. [*Who am I? The magic of driving and connecting forces in organizations*]

Gigch, J. P. van. (1991). *System design modeling and metamodeling.* New York: Springer Science and Business Media.

Ginneken, J. (2009). *De kracht van de zwerm. Zelfsturing in de organisatie.* Amsterdam: Business contact. [*The power of the swarm. Self-management in the organization*]

Gharajedaghi, J. (2011). *Systems thinking: Managing chaos and complexity: A platform for designing business architecture.* Burlington, MA: Morgan Kaufmann.

Gijzel, H., H. H. Nap, M. Herps, S. Mulder, M. van Klink, S. Schrijer-Snoeijs, K. Kuperus and M. Minkman (2017). *De wet langdurige zorg in de verzorging, verpleging en gehandicaptenzorg. Ervaringen uit de praktijk.* Amstelveen:

KPMG/Vilans. [*The law on long-term care in care, nursing and care for the disabled. Practical experiences.*]

Glaser, B. G. (1978). *Theoretical sensitivity. Advances in the methodology of Grounded Theory.* San Francisco: University of California Press.

Glaser, B. G. (1998). *Doing grounded theory: issues and discussions.* Mill Valley, CA: Sociology Press.

Glaudemans, M. (2015). Is er ruimte in de gevestigde orde. Essay over het individuele in organisatie, management en bestuur. Utrecht: Uitgeverij IJzer. [Is *there room in the established order? Essay on the individual in organization, management and governance.*]

Glaser, B. G. and A. L. Strauss. (1967). *The discovery of grounded theory. Strategies for qualitative research.* Chicago: Aldine.

Graham, B. and K. Thomas. (2008). Building knowledge. Developing a grounded theory of knowledge management for construction. *Electronic Journal of Business Research Methods,* vol. 6, issue 2, 115 – 122.

Glaser, B. G. and A. L. Straus (1967). *The discovery of grounded theory. Strategies for qualitative research.* Chicago: Aldine.

Gratton, L. (2011). *The shift. The future of work is already here.* London: Collins.

Groen, A. (2016). *Management control bij Buurtzorg Nijmegen-Oost: inspiratie in plaats van management en vertrouwen in plaats van control.* Bachelor thesis. Nijmegen: Radboud Universiteit Nijmegen. [*Management control at Buurtzorg Nijmegen-Oost: inspiration instead of management and trust in the place of control.*]

Groot, K. de, E. Mauritsen and A. Francke. (2018). Aantrekkelijkheid van het werken in de wijkverpleging: een online focusgroepstudie onder verpleegkundigen. *Verpleegkunde,* no. 2, 14-18. [Attractiveness of working in community nursing: an online focus group study among nurses. *Nursing*]

Groot, N. (2010). *Zelforganisatie en leiderschap. Een uitdagende paradox! Een complexiteitbenadering over het ontstaan van lokale verantwoordelijkheden en verbeterde resultaten.* Amsterdam: Mediawerf Uitgevers. [*Self-organization and leadership. A challenging paradox! A complexity approach to the emergence of local responsibilities and improved results*]

Guba, E. G. and Y. S. Lincoln. (1989). *Fourth generation evaluation.* Beverly Hills: Sage.

Gunsteren, H. R. van (1979). Complexiteit en cybernetische revolutie, M en O. *Tijdschrift voor Organisatiekunde en Sociaal Beleid*, vol. 33, no. 4: 324-339.

Gunsteren, H. van (2008). *Bouwen op burgers. Cultuur, preventive en de eigenzinnige burger.* Amsterdam: Van Gennep. [*Building on citizens. Culture, prevention and the wayward citizen.*]

Gupta, S. (2018). *Driving digital strategy. A guide to reimagining your business.* Boston, Mass.: Harvard Business Review Press.

Haan, E. de (2017). *Transities van sectoren. Systeemleren als succesfactor*. Amsterdam: Boom. [*Sector transitions. System learning as a success factor.*]

Hagel, J. III, J. S. Brown and L. Davison (2012). *The power of pull. How small moves, smartly made, can set big things in motion.* New York: Basic Books.

Hamel, G. (2007). *The future of management.* Boston, MA: Harvard Business School Press.

Harari, Y. N. (2016). *Homo Deus. A brief history of tomorrow*. London: Harvill Secker.

Hardjono, T., R. van Brakel and J. J. Kroon (2010). *Ketensamenwerking. Duurzaam werken in ketens en netwerken.* Leusden: C3. [*Chain collaboration. Working sustainably in chains and networks*.]

Hart, W. (2012). *Verdraaide organisaties. Terug naar de bedoeling*. Alphen a.d. Rijn: Vakmedianet. [*Twisted organizations. Back to the intention.*]

Hart, W. (2017). *Anders vasthouden. 9 sleutels voor het werken vanuit de bedoeling.* Alphen a.d. Rijn: Vakmedianet. [*Holding on differently. 9 keys for working from intent.*]

Harten, W. van and R. Schuring (2003). *Ondernemers in de zorg*. Assen: Koninklijke Van Gorcum. [*Entrepreneurs in healthcare.*]

Hauwert, S. (2018). *Ruimte voor eigen regie bij mensen met ernstige meervoudige beperkingen.* PhD thesis. Amsterdam: Vrije Universiteit Amsterdam. [*Room for personal control for people with severe multiple disabilities.*]

Have, S. ten, W. ten Have and B. Janssen (2009). *Het veranderboek. 70 vragen van managers over organisatieveranderingen.* Amsterdam: Mediawerf Uitgevers. [*The change book. 70 questions from managers about organizational change*.]

Have, W. ten (2011). *Beter presteren in de thuiszorg. Zelfsturende teams ter verbetering van efficiëntie en effectiviteit in de thuiszorg*. Master thesis. Tilburg: Universiteit van Tilburg. [*Better performance in home care. Self-managing teams to improve efficiency and effectiveness in home care.*]

Have, W. ten, A. B. Huijsmans, M. Otto and S. te Have (2018). *Verandermanagement veranderd. 18 populaire veranderideeën getoetst.* Amsterdam: Boom. [*Change management changed. 18 popular change ideas tested.]*

Heijnen, H. (2009). *Tien stappen op weg naar persoonlijk ondernemerschap.* Van Ierland Uitgeverij. [*Ten steps to personal entrepreneurship*.]

Heimans, J. and H. Timms (2018). *New power. Hoe macht verschuift en wat dat voor ons betekent.* Amsterdam: Business Contact. [*How power shifts and what that means for us.*]

Hepkema, W. (2012). *Stoppen met leidinggeven. Naar autonome en authentieke arbeidsrelaties.* Amsterdam: Boom/Nelissen. [*Stop leading. Towards autonomous and authentic employment relationships.*]

Heuvel, B. van den. (2014). *Netwerkzorg. Een nieuw organisatieconcept voor personen met een complexe, langdurige zorg- en ondersteuningsvraag*. Leuven: Acco.

[*Network care. A new organizational concept for people with complex, long-term care and support needs.*]

Hinssen, P. (2017). *The day after tomorrow. Hoe overleven in een tijd van radicale innovatie*. Leuven: Lannoo Campus. [*The day after tomorrow. How to survive in a time of radical innovation*.]

Hoebeke, L. (1994). *Making Work Systems Better: A Practitioner's Reflections.* Chichester, England: John Wiley & Sons Ltd.

Hoek, H. (2007). *Governance en gezondheidszorg. Private, publieke en professionele invloeden op zorgaanbieders in Nederland.* Assen: Van Gorcum. [*Governance and healthcare. Private, public and professional influences on care providers in the Netherlands.*]

Hoekstra, H. A. (2005). *Weten wat je wilt. Zelfregulatie en verandervermogen van individuen in organisaties.* Speech, Van Gorcum. [*Know what you want. Self-regulation and change capacity of individuals in organizations.*]

Hoffman, R. and B. Casnocha (2013). *The start-up of you. Adapt to the future, invest in yourself, and transform your career.* London: Random House.

Homan, T. (2005). *Organisatiedynamica. Theorie en praktijk van organisatieverandering.* The Hague: SDU Uitgevers. [*Organizational dynamics. Theory and practice of organizational change*.]

Homan, T. (2013). *Het et-cetera-principe. Een nieuw perspectief op organisatieontwikkeling*. Amsterdam: Boom Uitgevers. [*The et cetera principle. A new perspective on organizational development.*]

Hoogerwerf, L. (1998). *Opnieuw leren organiseren. Sociotechniek in actietheoretisch perspectief.* Utrecht: Lemma. [*Re-learn to organize. Sociotechnics in Action Theoretical Perspective.*]

Hooghiemstra, T. (2018). *Informationele zelfbeschikking in de zorg*. The Hague: SDU. [*Informational self-determination in healthcare.*]

Hoogveld, M. (2017). *Denk als een start-up. 9 manieren om slimmer en innovatiever te ondernemen.* Culemborg: Van Duuren Management. [*Think like a start-up. 9 ways to do business smarter and more innovatively.*]

Hoverstadt, P. (2008). *The fractal organization: creating sustainable organizations with the viable system model.* Chichester, England: John Wiley & Sons Ltd.

Huber, M. (2014). *Towards a new dynamic concept of health. Its operationalisation and use in public health and healthcare and in evaluating health effects of food.* PhD thesis, Universiteit van Maastricht.

Huguenin, P. and H. van Gestel (2007). *Verborgen orde. Systeemmanagement van organisaties*. Houten: Bohn Stafleu van Loghum. [*Hidden order. System management of organizations.*]

Huijsman, R. (2013). *Hoe slaagt de MOL? Management, organisatie en leiderschap voor toekomstige ouderenzorg*. Speech. Rotterdam: Erasmus Universiteit Rotterdam. [*How can the MOL succeed? Management, organization and leadership for future geriatric care.*]

Iansati, M. and K. R. Lakhani. (2020). *Competing in the age of AI. Strategy and leadership when algorithms and networks run the world.* Boston: Harvard Business Review.

Idenburg, P. J. and M. van Schaik (2010). *Diagnose 2015. Over de toekomst van de Nederlandse gezondheidszorg*. Schiedam: Scriptum. [*Diagnosis 2015. About the future of Dutch healthcare.*]

Idenburg, P. J. and M. van Schaik (2013). *Diagnose zorginnovatie. Over technologie en ondernemerschap*. Schiedam: Scriptum. [*Diagnosis healthcare innovation. About technology and entrepreneurship.*]

Idenburg, P. J. and S. Emonts. (2019). *Zorgenablers 2019. Technologische ontwikkelingen in de gezondheidszorg*. Utrecht: BeBright. [*Care enablers 2019. Technological developments in healthcare.*]

Illegems, J. (2017). *The internet of things in health care*. Master thesis. Ghent: Universiteit Gent.

Ismail, S. and Y. van Geest (2015). *Exponentiële organisaties. Waarom nieuwe organisaties tien keer beter, sneller en goedkoper zijn – en hoe jij dat ook wordt.* Amsterdam: Business Contact. [*Exponential organizations. Why new organizations are ten times better, faster and cheaper – and how you can be as well.*]

Ito, J. and J. Howe. (2016). *Whiplash. How to survive our faster future.* New York: Grand Central Publishing.

Iyawa, G. E., M. Herselman and A. Botha. (2016). Digital health innovation ecosystems: from systematic literature review to conceptual framework. *Procedia Computer Science* 100, 244 -252.

Jackson, M.C. (2003). *Systems Thinking, Creative holism for managers*. Chichester, England: John Wiley & Sons Ltd.

Jager, W. P. de (2001). *De evolutie van de democratie. Een verkennend onderzoek naar de betekenis van theorieën en modellen over de evolutie van complexe heterogene systemen voor de bedrijfs- en bestuurskunde*. Delft: Eburon. [*The evolution of democracy. An exploratory investigation into the meaning of theories and models about the evolution of complex, heterogenous systems for business administration and management.*]

Jager-Vreugdenhil, M. (2012). *Nederland participatieland? De ambitie van de Wet maatschappelijke ondersteuning (Wmo) en de praktijk in buurten, mantelzorgrelaties en kerken*, PhD thesis. Amsterdam: Universiteit van Amsterdam. [*The Netherlands land of participation? The aims of the Social Support Act (Wmo) and practice in neighbourhoods, informal care relationships and churches.*]

Jansen, T., G. van den Brink and J. Kole, eds. (2009). *Beroepstrots. Een ongekende kracht*. Amsterdam: Boom. [*Professional pride. An unprecedented power.*]

Jeninga, A. and H. Woldendorp (2004). Inrichting van vraagsturing in zorginstellingen: een opzet voor een kostprijsmodel, *Zorgspecial*, 2004, 39 – 42. [Set-up of demand management in healthcare institutions: a plan for a cost-price model, *Healthcare special.*]

Jeninga, A. and H. Woldendorp (2019). *Dit is waardegedreven zorg. Veranderen en waardegedreven zorg vanuit systemisch perspectief.* Amsterdam: Uitgeverij SWP. [*This is value-driven healthcare. Change and value-driven healthcare from the systemic perspective.*]

Jeurissen, P. (2016). *Steeds meer zorg, een betaalbare oplossing*? Speech. Nijmegen: Radboud Universiteit Nijmegen. [*Ever-more care, an affordable solution*?]

Jeurissen, P. H. Maarse and M. Tanke. (2018). *Betaalbare zorg*. The Hague: Sdu. [*Affordable care.*]

Jones, M. and J. Aloney. (2011). Guiding the use of grounded theory in doctoral studies. An example from the Australian film industry. *International Journal of Doctoral Studies,* vol 6, 95-114.

Jonge, E. de (2015). *Beelden van de professional. Inspiratiebronnen voor professionalisering*. PhD thesis. Utrecht: Universiteit Utrecht. [*Images of the professional. Sources of inspiration for professionalization.*]

Kane, G. C., A. N. Phillips, J. R. Copulsky and G. R. Andrus. (2019). *The technology fallacy. How people are the real key to digital transformation.* Cambridge, Mass.: The MIT Press.

Kanne, M. (2016). *Co-creatie van goede zorg. Ethische vragen, moreel beraad en normatieve professionalisering in de zorg en het sociaal werk*. PhD thesis. Utrecht: Universiteit voor Humanistiek. [*Co-creation of good healthcare. Ethical issues, moral considerations and normative professionalization in healthcare and social work.*]

Kanter, R. M. (2001), *Evolve! Succeeding in the digital of tomorrow*. Boston, Mass., Harvard Business School Press.

Kaplan, J. (2015). *Humans need not apply. A guide to wealth and work in the age of artificial intelligence*. New Haven, Conn.: Yale University Press.

Kawasaki, G. (2015). *The art of the start* 2.0. *The time-tested, battle-hardened guide for anyone starting anything*. London: Penguin.

Kay, K. (2015). *The spaghetti start-up. A tale of start-up survival or how to achieve radical growth with systems and design thinking.* Lasagnac.

Kelly, K. (2016). *The inevitable. Understanding the 12 technological forces that will shape our future*. New York: Viking.

Kerklaan, L. (2016). *De wendbare organisatie. Agility based strategy in de praktijk.* Deventer: Vakmedianet. [*The agile organization. Agility-based strategy in practice.*]

Kernick, D. (Ed.). (2004). *Complexity and healthcare organizations: a view from the street.* London, England: Radcliffe Medical Press.

Kessels, J. W. M. (2012). *Leiderschapspraktijken in een professionele ruimte*. Speech. Heerlen: Open Universiteit. [*Leadership practices in a professional space.*]

Kessener, B. and L. van Oss. (2019). *Meer dan de som der delen. Systeemdenken over organiseren en veranderen*. Deventer: Management Impact. [*More than the sum of the parts. System thinking about organizing and changing.*]

Kets de Vries, M. F. R. (2008). *Seks & Geld, Geluk & Dood. Mijmeringen uit het ondergrondse*. Amsterdam: Nieuwezijds. [*Seks & Money, Happiness & Death. Musings from the underground.*]

Kemperman, J., J. Geelhoed and J. op 't Hoog (2014). *Briljante businessmodellen in de zorg. Baanbrekende benaderingen voor beter en betaalbare zorg*. The Hague: Academic Service. [*Brilliant business models in care. Ground-breaking approaches to better, affordable care.*]

Kievit, J. (2017). *Zorg en kwaliteit: van individu, naar beide*. Valedictory speech. Leiden: Universiteit van Leiden. [*Care and quality: from individual to both.*]

Klink, A. (2012). *Toerusting in de arena van de gezondheidszorg. Waarom kostenbesparende innovaties de zorg duurder maken*. Speech. Amsterdam: Vrije Universiteit. [*Equipping in the arena of healthcare. Why cost-saving innovations make care more expensive.*]

Kolb, D. A. (1984). Experiential learning. *Experience as the source of learning and development.* Englewood Cliffs: Prentice Hall.

Kok, A. A. L. (2019). *How tough times become good times: studies on socioeconomic inequality, resilience, and succesful aging*. PhD thesis. Amsterdam: Vrij Universiteit.

Kool, R. B., L. M. Verhoef and J. A. M. Kremer (2014). *Explorerende studie over de toekomstige rol van het persoonlijk gezondheidsdossier*. Nijmegen: Radboud UMC. [*Exploratory study into the future role of the personal healthcare file.*]

Korsten, A. F. A. (2011). *Stelling nemen. Theorie als inspiratie en oriëntatiepunt voor bestuurskundig onderzoek*. Own publication. [*Taking a position. Theory as inspiration and orientation point for management theory research.*]

Kort, H. et al., eds. (2008) *Langdurige zorg en technologie*. Utrecht: Lemma. [*Long-term care and technology.*]

Koudstaal, M. (2016). *Common Wisdom Versus Facts: How Entrepreneurs Differ in their Behavioral Traits from other Occupational Groups*. PhD thesis. Amsterdam: Universiteit van Amsterdam.

Kraan, W. G. M. van der (2006). *Vraag naar vraagsturing. Een verkennend onderzoek naar de betekenis van vraagsturing in de Nederlandse gezondheidszorg*. PhD thesis. Rotterdam: Erasmus Universiteit Rotterdam. [*Demand for demand management. An exploratory study into the meaning of demand management in Dutch healthcare.*]

Kraaijeveld, K. (2018). *Hoe kunnen we de zorg blijvend (ont)regelen*? Amsterdam: De Argumentenfabriek. [*How can we permanently (de-)regulate care?*]

Kramer, B. (2001) *De bijdrage van strategische analyse aan strategievorming in de gezondheidszorg*. PhD thesis. Rotterdam: Erasmus Universiteit Rotterdam. [*The contribution of strategic analysis to strategy formation in healthcare.*]

Kremer, L. (2018). *Creatieve netwerken*. Speech. Amsterdam: Universiteit van Amsterdam. [*Creative networks.*]

Kreijveld, M. (2012). *Samen slimmer. Hoe de 'wisdom of crowds' onze samenleving zal veranderen*. The Hague: STT. [*Smarter together. How the 'wisdom of crowds' will change our society.*]

Kreijveld, M., J. Deuten and R. van Est (2014). *De kracht van platformen. Nieuwe strategieën voor innoveren in een digitaliserende wereld*. Deventer: Vakmedianet. [*The power of platforms. New strategies for innovation in a digitalizing world.*]

Kreukels, W. J. M. (1991). *Complexiteit, zelfsturing en dynamiek. Over management van complexe netwerken bij de overheid*. Speech. Alphen a.d. Rijn: Samson H.D./Tjeenk Willink. [*Complexity, self-management and dynamics. About management of complex networks for the government.*]

Krogt, F. J. van der (1995). *Leren in netwerken. Veelzijdig organiseren van leernetwerken met het oog op humaniteit en arbeidsrelevantie*. Utrecht: Lemma. [*Learning in networks. Versatile organization of learning networks with an eye to humanity and labour relevance.*]

Kromhout, M., N. Kornalijnslijper and M. de Klerk (2018). *Veranderde zorg en ondersteuning voor mensen met een beperking. Landelijke evaluatie van de Hervorming Langdurige Zorg*. The Hague: Sociaal en Cultureel Planbureau. [*Changed care and support for people with disabilities. National evaluation of the Reformation of Long-term Care.*]

Kuiper, H., R. van Amelsfoort and E. H. Kramer (2010). *Het nieuwe organiseren. Alternatieven voor de bureaucratie*. Leuven: Acco. [*New organization. Alternatives for bureaucracy.*]

Kurzweil, R. (2005). *De singulariteit is nabij. Het moment waarop de mensheid de grenzen van de biologie overstijgt*. Tilburg: De Wereld. [*The singularity is near. The moment at which humanity surpasses the limits of biology.*]

Kwakman. F. (2011). *Personal branding. Voor professionals die het verschil willen maken*. Amsterdam: Academic Service. [*Personal branding. For professionals who want to make a difference.*]

Kwakman, F. and R. Rosenmöller (2015). *Ik maak het verschil. De 7 strategieën om succesvol te zijn voor je klanten, je organisatie en jezelf*. Culemborg: Van Duuren Management. [*I make the difference. The 7 strategies for being successful for your customers, your organization and yourself.*]

Kwakman, F. and C. Zomerdijk (2012). *De ondernemende professional. Waarde creëren in een veranderende markt*. Culemborg: Van Duuren Management. [*The enterprising professional. Creating value in a changing market.*]

Laat, W. A. M., de (1983). *Vragen naar de onbekende weg*. Delft: Eburon. [*Asking about the unknown road.*]

Laat, de M. (2012). *Enabling professional development networks: how connected are you*? Speech. Heerlen: Open Universiteit.

Laeven, A. M. (2008) *Een gezonde blik naar buiten. Marktoriëntatie van ziekenhuizen*. Deventer: Kluwer. [*A healthy glance outside. Market orientation of hospitals.*]

Laloux, F. (2014). *Reinventing organizations. A guide to creating organizations inspired by the next stage of human consciousness*. Brussels: Nelson Parker.

Lambertz, M. (2016). *Freiheit und Verantwortung für intelligente Organisationen. Das Modell für lebensfähige Systeme nach Stafford Beer*. Own publication. [*Freedom and responsibility for intelligent organization. The viable system model of Stafford Beer.*]

Langer, E. J. (2010). *Counter clockwise. A proven way to think yourself younger and healthier*. London: Hodder and Stoughton, 2010.

Lanting, M. (2010). *Connect! De impact van sociale netwerken op organisaties en leiderschap*. Amsterdam: Business Contact, 2010. [*Connect! The impact of social networks on organizations and leadership.*]

Lanting, M. (2011). *Iedereen CEO. Netwerkleiderschap en de nieuwe organisatie*. Amsterdam: Business Contact. [*Everyone CEO. Network leadership and the new organization.*]

Lanting, M. (2013). *De slimme organisatie. De toekomst van werk, leiderschap en innovatie*. Amsterdam: Business Contact. [*The smart organization. The future of work, leadership and innovation.*]

Lanting, M. (2014). *Olietankers en speedboten. Wendbaar werken in de 21e eeuw*. Amsterdam: Business Contact. [*Oil tankers and speed boats. Agile work in the 21st century.*]

Lanting, M. (2017). *De disruptie paradox. In 5 stappen naar echte vernieuwing*. Amsterdam: Business Contact. [*The disruption paradox. Real innovation in 5 steps.*]

Lans, J. van der (2008). *Ontregelen. De herovering van de werkvloer*. Amsterdam: Uitgeverij Augustus. [*Deregulation. The re-taking of the workfloor.*]

La Porte, T. L., ed. (1975). *Organized social complexity: challenge to politics and policy*. Princeton.

Laurence, T. (2019). *Introduction to blockchain technology. The many faces of blockchain technology in the 21st century*. 's Hertogenbosch: Van Haren Publishing.

Leeuw, A. C. J. de (1984). *De wet van de bestuurlijke drukte. Over inspanning en resultaat van besturen*. Assen: Van Gorcum. [*The law of management pressure. About effort and results of management.*]

Leeuw, A. C. J. de (1994). *Besturen van veranderingsprocessen. Fundamenteel en praktijkgericht management van organisatieveranderingen*. Assen: Van Gorcum. [*Managing change processes. Fundamental and practice-oriented management of organizational change.*]

Leeuwen, Sj. Van (2007). *Zorgmarketing in de praktijk. Succesvol invoeren van marketing in de gezondheidszorg*. Assen: Van Gorcum. [*Care marketing in practice. Successful implementation of marketing in healthcare.*]

Ley, T. van der (2018). *Kwalitatief onderzoek naar hoe mensen een persoonlijke gezondheidsomgeving kiezen*. Utrecht: Nederlandse Patiëntenfederatie. [*Qualitative study into how people choose a personal healthcare environment.*]

Lindberg, C., S. Nash and C. Lindberg (2008). *On the edge. Nursing in the age of complexity*. Bordentown, New Jersey: PlexusPress.

Linders, L. (2019). *Op zoek naar houvast. Empowerment als handelingskader in de praktijk van zorg en welzijn*. Speech. Haarlem: Hogeschool Inholland. [*Looking for footing. Empowerment as an action framework in the practice of care and wellness.*]

Lockwood, T., ed. (2010). *Design thinking. Integrating innovation, customer experience, and brand value*. New York: Allworth Press.

Loo, M. van de (2014). *Persoonlijk ondernemerschap. Van speelbal naar sterspeler*. Amsterdam: Boom/Nelissen. [*Personal entrepreneurship. From football to star player.*]

Love, H. (2016). *The start-up J curve. The six steps to entrepreneurial success*. Austin, TX: Greenleaf Book Group.

Lucas, C. (2015). *Bewijsgestuurde zorg. Evidence based practice versus practice based evidence*. Speech, Universiteit van Amsterdam. [*Evidence-based care. Evidence-based practice versus practice-based evidence.*]

Luijkx, K. (2014). *Horen, zien en samen zorgen. Innovatie vanuit de leefwereld van ouderen*. Speech. Tilburg: Tilburg University. [*Hearing, seeing and caring together. Innovation from the experience of the elderly.*]

Maas, A. J. J. A. (1998). *Ongedefinieerde ruimten. Sociaal-symbolische configuraties. Een onderzoek naar theorie, methodologie en methode-ontwikkeling voor processen van organiseren*. Delft: Eburon. [*Undefined spaces. Social-symbolic configurations. A study into theory, methodology and method-development for processes of organization.*]

Machielse, A. (2016). *Afgezonderd of ingesloten. Over sociale kwetsbaarheid van ouderen*. Speech. Utrecht: Universiteit voor Humanistiek. [*Isolated or locked up. About social vulnerabiltiy of the elderly.*]

Madsbjerg, C. (2017). *Sensemaking. The power of the humanities in the age of algorithm*. New York: Hachette Books.

Maister, D. H. (1997). *Een echte professional*. Schoonhoven: Academic Service. [*A real professional.*]

Malby, B. and M. Anderson-Wallace. (2916). *Networks in healthcare: managing complex relationships*. Howard House, Bingley: Emerald.

Malik, F. (2006). *Managing, performing, living. Effective management for a new era*. Frankfurt/New York, Campus Verlag.

Malik, F. (2007). *Management. The essence of the craft*. Frankfurt/New York, Campus Verlag.

Malik, F. (2009). *Systemisches Management, Evolution, Selbstorganisation. Grundprobleme, Funktionsmechanismen und Lösungsansätze für komplexe Systeme*. Bern: Haupt Verlag. [*Systems of management, evolution, self-organization. foundational problems, functional mechanisms and possible solutions for complex systems.*]

Malik, F. (2011a). *Uncluttered management thinking. 46 Concepts for masterful management*. Frankfurt/New York: Campus Verlag.

Malik, F. (2011b). *Corporate policy and governance. How organizations self-organize*. Frankfurt/New York, Campus Verlag.

Malik, F. (2012). *The right corporate governance. Effective management for mastering complexity*. Frankfurt/New York, Campus Verlag.

Malik, F. (2015). *Navigieren in Zeiten des Umbruchs. Die Welt neu denken und gestalten*. Frankfurt/New York: Campus Verlag. [*Navigating in times of upheaval. Rethinking and redesigning the world.*]

Malik, F. (2016). *Strategy for managing complex systems. A contribution to management cybernetics for evolutionary systems*. Frankfurt/New York: Campus Verlag.

Malik, F. (2017). *Gefährliche Managementwörter*. Frankfurt: Campus Verlag. [*Dangerous management words.*]

Maljers, J., and W. P. M. Wansink (2009). *Alles is anders in de zorg: over bizarre budgetten, perverse regels en prima donna's*. Amsterdam, Nederland: Bert Bakker. [*Everything is different in care: about bizarre budgets, perverse rules and prima donnas.*]

Man, A. D. de, A. de Man and A. Stoppelenburg (2015). *Nieuwe business modellen in consulting: changing the game*. Amsterdam: Mediawerf Uitgevers. [*New business models in consulting: changing the game.*]

Marcus, G. and E. Davis. (2019). *Rebooting AI. Building Artificial Intelligence we can trust*. New York: Pantheon Books.

Marr, B. (2010). *The intelligent company. Five steps to success with evidence-based management*. Chichester: John Wiley & Sons.

Masselink, R. et al., eds. (2008). *Waarderend organiseren. Appreciative Inquiry: cocreatie van duurzame verandering*. Nieuwerkerk a.d. IJssel: Gelling Publishing. [*Dignifying organization. Appreciative inquiry: co-creation of lasting change.*]

Mastik, H. (2002). *Responsief simuleren. De speelruimte voor leren en sturen in meerduidige context*. Delft, Eburon. [*Responsive simulation. The space for learning and managing in an ambiguous context.*]

McAfee, A. and E. Brynjolfsson (2017). *Machine, platform, crowd. Harnesssing our digital future*. New York: W.W. Norton.

Mei, Jaap van der. *Fatale en vitale spiralen in de zorg. Zestien zorgeigen oplossingen.* VDM Projects, 2010. [*Fatal and vital spirals in care. Sixteen solutions unique to care.*]

Meadows, D. H. (2008). *Thinking in systems.* London; Chelsea Green Publishing.

Meurs, P. L. (2014). *Van regeldruk naar passende regels. Vertrouwen, veerkracht, verantwoordelijkheid en vrijheid.* Essay. Rotterdam: Erasmus Universiteiit CMDZ. [*From regulatory pressure to fitting rules. Trust, resiliance, responsibility and freedom.*]

Maso, I. and A. Smaling (2004). *Kwalitatief onderzoek: praktijk en theorie.* Amsterdam: Boom. [*Qualitative study: practice and theory.*]

Meeuwesen, A., P. van der Mast, H. Morhuis and R. Runhaar (2018). *Alternatieve financieringsvormen in het zorgstelsel.* Tilburg, TIAS, 22 February 2018. [*Alternative forms of financing in the care system.*]

Meijeren, L. van (2014). *'Shared decision making' at Buurtzorg.* Thesis. Ede: Christelijke Hogeschool.

Metz, R. (2016). *Independence or interdependence. A responsive evaluation on family group conferencing for older adults.* Thesis. Amsterdam: Hogeschool van Amsterdam.

Midgley, G. (2000). *Systemic intervention: philosophy, methodology and practice.* New York, NY: Kluwer Academic.

Minderhoud, L. (2017). *Van werknemer naar ondernemer. De winnaarsformule voor vrij ondernemen.* Utrecht: BigBusinessPublisher. [*From employee to entrepreneur. The winning formula for free enterprise.*]

Minkman, M., K. Ahaus and R. Huijsman (2010). Het ontwikkelingsmodel voor ketenzorg. Ketenkennis gebundeld in een generiek toepasbaar kwaliteitsmodel, *M&O. Tijdschrift voor Management en Organisatie*, no. 5, p. 26-44. [The development model for chain care. Chain expertise bundled in a generically applicable quality model, *M&O. Periodical for Management and Organization.*]

Minkman, M. (2012). *Developing integrated care. Towards a model for integrated care.* Thesis. EUR.

Minkman, M. (2017). *Innovatie van organisatie en governance van integrale zorg. 'Verlangen naar integraliteit'.* Speech. Tilburg: Tilburg University. [*Innovation of organization and governance of integrated care. 'Longing for integration.'*]

Minkman, M. Schaalverwarring in de regio. *Skipr* 9 January. [Scale confusion in the region.]

Mintzberg, H., B. Ahlstrand and J. Lampel (1998). *Strategy safari. A guided tour through the wilds of strategic management.* New York: The Free Press.

Modig, N. and P. Åhlström (2017). *This is lean. Resolving the efficiency paradox.* Stockhom: Rheologica Publishing.

Mohammadi, M. (2017). *Empatische woonomgeving*. Speech. Eindhoven: Technische Universiteit. [*Empathetic living environment.*]

Molenaar, C. (2017). *De kracht van platformstrategie. Het is buigen of barsten*. Amsterdam: Boom. [*The power of platform strategy. Bending or breaking.*]

Montfort, A. W. P. M. van (1986). *Economie en organisatie van de gezondheidszorg. Stand van zaken en perspectief*. Speech, Bohn, Scheltema & Holkema, Utrecht. [*Economy and organization of healthcare. State of affairs and prospects.*]

Montfort, A. W. P. M. van (1995). *Zorgverlening: een kwestie van instelling en ondernemen*. Speech. Rotterdam: Erasmus Universiteit Rotterdam. [*Care provision: a matter of attitude and enterprise.*]

Montfort, A. P. W. P. van (2011). *Technologie voor de zorg en zorg voor de technologie*. Speech. Universiteit Twente, Nederland. Obtained from http://doc.utwente.nl/79172/1/Oratieboekje_van_Montfort.pdf. [*Technology for care and care for technology.*]

Montfort, A. P. W. P. van (2016). *De ouderen pakken de lead in de zorg*! Valedictory speech. Universiteit Twente. [*The elderly taking the lead in care!*]

Montfort, A. W. P. M. van (2019a). *Reflecties op enkele thema's uit het boek van Tjeenk Willink*. Essay. [*Reflections on some themes from the book by Tjeenk Willink.*]

Montfort, A. W. P. M. van and R. van Wylick (2019b). *Zorg in perspectief van de cliënt. Essay 1. Het prosumentenmodel: van vóór via mét naar dóór de cliënt*. Amsterdam: Uitgeverij SWP. [*Care in the perspective of the client. Essay 1. The prosumer model: from for via with to by the client.*]

Montfort, A. W. P. M. and R. van Wylick. (2019c). *Zorg in perspectief van de cliënt. Ruimte voor realistische zorgfinanciering op maat. Essay 2*. Amsterdam: Uitgeverij SWP. [*Care in the perspective of the client. Space for realistic, customized care financing. Essay 2.*]

Moor, M. (2012). *Tussen de regels. Een esthetische beschouwing over geweld van organisatie*. Utrecht: Uitgeverij IJzer. [*Between the lines. An ethical consideration of the violence of organization.*]

Moore, G. (2014) *Crossing the chasm. Marketing and selling disruptive products to mainstream customers*. New York: HarperBusiness.

Morgan, G. (1986). *Images of organization*. Newbury Park: Sage.

Morgan, G. ed. (1983). *Beyond method. Strategies for social research*. Newbury Park: Sage.

Mulder, M. (2002). *Competentieontwikkeling in organisaties: perspectieven en praktijk*. 's Gravenhage: Elsevier. [*Competition development in organizations: perspectives and practice.*]

Mulje, M. (2013). D*ialectical systems thinking and the law of requisite holism concerning innovation*. Lichfield Park, AZ: Emergent Publications.

Nadella, S. (2017). *Hit refresh. De transformatie van Microsoft en de zoektocht naar een betere toekomst voor ons allemaal*. Amsterdam: A.W. Bruna Uitgevers. [*Hit refresh. The transformation of Microsoft and the search for a better future for all of us.*]

Nandram, S. S. (2015). *Organizational innovation by integrating simplification. Learning from Buurtzorg Nederland.* Heidelberg: Springer.

Nieuwenhof, R. (2005). *De taal van verandering. Veranderen in dialoog*. Schiedam: Scriptum. [*The language of change. Changing in dialogue.*]

Nies, H. L. G. R. (2012). *De zorg ontzorg/t. Veranderende rollen en resultaten in de langdurige zorg*. Speech. Amsterdam: Vrije Universiteit. [*Supporting supportive care. Changing roles and results in long-term care.*]

Njoku, G. U. (2015). *The impact of caring for seniors on the caregiver's stress level*. PhD thesis. Walden University.

Noddings, N. (2002). *Starting at home. Caring and social policy*. Berkeley: University of California Press.

Oldham, J. (2004). *The small book about large system change.* Chichester, UK, Kingsham Press.

Osterwalder, A., Y. Peigneur and P. van der Pijl (2010). *Business Model Generatie*. Alphen a.d. Rijn: Vakmedianet. [*Business model generation.*]

Osterwalder, A., Y. Peigneur, G. Bernarda and A. Smith (2014). *Waarde propositie ontwerp*. Alphen a.d. Rijn: Vakmedianet. [*Value proposition design.*]

Otto, M. and A. J. C. de Leeuw (1994). *Kijken, denken, doen. Organisatieverandering: manoeuvreren met weerbarstigheid*. Assen: Koninklijke Van Gorcum. [*Looking, thinking, doing. Organizational change: manoeuvring with resilience.*]

Pandit, N. R. (1996). The creation of theory: a recent application of the grounded theory method. *The Qualitative Report*, vol. 2, no. 4, 1 – 15.

Parker, G. G. et al. (2016). *Platform revolution. How networked markets are transforming the economy – and how to make them work for you*. New York/London: W.W. Norton & Company.

Peek, S. (2017). *Understanding technology acceptance by older adults who are again in place: a dynamic perspective.* PhD thesis. Tilburg: Tilburg University.

Peeters, P. H. and C. Cloïn (2012). *Onder het mom van zelfredzaamheid. Een journalistieke analyse van de nieuwe mantra in zorg en welzijn*. Eindhoven: Pepijn. [*Under the guise of self-reliance. A journalistic analysis of the new mantra in care and wellness.*]

Perez Ríos, J. (2012). *Design and Diagnosis for sustainable organizations.* Heidelberg, Germany: Springer.

Peters, F., A. Westerbeek and S. Tji (2014). *De kern van verpleegkundige en verzorgende beroepen.* Nijmegen: Kenniscentrum Beroepsonderwijs Arbeidsmarkt. [*The core of nursing and caring professions.*]

Peters, J. and R. Wetzels (2000). *Niets nieuws onder de zon en andere toevalligheden. Strategieontwikkeling door contextmanagement*. Amsterdam: Contact. [*Nothing new under the sun and other coincidences. Strategy development through context management.*]

Plochg, T., R. E. Juttman, N. S. Klazinga and J. P. Mackenbach, eds. (2007). *Handboek gezondheidszorgonderzoek*. Houten: Bohn Stafleu van Loghum. [*Handbook for healthcare research.*]

Poiesz, T. and J. Caris (2010). *Ontwikkelingen in de zorgmarkt. Een strategische analyse*. Deventer: Kluwer. [*Developments in the care market. A strategic analysis.*]

Pomeroy, L. (2018). *The evolution of knowledge transfer boundary networks in healthcare*. Dissertation. Londen: Imperial College.

Pomp, M. (2013). *Populatiebekostiging: panacee, hype of verkapt kartel? Een verkenning in opdracht van de Nederlandse Zorgautoriteit*. Utrecht: NZa. [*Population funding: panacea, hype or disguised cartel? An exploration at the behest of the Dutch Care Authority.*]

Pool, A., J. Mast and J. Keesom (2011). *Eerst buurten, dan zorgen: professioneel verplegen en verzorgen bij Buurtzorg*. The Hague: Boom Lemma Uitgevers. [*First neighbourhoods, then caring: professional nursing and caring at Buurtzorg.*]

Poortvliet, E. P., A. Vennekens and J. A. H. Heine (2011). *Evaluatie platform palliatieve zorg. Eindrapport*. Zoetermeer: Research en Beleid. [*Evaluation platform for palliative care. Final report.*]

Porter, M. E. and E. O. Teisberg (2006). *Redefining health care. Creating value-based competition on results.* Boston, Massachusetts: Harvard Business School Press.

Porter, M. E., and C. Guth (2012). *Redefining German health care. Moving to a value-based system.* Heidelberg, Duitsland: Springer.

Postma, J. P. (2015). *Scaling care: an analysis of the structural, social and symbolic dimensions of scale in healthcare*. PhD thesis. Rotterdam: Erasmus Universiteit Rotterdam.

Putters, K. (2017). *Was getekend. Op weg naar een vernieuwd social contract in de zorg*. Speech. Rotterdam: Erasmus Universiteit Rotterdam. [*Signed. En route to an innovative social contract in care.*]

Qualman, E. (2009). *Socialnomics. How social media transforms the way we live and do business*. Chichester, England: John Wiley & Sons Ltd.

Raak, R. van (2015). *Transition policies. Connecting system dynamics, governance and instruments in an application to Dutch healthcare*. PhD thesis. Rotterdam: Erasmus Universiteit Rotterdam.

Rademakers, J. (2016). *De actieve patiënt als utopie*. Speech. Maastricht: Universiteit Maastricht. [*The active patient as utopia.*]

Ragin, C. C. (2000). *Fuzzy-set social science*. Chicago: University of Chicago Press.

Ramo, J. C. (2016) *The seventh sense. Power, fortune and survival in the age of networks*. Boston, Massachusetts: Little, Brown and Company.

Razeghi, A. (2014). *Bend the curve. Accelerate your start-up's success*. Techstars Series.

Reijerse, C. H. and H. Woldendorp (2000). *Prestaties en competenties managen. Organisatieverandering en gedragsverandering*. Van Gorcum: Assen. [*Managing performance and competencies. Organizational change and behavioural change.*]

Ridder, W. P. de (2016). *Digital by default. Strategisch management in de onvermijdelijke digitale transformative*. Mijnmanagemenboek. [*Digital by default. Strategic management in the unavoidable digital transformation.*]

Ries, E. (2011). *The lean start-up*. London: Penguin Books.

Ries, E. (2017). *The start-up way. How entrepreneurial management transforms culture and drives growth*. London: Penguin.

Rifkin, J. (2014). *The zero marginal cost society. The internet of things, the collaborative commons, and the eclipse of capitalism*. New York: Palgrave MacMillan.

Risseeuw, M. (2004). *Managen alleen als het leuk is*. Twynstra Gudde. [*Managing only when it is fun.*]

Robertson, B. (2015). *Holacracy. De nieuwe manier van werken in een snel veranderende wereld*. Amsterdam: Business Contact, 2015. [*Holacracy. The new way of working in a rapidly changing world.*]

Roobeek, A. J. M. (2005). *Netwerklandschap. Een routeplanner voor transformaties naar netwerkorganisaties*. MeetingMoreMinds. [*Network landscape. A route planner for transformation to network organizations.*]

Roozendaal, A. (2008). *Contextueel leiderschap. Diagnose en ontwikkeling met behulp van de referentiemethode*. Assen: Van Gorcum. [*Contextual leadership. Diagnosis and development with the help of the reference method.*]

Rosmalen, B. van (2016). *Muzische professionalisering. Publieke waarden in professioneel handelen*. Utrecht: IJzer. [*Musical professionalization. Public values in professional action.*]

Rosnow, R. L. ed. (1986). *Contextualism. An understanding in behavioral science. Implications for research and theory*. Praeger, New York.

Ross, A. (2016). *The industries of the future*. London: Simon & Schuster.

Rossen, L. and C. Ramakers (2013). *Zingeving en duurzame inzetbaarheid van vrijwilligers in de zorg voor ouderen*. [*Sense-making and sustainable deployability of volunteers in care of the elderly.*]

Rotmans, J. (2012). *In het oog van de orkaan. Nederland in transitie*. Boxtel: Aenas. [*In the eye of the storm. The Netherlands in transition.*]

Rotmans, J. (2014). *Verandering van tijdperk. Nederland kantelt*. Boxtel: Aenas. [*Changing eras. The Netherlands shifts.*]

Rotmans, J. (2017). *Omwenteling. Een kantelende samenleving en economie*. Amsterdam: de Arbeiderspers. [*Upheaval. A shifting society and economy.*]

Rummler, G. A. and A. P. Brache (2013). *How to manage the white space on the organization chart.* London: John Wiley & Sons.

Ruijters, M. (2006). *Liefde voor leren. Over diversiteit van leren en ontwikkelen in en van organisaties.* Deventer: Kluwer. [*Love of learning. About diversity of learning and development in and of organizations.*]

Ruijters, M. and I. Veldkamp (2012). *Drie. Vormgeven aan organisatieontwikkeling.* Deventer: Kluwer. [*Three. Realizing organizational development.*]

Ruwaard, D. (2012). *De weg van nazorg naar voorzorg: buiten de gebaande paden.* Speech. Maastricht:Universiteit Maastricht. [*The road from aftercare to pre-care: off the beaten paths.*]

Sacolick, I. (2017). *Driving digital. The leader's guide to business transformation through technology.* New York: Amacom.

Sahota, N. and M. Ashley. (2019). *Own the A. I. revolution. Unlock your artificial intelligence strategy to disrupt your competition.* New York: McGrawHill.

Schagen, van B. and H. Woldendorp (2003). Naar een all care marketingstrategie voor zorginstellingen. *Zorgspecial*, no. 8, 12-13. [To an all-care marketing strategy for care institutions. *Care special.*]

Schaick, R. van and W. Peul. (2012). *Besturingsfilosofgie complexe zorgnetwerken. Coöperatief organiseren van regionaal geordende waardenetwerken voor concentratie en spreiding neurochirurgie.* MBA Thesis. Rotterdam: Erasmus Universiteit. [*Management philosophy for complex care networks. Cooperatively organizing regionally organized value networks for concentration and distribution of neurosurgery.*]

Schatzki, T. R. (2008). *Social practices. A Wittgensteinian approach to human activity and the social.* Cambridge: Cambrige University.

Schaveling, J., B. Bryan and M. Goodman (2012). *Systeemdenken. Van goed bedoeld naar goed gedaan.* The Hague, Nederland: Academic Service. [*System thinking. From good intentions to well done.*]

Schein, E. H. (1987/1988). Process consultation I and II. Reading, MA: Addison Wesley.

Schnelle, W. (2008). *A discursive approach to organizational and strategy consulting.* Quickborn: Metaplan.

Schrijvers, G. (2017). *Integrated care. Better and cheaper.* The Hague: SDU uitgevers.

Schwab, K. (2016). *The fourth industrial revolution.* New York: Currency.

Schwab, K. (2018). *Shaping the future of the fourth industrial revolution.* New York: Currency.

Senge, P. (1992). *The fifth discipline. The art and practice of the learning organization.* London: Century Business, 1992.

Senge, P., et al. (2015). *Presence. Een ontdekkingsreis naar diepgaande verandering in mensen en organisaties.* Amsterdam: Academic service. [*Presence. An exploration of deep change in people and organizations.*]

Sennett, R. (2013). *Respect in een tijd van sociale ongelijkheid.* Amsterdam: Byblos. [*Respect in a time of social inequality.*]

Sennett, R. (2016). *Samen. Een pleidooi voor samenwerken en solidariteit.* Amsterdam: Meulenhoff. [*Together. A plea for collaboration and solidarity.*]

Serrurier Schepper, M. and T. Hiddink. (2019). *Artificial intelligence in action. AI oplossingen bedenken en implementeren.* Culemborg: Van Duuren Management. [*Artificial intelligence in action. Devising and implementing AI solutions.*]

Sherwood, D. (2002). *Seeing the forest for the trees. A manager's guide to applying systems thinking.* London: Nicholas Brealey Publishing.

Shirky, C. (2009). *Here comes everybody. How change happens when people come together.* London: Penguin.

Shirkey, C. (2010). *Cognitive surplus. Creativity and generosity in a connected age,* London: Allen Lane.

Sidhu, I. (2016). *The digital revolution. How connected digital innovations are transforming your industry, company and career.* Old Tappan, NJ: Pearson Education, Inc.

Siebel, T. M. (2019). *Digital transformation. Survive and thrive in an era of mass extinction.* New York: Rosetta Books.

Simon, F. (2015). *Rumbling on performativity: the complex practice of policy development in a University of Applied Sciences.* PhD thesis. Heerlen: Open University.

Simon, F. (2017). De onderzoeker in een responsieve complexiteitsbenadering. *Kwalon,* 22, no 2, 12 - 20. [The researcher in a responsive complexity approach.]

Slaets, J. (2017). *Kwaliteit van zorg: wie mag het zeggen*? Vijfde Els Borst Lezing. Centrum voor Ethiek en Gezondheid. [*Quality of care: who has the say?* Fifth Els Borst Lecture.]

Smaling, A. (2008). *Dialoog en empathie in de methodologie.* Speech. Utrecht: Universiteit voor Humanistiek. [*Dialogue and empathy in methodology.*]

Smid, G. A. (2001). *Professionals opleiden. Over het ontwerpen van competentiegericht vervolgonderwijs voor hoger opgeleiden.* Academic Service. [*Training professionals. About designing competency-focused continued education for the highly educated.*]

Snijders, F. (1985). *Procesdenken: argumenten voor een interactieve opvatting van de werkelijkheid.* Utrecht: H. en S. [*Process thinking: arguments for an interactive view of reality.*]

Spil, T. and M. Michel-Verkerke (2012). *De waarde van informatie in de gezondheidswereld.* Delft: Eburon. [*The value of information in the healthcare world.*]

Sprenger, C., (2001). *Leerpraktijken. Lerend werken aan organisatieverandering.* Alphen a.d. Rijn, Samson. [*Learning practices. Agile work on organizational change.*]

Stacey, R. D. (1996). *Complexity and creativity in organizations*. San Francisco, CA: Berrett-Koehler Publishers.

Stacey, R. and D. Griffin. (2005). *A complexity perspective on researching organizations: taking experience seriously*. Abingdon: Routledge.

Stadhouders, N. W. (2019). *Effective healthcare cost-containment policies. Using the Netherlands as a case study*. PhD thesis. Nijmegen: Radboud University Nijmegen.

Stoopendaal, A. and R. Bouwman. (2018). *Ruimte voor vertrouwen. De dynamiek van vertrouwen in het toezicht op zorg*. Rotterdam: ESHPM. [*Space for trust. The dynamics of trust in the oversight of care.*]

Stowell, F. and C. Welch (2012). *The manager's guide to systems practice. Making sense of complex problems*. Chichester, England: John Wiley and Sons.

Strauss, A. and J. Corbin. (1998). *Basics of qualitative research: techniques and procedures for developing grounded theory*. (2nd ed.). Thousand Oaks, CA: Sage.

Strien, P. J. van (1986). *Praktijk als wetenschap. Methodolgie van het social-wetenschappelijk handelen*. Assen: Van Gorcum. [*Practice as science. Methodology of social-scientific action.*]

Strikwerda, H. (2014). *Bespiegelingen over governance, bestuur, management en organisatie in de 21e eeuw*. Assen: Koninklijke Van Gorcum. [*Reflections on governance, direction, management and organization in the 21st century.*]

Strikwerda, H. and J. ten Wolde (2017). *Verplichte literatuur voor bestuurders en commissarissen. Professionaliteit in governance*. Deventer: Vakmedianet. [*Required literature for directors and commissioners. Professionalism in governance.*]

Susskind, R. and D. Susskind (2017). *The future of professions. How technology will transform the work of human experts.* Oxford University Press.

Taleb, N. N. (2007). *The black swan. The impact of the highly improbable.* London: Random House.

Taleb, N. N. (2012). *Antifragile. How to live in a world we don't understand.* London: Pearson.

Taleb, N. (2018). *Skin in the game. Hidden asymmetries in daily life*. New York: Random House.

Tegmark, M. (2017). *Life 3.0. Being human in the age of artificial intelligence*. London: Allen Lane.

Teisman, G. R., A. van Buuren and L. Gerrits (eds.) (2009). *Managing Complex Governance Systems: Dynamics, Self-Organization and Coevolution in Public Investments.* New York: Routledge.

Termeer, C. J. A. M. and M. J. W. van Twist (1991). De configuratiebenadering: een procestheorie voor sturingsvraagstukken. *Beleid en maatschappij*, vol. 5, no. 4, 185-195, 205. [The configuration approach: a process theory for management issues. *Policy and society.*]

Thiecke, M. and B. van der Zeeuw (2013). *Systemisch transitiemanagement. Neem voor de verandering de makkelijke weg*. Amsterdam: Boom/Nelissen. [*Systemic transition management. Take the easy way for a change.*]

Thomas, J. B., S. M. Clark and D. A. Goia. (1993). Strategic sensemaking and organizational performance: linkages among scanning, interpretation, action and outcomes. *Academy of Management Journal*, vol. 36, 239 – 270.

Tjeenk Willink, H. (2018). *Groter denken, Kleiner doen. Een oproep.* Amsterdam: Prometheus. [*Think bigger, act smaller. A summons.*]

Tonkens, E., J. van den Broeke and M. Hoijtink (2008). *Op zoek naar weerkaatst plezier. Samenwerking tussen mantelzorgers, vrijwilligers, professionals en cliënten in de multiculturele stad.* The Hague: Nicis Institute. [*Looking for reflected enjoyment. Collaboration between informal caregivers, volunteers, professionals and clients in the multicultural city.*]

Tonkens, E. (2004). *Mondige burgers, getemde professionals. Marktwerking, vraagsturing en professionaliteit in de publieke sector.* Utrecht: NIZW, 2004. [*Vocal citizens, timid professionals. Market effect, demand management and professionalism in the public sector.*]

Topol, E. (2012). *The creative destruction of medicine. How the digital revolution will create better health care.* New York: Basic Books.

Topol, E. (2015). *The patient will see you now. The future of medicine is in your hands.* New York: Basic Books.

Topol, E. 2019). *Deep medicine. How artificial intelligence can make healthcare human again.* New York: Basic Books

Trusko, B. E. (2007). *Improving healthcare quality and cost with Six Sigma.* Upper Saddle River, N.J.: FT Press.

Twist, M. van (1991). *Organiseren: configupraatjes en autopoëzie*. Rotterdam: Erasmus Universiteit. [*Organizing: configuration talks and self-poetry.*]

Twist, M. van (2018). *Woorden wisselen. Werken aan een hertaling van besturen, organiseren en adviseren*. Deventer: Vakmedianet. [*Exchanging words. Working on a rewording of management, organizing and consulting.*]

Ubbink, D. (2018). *Juweeltjes in de zorg*. Speech. Amsterdam: Universiteit van Amsterdam. [*Gems in care.*]

Valentijn, P. P. (2015). *Rainbow of chaos. A study into the theory and practice of integrated primary care*. Thesis. Tilburg: Tilburg University.

Veen, M. v.d., I. Wakkee and L. van Nispen (2016). *Ondernemerschap: een persoonlijke keuze. Een onderzoek naar kenmerken en behoeften van aspirantondernemers.* Utrecht: Kamer van Koophandel. [*Entrepreneurship: a personal choice. A study of characteristics and needs of aspiring entrepreneurs.*]

Veen, N. et al. (2015). *Cultuursensitief addendum bij de Mulktidisciplinaire Richtlijn (MDR). Schizofrenie*. Utrecht: Trimbos Instituut. [*Culturally sensitive addendum to the Multidisciplinary Guideline (MDR). Schizophrenia.*]

Veer, A. J. E. de, H. E. Brandt, F. G. Schellevis and A. L. Francke (2008). *Buurtzorg: nieuw en toch vertrouwd. Een onderzoek naar de ervaringen van cliënten, mantelzorgers, medewerkers en huisartsen*. Utrecht: Nivel. [*Buurtzorg: new and yet familiar. A study into the experiences of clients, informal caregivers, employees and general practitioners.*]

Veltenaar, R. and L. Zevenbergen. (2020). *Once upon a future*. Haarlem: Bertram en De Leeuw Uitgevers.

Verborg, F. (2016). *Meer ik, meer moraal. Persoonlijk leiderschap in de georganiseerde samenleving*. Zoetermeer: Klement. [*More me, more moral. Personal leadership in the organized society.*]

Verhees, G. (2013). *Publiek-private samenwerking: adaptieve planning in theorie en praktijk*. PhD thesis. Groningen: Rijksuniversiteit Groningen. [*Public-private cooperation: adaptive planning in theory and practice.*]

Verhoeven, H. (2017). *Werkmakers. Van solliciteren naar werk creëren, van werkzoeker naar werkmaker*. Culmeborg: AnderZ. [*Work-makers. From applying for to creating work, from applicant to work-maker.*]

Vermaak, H. (2009). *Plezier beleven aan taaie vraagstukken. Werkingsmechanismen van vernieuwing en weerbarstigheid*. Deventer: Kluwer. [*Experiencing pleasure from tough issues. Effect mechanisms of innovation and resilience.*]

Vermeulen, H. (2019). *Beter laten, beter maken, beter doen*. Speech. Nijmegen: Radboud Universiteit. [*Better facilitation, better creation, better action.*]

Versleijen, M. (2012). *Populatiebekostiging: geld volgt zorg?! Randvoorwaarden van populatiebekostiging in het Nederlandse zorgstelsel*. Master thesis. Wageningen:, Wageningen University. [*Population funding: does that apply for care?! Preconditions for population funding in the Dutch care system.*]

Verver, D., H. Merten and C. Wagner (2016). *Eindrapport 'Toezicht op zorgnetwerken van thuiswonende kwetsbare ouderen'*. Amsterdam: VU: EMGO Instituut. [*Final report 'Oversight of care networks for vulnerable elderly persons living at home.*]

Vester, F. (2012). *The art of interconnected thinking: ideas and tools for a new approach to tackling complexity*. Munich, Germany: MCB-Verlag.

Veuger, J. (2014). *Materieel immaterieel. Besturing van woningcorporaties in samenhang met maatschappelijke waarden*. PhD thesis. Rotterdam: Erasmus Universiteit Rotterdam. [*Materially immaterial. Management of housing corporations in connection with social values.*]

Veuger, J. (2017). *Een wendbare vastgoedeconomie met disruptie & blockchain*. Lectoraat Hanze Hogeschool, Groningen. [*An agile real estate economy with disruption & blockchain.*]

Veuger, J. (2020). *Blockchain convergentie.* Speech. Saxion University of Applied Sciences. [*Blockchain convergence.*]

Veuger, J. and H. Woldendorp. (2021). *Blockchain in de zorg.* Assen: Koninklijke Van Gorcum. [*Blockchain in care.*]

Vickers, J. (2016). *Exploring engagement: a grounded theory study of young people's interactions with healthcare professionals.* Ph.D. thesis. Salford: University of Salford.

Viki, T., D. Toma and E. Gons (2017). *De corporate start-up. Hoe je als gevestigd bedrijf een succcesvol ecosysteem voor innovatie creëert.* Deventer: Vakmedianet. [*The corporate start-up. How you create a successful ecosystem for innovation as an established company.*]

Vincent, A. (2017). *Jobmarketing 3.0. Jouw arbeidsmarkt: nu vindbaar, straks nieuw werk.* Houten: Het Spectrum. [*Job marketing 3.0. Your labour market: searchable now, new work later.*]

Visser, S., J. Kremer, R. Westendorp and A. Klink (2012). *Kwaliteit als medicijn. Aanpak voor betere zorg en lagere kosten.* Booz & Co. [*Quality as medicine. Approach for better care and lower costs.*]

Vissers, J. and G. de Vries (2005). *Sleutelen aan zorgprocessen. Een visie op zorglogistieke bedrijfsvoering.* Speech. Rotterdam: Erasmus Universiteit Rotterdam. [*Keys to care processes. A view of the care logistics business.*]

Vlugt, E. de. (2016). *Robots: who cares? Technologie als verlengstuk.* Speech. The Hague: Haagse Hogeschool. [*Robots: who cares? Technology as an extension.*]

Voigt, R. J. (1990). Beleidsmakers als meesters in het spel der ficties. *Bestuur. Maandblad voor Overheidskunde*, vol. 9, no. 2. [Policymakers as masters in the game of fictions. *Management. Monthly periodical for governance.*]

Volberda, H. W. (1998). *Blijvend strategisch vernieuwen: concurreren in de 21e eeuw.* Deventer: Kluwer. [*Continuously innovating strategically: competition in the 21st century.*]

Voogt, T. (1990). *Managen in een meervoudige context. Naar een methode voor het ontwikkelen en veranderen van sociaal-cognitieve configuraties.* Delft: Eburon. [*Managing in an ambiguous context. Towards a method for developing and changing social-cognitive configurations.*]

Vos, C. de (2014). *Kwaliteit, disciplinering en sturing. Een historisch sociologisch onderzoek naar de vormgeving van kwaliteit van zorg in ziekenhuizen.* PhD thesis. Rotterdam: Erasmus Universiteit Rotterdam. [*Quality, discipline and management. A historical-sociological study into the design of quality of care in hospitals.*]

Vos, J. (2010). *De Münchhausenbeweging: beweging voor samenwerking.* Deventer: Kluwer. [*The Münchhausen movement: movement for collaboration.*]

Vries, G. de (1977). *Sociale orde, regels en sociologie: een wetenschapsfilosofisch onderzoek naar theorievorming in de sociologie*. Meppel: Boom. [*Social order, rules and sociology: a scientific-philosophical study into theory formation in sociology.*]

Vries, T. de (2005). *Technologie en zorg. Wie wordt er beter van*? Speech. Humanistic University Press. [*Technology and care. Who benefits?*]

Waal, S. P. M. de et al. (2003). Maatschappelijk ondernemerschap in de zorg, in W. van Harten & R. W. Schuring (eds.), *Ondernemen in de zorg*, Koninklijke van Gorcum, 2003, p. 39. [Social entrepreneurship in care, in *Entrepreneurship in care.*]

Waal, S. P. M. de (2008). *Strategisch management voor de publieke zaak. Hoe burgers, bedrijven, non- profitorganisaties en overheid gezamenlijk problemen oplossen.* Lemma. [*Strategic management for public matters. How citizens, companies, non-profit organizations and government collectively solve problems.*]

Wachter, R. M. (2017). *The digital doctor. Hope, hype, and harm at the dawn of medicine's computer age.* New York: McGrawHill Education.

Waldock, B. (2015). *Being agile in business. Discover, faster, smarter, leaner ways to work.* Harlow: Pearson.

Wallin, A. J. (2018). *Rethinking digital transformation of healthcare. The role of technology and institutions in service innovation.* Dissertation. Helsinki: Aalto University.

Walstra, J. (2011). *Klantgericht innoveren.* Amsterdam: Pearson AddisonWesley. [*Customer-oriented innovation.*]

Wanrooy, M. J. (2008). *Het spel en de knikkers. Besturing van professionele organisaties.* Schiedam: Scriptum Management. [*The game and the marbles. Managing professional organizations.*]

Water, R. van de and M. Weggeman (2017). *Stagnatie van professionals. Voorkomen en aanpakken.* Schiedam: Scriptum Management. [*Stagnation of professionals. Prevention and approach.*]

Watzlawick, P. (1976). *Is 'werkelijk' waar? Spraakverwarring, zinsbegoocheling en onvoorstelbare werkelijkheid.* Deventer: Van Loghum Slaterus. [*Is 'reality' true? Linguistic confusion, sensory tricks and unimaginable reality.*]

Watzlawick, P. (1984). Components of ideological 'realities,' in: P. Watzlawick, ed. *The invented reality. How do we know what we believe we know? Contributions to constructivism.* New York: Norton, p. 206-249.

Watzlawick, P. (1989). *Münchhausens ladder en Wittgensteins ladder. Uit de greep van de werkelijkheid.* Deventer: Van Loghum Slaterus. [*Münchhausen's ladder and Wittgenstein's ladder. Out of the grip of reality.*]

Watzlawick, P., J. Helmet Beavin and D. D. Jackson (1970). *De pragmatische aspecten van de menselijke communicatie.* Deventer: Van Loghum Slaterus. [*The pragmatic aspects of human communication.*]

Watzlawick, P., J. H. Weakland and R. Fisch (1974). *Het kan anders. Over het onderkennen en oplossen van menselijke problemen*. Deventer: Van Loghum Slaterus. [*It can be different. About exploring and solving human problems.*]

Weber, W. W., et al., eds. (2010). *Peter F. Drucker's Next management: New institutions, new theories and practices*. Göttingen, Verlag Sordon.

Weber, W. (2007). *Complicate your life*. Göttingen: Sordon.

Weggeman, M. (2003). *Provocatief adviseren. Organisaties mooier maken*. Schiedam, Scriptum. [*Provocative consulting. Making organizations more beautiful.*]

Weggeman, M. (2015). *Essenties van leidinggeven aan professionals*. Schiedam: Scriptum Management. [*Essences of leading professionals.*]

Weick, K. E. (1969) *The social psychology of organizing*, Addison-Wesley Publishing Company, California.

Weick, K. E. (1995). *Sensemaking in organizations*. Thousand Oaks, CA: Sage

Weick, K. E., K. M. Sutcliffe and D. Obstfeld. (2005). Organizing and the process of sensemaking and organizing. *Organization Science*, vol. 16, nr. 4, 409 - 421.

Weisbord, M. R. (1991). *Productive workplaces. Organizing and managing for dignity, meaning and community*. San Francisco: Jossey-Bass.

Werkman, R. A. (2006). *Werelden van verschil. Hoe actoren in organisaties vraagstukken in veranderprocessen hanteren en creëren*. PhD thesis. Amsterdam: Universiteit van Amsterdam. [*Worlds of difference. How actors in organizations use and create issues in change processes.*]

West, G. (2017). *Scale. The universal laws of growth, innovation, sustainability, and the pace of life in organisms, cities, economies, and companies.* New York: Penguin Press.

Wester, F. (1995). *Strategieën voor kwalitatief onderzoek*. Bussum: Coutinho. [*Strategies for qualitative research.*]

Westerman, G., D. Bonnet and A. McAfee (2014). *Leading digital. Turning technology into business transformation*. Boston: Harvard Business Review Press.

Wheatley, M. J. and M. Kellner-Rogers. (1999). *A simpler way*. San Francisco: Berrett-Koehler.

Wheatley, M. J. (2017). *Who do we choose to be? Facing reality, claiming leadership, restoring sanity*. Oakland, CA: Berrett-Koehler.

Wielinga, E. en S. Robijn. (2018). *Netwerken met energie. Gereedschap voor co-creatie*. Schiedam: Schriptum. [*Networking with energy. Tool for co-creations.*]

Wierdsma, A. (1999). *Co-creatie van verandering*. Delft: Eburon. [*Co-creation of change.*]

Wieringen, M. van et al. (2014). *Hoe thuiszorgorganisaties samenwerking organiseren: visies, praktijken en dilemma's. Rapportage over de samenwerking van thuiszorgmedewerkers met mantelzorgers en andere organisaties*. Amsterdam: Vrije Universiteit. [*How home care organizations organize collaboration: visions, practices and dilemmas. Report on the collaboration of home care employees with informal caregivers and other organizations.*]

Wijdeven, T. van de (2012). *Doe democratie. Over actief burgerschap in stadswijken.* Delft: Eburon. [*Do democracy. About active citizenship in urban neighbourhoods.*]

Willems, N., R. Linck and E. Kaats, eds. (2018). *Organiseren in en met netwerken.* Deventer: Vakmedianet. [*Organizing in and with networks.*]

Williams, S. P. (2019). *Blockchain: the next everything.* London: Simon & Schuster.

Winch, P. (1958). *The idea of a social science and its relation to philosophy.* New York: Humanities Press.

Winters, S. (2014). *Trinity of quality improvement. Studies on structure, process and outcome related to quality improvement in long-term care in the Netherlands between 2007 and 2011.* PhD thesis. Rotterdam: Erasmus Universiteit Rotterdam.

Wit, E. et al. (2007). *De autonome mens. Nieuwe visies op gemeenschappelijkheid.* Amsterdam: SUN. [*The autonomous person. New views of commonality.*]

Witte, Luc P. de (2008). *Technologie, mij (') zorg! Over langdurige zorg, technologie en innovatie.* Speech. Maastricht: Universiteit van Maastricht. [*Technology, me (') care! About long-term care, technology and innovation.*]

Wittgenstein, L., (1992). *Filosofische onderzoekingen.* Meppel: Boom, 1953. [*Philosophical studies.*]

Wirtz, F. D. (1990). *Metamanagement. Achtergronden en ontwikkelingen, mogelijkheden en veranderingen in theorie en praktijk van het organiseren. Deel 1 Achtergronden en ontwikkelingen.* Baarn: Nelissen. [*Metamanagement. Backgrounds and developments, possibilities and changes in the theory and practice of organization. Part 1 Backgrounds and developments.*]

Wirtz, F. D., (1992). *Metamanagement. Achtergronden en ontwikkelingen, mogelijkheden en veranderingen in theorie en praktijk van het organiseren. Deel 2 Standaardbeelden en perspectieven.* Baarn: Nelissen. [*Metamanagement. Backgrounds and developments, possibilities and changes in the theory and practice of organization. Part 2 Standard views and perspectives.*]

Woldendorp, H. (1997). Drukte of druktemakers, in: A. van Dijk, ed., *De ladder op omlaag? Een psychologie van besturen.* Assen: Van Gorcum. [Pressure or pressure-makers, in *Down the ladder? A psychology of managing.*]

Woldendorp, H. (2006). Een businessmodel voor de ouderenzorg. *Zorgspecial*, no. 5, 6 – 9. [A business model for geriatric care. *Care special.*]

Woldendorp, H. (2018). *Toekomstbestendige zorgprofessionals en zorgorganisaties. De consequenties van platformtechnologie voor de ouderenzorg.* Assen: Koninklijke Van Gorcum. [*Future-proof care professionals and care organizations. The consequences of platform technology for geriatric care.*]

Woldendorp, H. (2021). *Technologische en sociale innovatie in de ouderenzorg. The impact of COVID-19.* Amsterdam: Uitgeverij SWP. [*Technological and social innovation in geriatric care. The impact of COVID-19.*]

Woldendorp, H. and A. Jeninga (2018). *Organisaties ontwarren. Systemisch kijken, denken en doen binnen de gezondheidszorg.* Amsterdam: Uitgeverij SWP. [*Detangling organizations. Systemic viewing, thinking and acting within healthcare.*]

Woldendorp. H. and T. Woldendorp (2019). *De start-up professional. Ondernemen als loopbaanstrategie.* Amsterdam: Uitgeverij SWO. [*The start-up professional. Entrepreneurship as a career strategy.*]

Woldendorp, H. and J. Hoekman (2019). *Een evolutietheorie van het sociaal domein: de weerbarstige praktijk.* Amsterdam: Uitgeverij SWP. [*An evolutionary theory of the social domain: the resilient practice.*]

Womack, J. P., D. T. Jones, D. Roos and D. Sammons (1990). *The machine that changed the world.* New York: MacMillan.

Wouden, R. van der (1990). *De dynamiek van beleid. Onbetaalde arbeid en theorieën over beleid.* PhD thesis. Amsterdam: Universiteit van Amsterdam. [*The dynamics of policy. Unpaid labour and theories about policy.*]

Wulven, van G. (2017). *Innoveer jezelf. In 6 stappen innovatief in je werk.* Culemborg: Maven. [*Innovate yourself. Innovating in your work in 6 steps.*]

Yin, R. K. (2009). *Case study research. Design and methods.* Los Angeles: Sage.

Zegveld, C. (2018). *Netwerkaansprakelijkheid voor gebrekkige samenhangende zorg.* PhD thesis. Tilburg: Universiteit Tilburg. [*Network liability for defectively coherent care.*]

Zerubavel, E. (2018). *Taken for granted. The remarkable power of the unremarkable.* Princeton: Princeton University Press.

Zijderveld, A. C. (1974). *De relativiteit van kennis en werkelijkheid. Inleiding tot de kennissociologie.* Meppel: Boom. [*The relativity of knowledge and reality. Introduction to knowledge sociology.*]

Zohar, D. (2017). *Quantum leiderschap.* Amsterdam: Business Contact. [*Quantum leadership.*]

Zorggroep Almere (2013). *Maatschappelijke Businesscase Verpleegkundige Praktijk.* [*Social business case for nursing practice.*]

Zulauf, C. (2001). *The big picture. A systems thinking story for managers.* Lexington: Linkage Press.

Zuyderhoudt, R. (2007). *Op zoek naar synergie. Omgaan met onoplosbare problemen.* PhD thesis. Amsterdam: Universiteit van Amsterdam. [*Looking for synergy. Handling unsolvable problems.*]

Zwakhalen, S. M. G. (2018). *De zorg voor ouderen thuis: veel spreiding, niet gemiddeld.* Speech. Maastricht: Universiteit van Maastricht. [*The care for the elderly at home: a lot of spread, not average.*]

Zwart, C. and B. Middel (2005). *Omvormen van jezelf en de wereld om je heen. Een uitnodiging tot de ontwikkelkunde*. Assen: Van Gorcum. [*Transforming yourself and the world around you. An invitation to development.*]

Zwart-Olde, I., M. Jacobs and M. Broese van Groenou (2013). *Zorgnetwerken van kwetsbare ouderen*. Amsterdam: Vrije Universiteit. [*Care networks of vulnerably elderly people.*]

POLICY DOCUMENTS AND REPORTS (2004 – 2021)

Actiz, BTN, Patiëntenfederatie Nederland, Verenso, V &VN. (2016). *Kwaliteit in dialoog. Kwaliteitskader ouderenzorg*. Cover note. [*Quality in dialogue. Quality framework for geriatric care.*]

Actiz en Hogeschool Utrecht. (2019). *Opschalen van technologie in de wijk*. Utrecht: Avctiz. [*Scaling up technology in the neighbourhood.*]

Audit Commission (2004). *Older people – independence and well-being. The challenge for public services*.

Berenschot. (2019). *Naar werkende governance op blockchain in de zorg. Kaders voor verstandige toepassing en ontwikkeling*. Utrecht: Berenschot. [*To working governance on blockchain in care. Frameworks for intelligent application and development.*]

CEG. (2019). *Veilige zorg, goede zorg*? The Hague: Centrum voor Ethiek en Gezondheid. [*Safe care, good care?*]

Chapman, S., J. Miller and J. Spetz. (2019). *The impact of emerging technologies on long-term care and the health workforce*. San Francisco: University of California. Research report.

Commissie Toekomst Zorg Thuiswonende Ouderen. *Oud en zelfstandig in 2030. Een reisadvies*. The Hague: 2020. [*Old and independent in 2030. Travel advice.*]

Deloitte. (2017). *Personalized health. Preparing for tomorrows healthcare*.

Denktank IZO. (2019). *Met elkaar in gesprek over de toekomst*. Vision document. [*Talking with each other about the future.*]

Eindevaluatie experiment regelarme instelling. (ERAI). (2016). The Hague: Ministerie van VWS. [*Final evaluation of experiment on low-regulation institution.*]

Equalis. (2019). *Samen beslissen in de praktijk. Hoe wordt Samen Beslissen toegepast in de praktijk en welke rol speelt uitkomstinformatie hierbij*? Amsterdam: Vrije Universiteit. [*Deciding together in practice. How Deciding Together is applied in practice and what role dies outcome information play?*]

EZK. (2018). *Nederlandse digitaliseringsstrategie. Hier kan het. Hier gebeurt het*. The Hague: Ministerie van Economische Zaken en Klimaat. [*Dutch digitalization strategy. It's possible here. It's happening here.*]

FME. (2018) *Betere zorg door technologie. FME agenda zorgtechnologie*. Zoetermeer: FME. [*Better care through technology. FME agenda for care technology.*]

FMS. (2017). *Visiedocument Medisch Specialist 2025. Ambitie, vertrouwen en samenwerken*. Utrecht: Federatie Medisch Specialisten. [*Vision document, Medical Specialist 2025. Aims, trust and collaboration.*]

FWG. (2017). *FWG trendrapport. De zorg, ongelijk voor iedereen*. Utrecht: October 2017. [*FWG trend report. Care, unequal for everyone.*]

Idenburg, P. J. and S. Emonts. (2019). *Zorg enablers 2019. Technologische ontwikkelingen in de gezondheidszorg*. Utrecht: BeBright. [*Care enablers 2019. Technological developments in healthcare.*]

IGJ. (2018). *Goede zorg in zorgnetwerken.* Utrecht: Inspectie Gezondheidszorg en Jeugd. [*Good care in care networks.*]

Jester Strategy. (2019). *Technologie in de verpleeghuiszorg*. Amersfoort: Jester Strategy. [*Technology in nursing home care.*]

KPMG (2013). *Integrale zorg. Naar nieuwe coalities in de zorg*. [*Integrated care. To new coalitions in care.*]

KPMG (2014a). *The primary care paradox. New designs and models.*

KPMG (2014b). *Applicability of consumer directed care principles in residential aged care homes.*

KPMG (2014c). *An uncertain age*: *reimagining long term care in the 21st century.*

KPMG (2016a). *What works. Staying power. Success stories in global healthcare.*

KPMG (2016b). *Digital health*: *heaven or hell. How technology can drive or derail the quest for efficient, high quality healthcare.*

KPMG (2017a). *The MedTech market in the Netherlands.*

KPMG (2017b). *Mag het een ietsje meer zijn. De true value van de digitale economie.* [*Can it be just a bit more. The true value of the digital economy.*]

KPMG. (2018). *Juiste zorg op de juiste plek. Onderzoek naar condities en consequenties.* [*The right care in the right place. Research into conditions and consequences.*]

KPMG. (2019).*Wie doet het met wie. Het verbonden zorglandschap*. [*Who does it with whom? The connected care landscape.*]

Linschoten, C. P. and B. te Velde. (2016). *Inventarisatie en analyse van multidisciplinaire zorg voor ketsbare ouderen*. Groningen: Argo. [*Inventory and analysis of multidisciplinary care for vulnerable elderly persons.*]

LUMC. (2020). *Gezond lang thuis wonen in Den Haag: de IZI pilots*. The Hague: LUMC-Campus. [*Living healthy at home for a long time in The Hague.*]

Morgens. (2019). *De ouderenzorg van morgen. Vergrijzing vraagt om ingrijpende veranderingen*. [*Tomorrow's geriatric care. Population aging requires drastic changes.*] Leiden: Morgens.

NDSD (2016). *De rol van populatiebekostiging in het sociaal domein. Verder komen met 'de bedoeling centraal'*. The Hague: Netwerk directeuren Sociaal Domein. [*The role of population funding in the social domain. Moving forward with 'the intention central'.*]

Neomax. (2017). *De digitale transformatie.* Amersfoort: Neomax. [*The digital transformation.*]

Nictiz (2017). *Evaluatie van eHealth-technologie in de context van beleid.* The Hague: Nictiz. [*Evaluation of eHealth technology in the context of policy.*]

Nictiz (2019). *Artificial intelligence in de zorg. Begrippen, praktijkvoorbeelden en vraagstukken.* The Hague: Nictiz. [*Artificial intelligence in care. Terms, examples from practice and issues.*]

Nictiz and Nivel. (2019). *Samen aan zet! eHealth monitor 2019.* The Hague: Nictiz. [*It's our move! eHealth monitor 2019.*]

Nies, H. et al. (2019). *Ouderen- en gehandicaptenzorg in Scandinavië. Op zoek naar bronnen voor duurzame vernieuwing.* Utrecht: Vilans. [*Geriatric and handicapped care in Scandinavia. Looking for sources for sustainable innovation.*]

Niezen, M.G.H. and P. Verhoef (2018). *Digitale gezondheidsregie – meer gegevens, meer grip?* Rathenau Instituut. The Hague: Rathenau Insituut. [*Digital health control – more data, more grip?*]

Nivel. (2014). *Ouderen van de toekomst. Verschillen in de wensen en mogelijkheden voor wonen, welzijn en zorg.* Utrecht: Nivel. [*The elderly of the future. Differences in preferences and possibilities for living, wellness and care.*]

NZa (2018). *Monitor. Zorg voor ouderen 2018.* Utrecht: Nederlandse Zorgautoriteit. [*Monitor. Care for the elderly 2018.*]

NZa (2019). *Voortgangsrapportage doorontwikkeling Wijkverpleging.* Utrecht: Nederlandse Zorgautoriteit. [*Progress report on further development of District nursing.*]

ParkinsonNet (2019). *Handreiking aandoeningsspecifieke netwerken.* [*Manual for condition-specific networks.*]

PBL (2019). *Zelfstandig thuis op hoge leeftijd.* The Hague: Planbureau voor de Leefomgeving. [*Independent at home at a later age.*]

PinkRoccade Healthcare (2013). *Het stormt in de polder. Een anticiperende kijk op het zorglandschap.* PinkRoccade. [*It's storming in the polder. An anticipatory look at the care landscape.*]

PWC. (2017). *Sherlock in Health: How artificial intelligence may improve quality and efficiency, whilst reducing healthcare costs in Europe.*

Rathenau Instituut. (2019). *Een missiegerichte aanpak voor slimme zorg en e-health.* The Hague: Rathenau Instituut. [*A mission-oriented approach to smart care and e-health.*]

RIVM (2014). *Burgers en gezondheid. Themarapport Volksgezondheid. Toekomst Verkenning 2014.* Bilthoven: Rijksinstituur voor Volksgezondheid en Milieu. [*Citizens and health. Theme report on public health. Future exploration 2014.*]

RIVM. (2018). *Robotisering. Themarapport Volksgezondheid Toekomstverkenning. 2018*. Bilthoven: Rijksinstituur voor Volksgezondheid en Milieu. [*Robotization. Theme report on public health. Future exploration 2018.*]

Roland Berger. (2016). *Digital and disrupted: all change for healthcare. How can pharma companies flourish in a digitized healthcare world?*

RVS. (2010). *Gezondheid 2.0*. The Hague: Raad voor Volksgezondheid en Samenleving. [*Health 2.0.*]

RVS. (2017a). *Zorgrelatie centraal. Partnerschap leidend voor Zorginkoop*. The Hague: Raad voor Volksgezondheid en Samenleving. [*Care relationship central. Partnership leading for care procurement.*]

RVS (2017b). *Heft in eigen hand. Zorg en ondersteuning voor mensen met meervoudige problemen*. The Hague: Raad voor Volksgezondheid en Samenleving. [*In control. Care and support for people with multiple problems.*]

RVS (2019a). *Blijk van vertrouwen. Anders verantwoorden voor goede zorg*. The Hague: Raad voor Volksgezondheid en Samenleving. [*Look of trust. Accounting differently for good care.*]

RVS. (2019b). *Samen maken we de zorg (beter)*. The Hague: Raad voor Volksgezondheid en Samenleving. [*Together, we make care (better).*]

RVS. (2019c). *(Waarde(n)volle zorgtechnologie. Een verkennend advies over de kansen en risico's van kunstmatige intelligentie in de zorg*. The Hague: Raad voor Volksgezondheid en Samenleving. [*Valuable care technology. An exploratory recommendation on the opportunities and risks of artificial intelligence in care.*]

RVS. (2019d). *Complexe problemen, eenvoudige toegang. Botsende waarden bewuster afwegen*. Essay. The Hague: Raad voor Volksgezondheid en Samenleving. [*Complex problems, easy access. Weighing conflicting values more deliberately.*]

RVS. (2020). *De derde levensfase: het geschenk van de eeuw*. The Hague: Raad voor Volksgezondheid en Samenleving. [*The third life phase: the gift of the century.*]

RVS. (2020). *Zorg op afstand dichterbij? Digitale zorg na de coronacrisis*. The Hague: Raad voor Volksgezondheid en Samenleving, August 2020. [*Remote care closer? Digital care after the corona crisis.*]

RVZ (2014a). *De stem van de verzekerden. Advies over de legitimiteit en de governance van zorgverzekeraars*. The Hague: Raad voor Volksgezondheid en Zorg. [*The voice of the insured. Advice on the legitimacy and governance of healthcare insurers.*]

RVZ (2014b). *Patiënteninformatie, informatievoorziening rondom de patiënt*. The Hague: Raad voor de Volksgezondheid en Zorg. [*Patient information, information provision around the patient.*]

RVZ. (2015). *Consumer eHealth*. The Hague: Raad voor Volksgezondheid en Samenleving.

RVZ (2017). *No evidence without context. About the illusion of evidence-based practice in healthcare*. The Hague: Raad voor Volksgezondheid en Zorg.

SCP. (2011). *Kwetsbare ouderen*. The Hague: Sociaal en Cultureel Planbureau. [*Vulnerable elderly.*]

SCP (2016a). *Wel Thuis*? The Hague: Sociaal en Cultureel Planbureau. [*At Home?*]

SCP. (2016b). *De toekomst tegemoet. Leren werken, zorgen, samenleven en consumeren in het Nederland van later*. The Hague: Sociaal en Cultureel Planbureau. [*Facing the future. Agile working, caring, society and consumers in the Netherlands of later.*]

SCP. (2018). *Kwetsbaar en eenzaam? Risico's en bescherming in de ouder wordende bevolking*. The Hague: Sociaal en Cultureel Planbureau. [*Vulnerable and lonely? Risks and protection in the aging population.*]

SCP. (2019a). *Wat als de zorg wegvalt. Een simulatie van alternatieven voor zorg en ondersteuning voor mensen met een gezondheidsbeperking*. The Hague: Sociaal en Cultureel Planbureau. [*What if care goes away. A simulation of alternatives for care and support for people with a health limitation.*]

SCP. (2019b). *Zorgen voor thuiswonende ouderen. Kennissynthese over de zorg voor zelfstandig wonende 75 plussers, knelpunten en toekomstige ontwikkelingen*. The Hague: Sociaal en Cultureel Planbureau. [*Caring for the elderly living at home. Knowledge synthesis of care for independently living 75-plussers, bottlenecks and future developments.*]

SCP. (2019c). *Mantelzorgers in het vizier. Beleidssignalement mantelzorg*. The Hague: Sociaal en Cultureel Planbureau. [*Informal caregivers in view. Policy description of informal care.*]

SiRM. (2019). *Scenario's ouderenzorg in beeld. Sectorbeeld ouderenzorg naar 2030 – 2040*. Utrecht: Strategies in Regulated Markets. [*Scenarios in elderly care in view. Sector view of elderly care to 2030 – 2040.*]

Smelik, J. and I. Bardoel. (2018). *Actieprogramma zorgzame gemeenschappen: Nederland Zorgt Voor Elkaar*. Maarn: NLZVE. [*Action programme for caring communities: The Netherlands caring for each other.*]

Stichting Lezen en Schrijven (2018). *Feiten en cijfers laaggeletterdheid*. The Hague: Stichting Lezen en Schrijven. [*Facts and figures illiteracy.*]

Swedish society of nursing. (2012). *eHealth. A strategy for nurses*. Stockholm: Swedish Society of Nursing.

Taskforce De juiste zorg op de juiste plek (2018). *De juiste zorg op de juiste plek. Wie durft?* [*The right care in the right place. Who dares?*]

TD Connect. (2018). *AI en gezondheidszorg. Feiten en cijfers*. [*AI and healthcare. Facts and figures.*]

TNO (2012). *Ruimte voor professionals. Lessen op basis van drie organisaties die een publieke taak uitvoeren*. Nijmegen: Radboud Universiteit, ITS. [*Space for professionals. Lessons based on three organizations that carry out a public task.*]

TNO (2019). *Prognose capaciteitsontwikkeling verpleeghuiszorg*. Delft: TNO. [*Prognosis for capacity development of nursing home care.*]

Transitieprogramma in de langdurige zorg (2009). *Maatschappelijke Business case Buurtzorg Nederland.* [*Social business case: Buurtzorg Nederland.*]

Vilans (2007). *Factsheet zelfmanagement bij ouderen*. Utrecht: Vilans. [*Factsheet on self-management for the elderly.*]

Vilans (2014). *Implementatie van Ambient Intelligent Technology/slimme zorgtechnologie in Nederland*. Presentation. Utrecht: Vilans. [*Implementation of Ambient Intelligent Technology/smart care technology in the Netherlands.*]

Vilans (2016a). *Met eHealth zorgen dat de zorg beter werkt*. Utrecht: Vilans. [*Ensuring with eHealth that care works better.*]

Vilans (2016b). *Een integraal zorgsysteem, vraagstuk of prachtstuk*? Utrecht: Vilans. [*An integrated care system, issue or centrepiece?*]

Vilans (2018). *12 technologische ontwikkelingen in de zorg*. Utrecht: Vilans. [*12 technological developments in care.*]

Vilans (2019). *Technologie voor zorg en ondersteuning in de wijk. Inspiratie en mogelijkheden*. Utrecht: Vilans. [*Technology for care and support in the neighbourhood. Inspiration and possibilities.*]

VWS. (2017). *Actieplan (Ont)regel de zorg*. The Hague: Ministerie van VWS. [*Action plan for (De-)regulation of care.*]

WeCare Health. *Kwaliteitskader*. TÜV Rheinland Quality. [*Quality framework.*]

Wind, A. and B. te Velde. (2019). *Handreiking kwetsbare ouderen thuis. Handreiking voor integrale zorg en ondersteuning in de wijk*. [*Manual for vulnerable elderly at home. Manual for integrated care and support in the neighbourhood.*]

WRR. (2017). *Weten is nog geen doen. Een realistisch perspectief op redzaamheid*. The Hague: Wetenschappelijke Raad voor het Regeringsbeleid. [*Knowing is not doing. A realistic perspective of sufficiency.*]

ZonMw and Zorginstituut Nederland. (2015). *Het in beeld brengen van kwaliteit van leven in de sector Verpleging en Verzorging. Inventarisatie van het gebruik van methoden die kwaliteit van leven in beeld brengen*. The Hague: ZonMw. [*Mapping quality of life in the Nursing and Care sector. Inventorying the use of methods that visualize quality of life.*]

Zorginstituut Nederland. (2017) *Kwaliteitskader verpleeghuiszorg. Samen leren en verbeteren*. Diemen: Zorginstituut Nederland. [*Quality framework for nursing home care. Learning and improving together.*]

Zorginstituut Nederland. (2018a). *Meer patiëntregie door uitkomstinformatie in 2022*. Diemen: Zorginstituut Nederland. [*More patient control through outcome information in 2022.*]

Zorginstituut Nederland. (2018b). *Naar integrale zorg voor kwetsbare ouderen thuis. Startnotitie.* Diemen: Zorginstituut Nederland. [*To integrated care for vulnerable elderly at home. Start note.*]

Zorgpact. (2017). *De samenwerking dient de mens. Inzichten en voorbeelden van innovatieve partnerschappen in het Zorgpact*. [*The collaboration serves people. Insights and examples of innovative partnerships in the Care Pact.*]

Editor's Contact Information

Jan Veuger, PhD, MRE, BBA, FRICS

Professor of Blockchain, Saxion University of Applied Sciences,
School of Finance and Accounting,
School of Creative Technology,
School of Governance, Law and Urban Development,
Hospitality Business School,
School of Commerce and Entrepeneurship,
School of People and Society,
The Netherlands
j.veuger@saxion.nl

INDEX

A

B

C

D

E

L

M

N

O

P

Q

R

S

T

V

W